D0918631

**PSROs: The Law
and the Health
Consumer**

PSROs: The Law and the Health Consumer

Alice Gosfield, J.D.

Ballinger Publishing Co. • Cambridge, Mass.
A Subsidiary of J. B. Lippincott

The basic research for this book was supported by research grant number 1 R18 HSO1547–01 from the Public Health Service of the Department of Health, Education and Welfare. The opinions in this book are those of the author and should not be considered the opinions or policies of any agency of the United States Government.

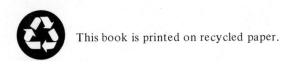 This book is printed on recycled paper.

International Standard Book Number: 0–88410–123–1

Library of Congress Catalog Card Number: 75–13340

Printed in the United States of America

Library of Congress Cataloging in Publication Data

Gosfield, Alice.
   PSROs: the law and the health consumer.

   Includes bibliographical references.
   1. Professional standards review organizations (Medicine) — Law and legislation — United States.
I. Title.
KF3827.P7G67   344'.73'041   75-13340
ISBN 0-88410-123-1

To My Parents

Contents

Preface   ix

Chapter One
Introduction   1

Is a Consumer Perspective Different?   4
The Law Summarized   8
Why Examine PSROs?   10
Notes for Chapter One   19

Chapter Two
Norms   29

Statutory Requirements   34
Selecting and Applying Norms   36
The Process of Review   38
Incentives to Use Norms   43
Systemic Implications of 'Standardized' Review   44
Notes for Chapter Two   50

Chapter Three
PSROs and Institutional Review   67

Delegating Case by Case Review   71
PSROs and HMOs   89
PSROs and State Medicaid Agencies   94
Notes for Chapter Three   97

Chapter Four
PSROs and Paying Agents   109

Prior Problems, Present Resolutions   112
Paying Agents in the PSRO Program   121
Notes for Chapter Four   127

Chapter Five
Hearings and Review   137

Medicaid   139
Medicare   141
PSRO Provisions   144
Notes for Chapter Five   158

Chapter Six
Accountability   173

The Theory   174
Legislative and Regulatory Process   178
Making the System More Responsive   182
Consumer Participation   200
Notes for Chapter Six   209

Chapter Seven
Sanctions and Enforcement   229

Liability   231
Malpractice Exemption   235
Rotation   238
Other Enforcement Issues   247
Notes for Chapter Seven   250

Index   261

About the Author   265

Preface

Most of the voluminous literature analyzing health care policies can be divided into two categories: (1) academic, scholarly, and professional analysis aimed at policymakers, legislators, planners, administrators, and practitioners, and, (2) manuals, guides, and handbooks written to help patients—consumers— understand the increasingly complex health care delivery system which operates for their benefit. The scholarly literature, while regarded seriously by those who operate and control health care delivery, often deals little, if at all, with the effects on patients of the policies it analyzes. By the same token, the consumer-oriented material, of much smaller volume, is often simplistic when written for consumers themselves, and is considered polemical and frivolous when aimed at policymakers. This study of a specific health care problem, through in depth examination of one program, is my attempt to bridge the division between the two styles of analysis, and at the same time to eliminate some of the deficiencies in each.

This book is not a PSRO manual; yet it explains the program and contains what I hope are practical recommendations of policies and actions which would benefit the patients who are only one group of participants in the health care delivery system. It is written in nontechnical language, although some of the problems it discusses are among the most complex of public policy issues. (It is for simplicity that some of the illustrations of medical problems in the text focus on common disorders which a lay reader will recognize, but which may not be the best examples of medical problems illustrating each proposition.)

In addition, the book has many footnotes to document its assertions and to bring together diverse and widely scattered source material for the reader who seeks to go further on any single issue. And, with my apologies to some, the footnote style is closest to a legal style and, therefore, perhaps more dense than that of other disciplines. To the consumer-reader unaccustomed to this style of writing I would say if the footnotes serve your purposes use them as a resource. But the arguments and analyses in the text are complete, and you will not miss some central proposition if you choose to use the footnotes selectively or not at all.

One final word about footnotes: the PSRO program is in its initial stages of implementation at this writing. The boundaries of its operation have been broadly set by the statute and those regulations which have been issued. The footnotes documenting these choices (and other material) are current as of March 1975. There will be further developments in the program in the near future which this book does not directly cite. However, the issues and policies among which choices will be made are set forth and it is unlikely something radically different from the scope presented here will arise.

Balancing the needs for cost control with quality assurance of medical care has been one of the most difficult areas of health care policy. As a subject for study it is usually reserved to physicians and medical economists because their technical expertise best qualifies them to analyze the implications of the dynamic between those needs. Yet, as I hope this book demonstrates, many of the problems created by those inherent conflicts are *not* technical problems, but policy choices in which others—traditionally viewed as "non-experts"—can and must participate. Public financing of health care has required nonmedical legislators to enter the arena of these formerly exclusively scholarly debates. Their entry has opened the field to everyone concerned about and affected by the many laws now governing health care delivery. This book is an attempt to further expand the field to include, in a meaningful way, the participation and interests of consumer-patients.

The principal writing and research for this book was supported by a grant from the Department of Health, Education and Welfare to the Health Law Project of the University of Pennsylvania, where I was previously employed as an attorney. Edward V. Sparer of the University of Pennsylvania Law School was the director and founder of the Health Law Project.

I would like to thank William P. Scott, who as a second year student under my direction did the basic research, analysis, and writing on Chapter Four, "PSROs and Paying Agents." His probing questions often helped me to clarify my own thoughts. I owe thanks to Lotte Gottschlich and her assistant Pat Fisher for keeping the Project organized and helping me to amass the enormous quantity of literature I requested. Bobbi Haas provided special assistance by reading hundreds of article abstracts to help me find those of special interest. Beverly Wentzel performed a valuable service in her common-sense reading of the first major draft. I would like also to acknowledge the assistance of the dozen or so typists who helped to produce the several drafts of the manuscript.

My thanks go to Faith Rafkind for her substantive comments, her ready ear, and her willingness to discuss issues. My special thanks go to Ed Shay for his substantive help based on his own expertise, and for his constant support. Without him this book would not have been written.

Alice Gosfield
Philadelphia
March, 1975

PSROs: The Law and the Health Consumer

Chapter One

Introduction

Major changes in this country's health care system will result from a little-known federal law passed in 1972.[1] This law gives the federal government—through HEW—the responsibility to implement a system to control costs and review the quality of medical care given to the aged (Medicare beneficiaries) and the poor (Medicaid recipients) and those receiving Maternal and Child Health and Crippled Children's Services, the costs of whose care is reimbursed by government funds.[2] Physician groups called Professional Standards Review Organizations (PSROs) are empowered under the law to organize and administer 203 local organizations across the country to monitor and control patient utilization of governmentally paid for medical services. The program requires the use of physician-established norms to check individual services for medical necessity, appropriateness, and quality.[3]

There are two essential paradoxes in the present PSRO law: (1) although regulation of fees and services by law has traditionally been anathema to physicians, they will develop and operate the PSRO system; and (2) despite the law's apparent concern for the quality of services rendered to the patients whose health care PSROs will review, there are provisions excluding patients from the processes that will determine what health care they receive. With the recent focus of the ongoing health care debate on national health insurance, the basic issues raised by the PSRO program will become of greater concern to most Americans because almost all the insurance proposals contain some mechanism to control costs and assure quality of care; and in the principal proposals before Congress, PSROs are given the responsibility to monitor and control care for all covered patients.[4]

The principal issues raised by the PSRO system are those of (1) defining good quality care, and (2) achieving a balance between the implementation of that definition and the control of health care costs. The policy choices determining the program's operation will affect every element of the American health care delivery system: hospitals and nursing homes, health maintenance organizations and physicians, fiscal intermediaries and carriers (Blue Cross and Blue Shield primarily), state agencies administering Medicaid, and, most significantly, the patients whose health care PSROs review. Those patients (at present, Medicare, Medicaid, and Title V beneficiaries) are the people who will be most directly affected by PSRO activities, because, under the PSRO scheme, no federal money can be paid for their care unless a PSRO has approved the care. Consequently, patients may be denied care because a health care provider fears PSRO disapproval, or patients may be forced to absorb costs which they assumed, because of their participation in a government funded program, would be covered by the government. Because of the financial power of PSROs, health care providers will be influenced to act within PSRO guidelines and the day to day practice of medicine may be considerably altered as a result. Although the PSRO program represents an unprecedented, major intervention of government in regulation of the actual delivery of medical services to large segments of the population, the consumer-patients whose lives will bear the impact of the program have been exluded both from participation in the actual structure of the PSRO system and from the policy discussions formulating its functions.

Since the PSRO concept was first introduced in 1970,[5] it has been the subject of a barrage of criticism, charges, and countercharges from widely divergent sources: from the program's staunchest proponents headed by Senator Wallace Bennett (R–Utah), the sponsor of the legislation,[6] to the few medical organizations which offered early, qualified support for the program,[7] to legislators seeking its repeal[8] and opponent physicians who claim the program "will change the practice of medicine as we know it."[9] The controversy has encompassed a wide variety of positions and has considered the interests of most participants in the health care delivery system—except the interests and perspectives of the patients for whom the health care system operates. Among the published considerations of the program's implications there is not only little evidence of objective and critical analysis, but there is also lacking a comprehensive examination of the program considering the perspective of the consumer-patient.[10]

This study examines and analyzes the structure and functions of the PSRO system. It considers its effects on the other components of the national and local health delivery scenes and presents the significance and implications of those findings for consumers. Initially, this book demonstrates the difference between a *consumer's* perspective and a *taxpayer's* perspective (often called "public interest"), including areas of conflict between those points of view (Chapter One). The analysis then focuses on the interaction between PSROs and the other elements of the health care delivery system.

Because the law prescribes the use of "norms" as a standardized methodology for reviewing medical necessity, quality, and appropriateness of services,[11] the use of these norms will influence the activites of medical care practitioners (e.g., doctors, nurses, dentists, physical therapists, social workers). The chapter on "Norms" (Chapter Two) analyzes the methodology which will be used to scrutinize medical practices, and, using examples, demonstrates the need for and value of consumer participation in the norms-setting process, where appropriate. Because the use of norms will standardize medical practice and review of it, it will also have implications for health care financing. These issues are considered.

Chapter Three, "PSROs and Institutional Review," analyzes the relationship between PSROs and the health care institutions (hospitals, nursing homes) over which they have jurisdiction. Utilization review committees were required to be established in each hospital participating in Medicare and Medicaid.[12] They were charged with the responsibility of reviewing medical services rendered in their institutions. Their failure led directly to the creation of PSROs. These committees will, however, continue to operate as part of the PSRO system.[13] Chapter Three analyzes the interaction between these committees and PSROs and discusses the incentives to them to seek autonomy within the system. It also discusses the relationships of PSROs with health maintenance organizations (HMOs)[14] and state government agencies administering Medicaid programs.

Chapter Four, "PSROs and Paying Agents," examines the activities of the insurance companies (primarily Blue Cross and Blue Shield) which have been used in Medicare and Medicaid to administer the payment of government health care benefits[15] as "carriers," "intermediaries," and "fiscal agents." As part of that function, under prior law, they were supposed to review services to control costs. They, too, were unsuccessful, and PSROs will in large part absorb the functions these paying agents failed to perform. Chapter Four examines the performance failures of these insurance companies and considers how and whether PSROs can confront those failures successfully. Throughout the book the importance to consumers of the PSROs' relationships with other activities and the courses their development can take are presented. Where regulations and policy decisions determining these interactions have already been made, the study discusses whose interests prevailed and what incentives led to those choices. Where policy has not yet been established, the options available under the law are presented and choices are suggested which would make the PSRO program more responsive to consumer-patients' needs.

Having analyzed the relationship of PSROs to the other components of the health care scene, the study considers the operation of PSROs as a regulatory system. The following three chapters focus on that aspect of the program which can be considered its "accountability." The law provides a mechanism—the hearings and review process[16]—for ensuring the accountability of the program to individuals affected by it. The procedures under this provision are the means for dissatisfied participants to obtain review of PSRO determinations adverse to them. The chapter "Hearings and Review" (Chapter Five) examines the previously existing Medicare and Medicaid review processes and analyzes the effect of the PSRO provisions on rights which were established under the old mechanisms. The legal and constitutional implications of the changes are discussed. The next chapter, "Accountability" (Chapter Six), presents a theory of consumer accountability often overlooked in consumer-oriented policy analyses. It defines the concept, establishes its importance in government programs, and, finally, distinguishes consumer accountability from other types of program responsiveness (taxpayer accountability, or responsiveness to Congress and HEW, for example). The test of the theory, examining those provisions which could reveal the extent of program accountability, proves that PSROs are essentially unaccountable as a system to their consumers. Despite this inherent defect, specific techniques for making the system more responsive to consumer needs are presented. Finally, Chapter Seven, "Sanctions and Enforcement," confronts the question of the accountability of the participants in the program to the system itself. How will the program guarantee its own existence in the face of concerted opposition from the very physicians who must be its administrators? The last chapter examines the sanctions and incentives created by law to ensure that the program will work and analyzes how and whether they can be effective.

IS A CONSUMER PERSPECTIVE DIFFERENT?

The PSRO system of "peer review," in which only physicians evaluate other physicians to control costs and assure quality of medical services, has been described incorrectly by several nonconsumer commentators as a program finding its impetus in consumerism.[17] The program's consumers are the patients whose care is reviewed. PSROs may hold the promise of a beneficial effect to the nonpatient public through contained costs and therefore contained taxes, but the program's only consumer orientation lies in its professed goal of assuring quality medical care.

These dual foci of PSRO review activities—cost and quality—create the primary tension in the program. That the PSRO law was conceived initially as a cost control measure is unquestionable.[18] In July 1970, while discussing the need for a better system to control spiraling medical costs, Senator Bennett said, "The American people are justifiably concerned over the tremendous cost of health care."[19] When he introduced his bill as an amendment (No. 851) to H.R. 17550 (then the Social Security Amendments of 1969), he said:

> We have learned from long, hard, and costly experience that the Federal Government and its various public and private agents generally have been unable effectively to monitor and assure economical and efficient use of properly provided health care services in Medicare and Medicaid.[20]

And later that year, clarifying his original proposal, he emphasized:

> The taxpayers—the average citizen and his employer—are on a treadmill when it comes to financing Medicare and Medicaid. They are asked to pay more and more simply to maintain present benefit levels.
>
> My amendment to establish professional standards review organizations was intended as a responsible effort to establish a comprehensive commonsense means of slowing down—perhaps even stopping—that taxpayers' treadmill.[21]

Although the bill passed the Senate, the Senate and House conferees could not agree on the amendment before the end of the 91st Congress. It was reintroduced with some modifications on January 25, 1972 as Amendment No. 823 to H.R. 1, the Social Security Amendments of 1971.[22] It was at that time that Bennett's recognition of the inter-relation between cost control and quality assurance was first expressed:

> . . . [R]ising health care costs fall disproportionately on those who have the greatest need for health care services—the chronically ill, the aged, and the poor. . .
>
> In addition to the rapidly rising cost of health care, a problem exists with respect to the quality of that care. The Committee on Finance held two extensive series of hearings on health care in 1970. In the spring of 1970, we held oversight hearings on the social security amendments which contained many medicare changes. During the course of those hearings, disturbing testimony was heard bearing on the quality of health care. We heard practicing physicians testify to the effect that in many areas of the country a good deal of unnecessary and avoidable surgery was being performed and excessive and inappropriate health care services provided. We learned of significant variations between sections of the country in the lengths of hospitalization for similar patients having a given illness.
>
> As these problems of rising costs, unnecessary services and uneven quality became apparent, the most disturbing fact was that in most areas of the country no effective review mechanism exists whereby practicing physicians can in organized and publicly accountable fashion, determine on a comprehensive and ongoing basis if services are medically necessary and if they meet quality standards. This amendment would go a long way toward correcting that intolerable situation.[23]

The quality problems to which Senator Bennett refers are problems of overutilization, the use of more services than are necessary to achieve desired results.[24] According to his analysis, eliminating overutilization and unnecessary services would lower the cost of health care. The concerns he was advocating are those of taxpayers who do have an interest in having approved the least expensive (but presumably still effective) medical services, in order to lower overall costs of health care thereby lessening their individual tax burdens. But because Medicare and Medicaid patients represent only 38 to 40 percent of the population of this country,[25] there are more taxpayers who do not receive Medicare and Medicaid benefits than those who are consumers of those services. Because of their numerical majority in the population, the taxpayers to whom Bennett had originally addressed the lowered cost impact of this program are often called the general public, and their interests, the public interest. As the financers of government, their interests in the PSRO program often will be those expressed by Senator Bennett as well as those reflected in Department of Health, Education and Welfare actions implementing and administering the program.[26]

In contrast, the consumers whose health care this program will review have an interest in obtaining all those medical services necessary to their achieving the best health status possible for them. Indeed, that desire for the best possible care is common to all patients (not just government funds recipients) when they are ill and undergoing diagnosis or treatment; and, in most cases, it is tempered by the ability to buy available services and the willingness of health care professionals and institutions to provide them. In the PSRO system there will be a point in the review of many kinds of care when the consumers' interest in the best quality care and the taxpayers' interest in lowered costs will conflict. For example, in the treatment of some cancers it may be less expensive in the long run to perform a major surgical procedure to remove a tumor than to give X-ray treatments over a long period of time with additional treatment for the side effects of the X-rays. Similarly, a procedure which can be performed competently either on an in-patient basis or an out-patient basis (during a stay in the hospital as opposed to during a short visit to a clinic or a physician's office) may be chosen by the consumer and his physician to be performed on the more expensive in-patient basis because of lowered risk of infection there and better backup care in the event of an emergency.[27] Where care is being reviewed for a condition about which there is significant medical and scientific controversy as to the treatment of choice (e.g., inflamed tonsils, breast cancer, or gastric ulcers), because of the goal of lowered costs, will PSROs necessarily approve only the least expensive care?[28] The role of the conflicting interests of cost and quality, representing the taxpayer and consumer interests respectively, in each of the 203 areas nationwide will be expressed in the balance between two factors: (1) the extent to which physicians establishing and applying norms accede to cost control needs and (2) the level of stringency exercised by the Secretary in controlling PSROs or the discretion he grants to local groups.[29]

There are other areas where the consumer perspective and the perspective of other actors in the PSRO system will conflict. There may be tension between the patient's right to the confidentiality of his medical history and the PSRO system's need to develop statistics on health care delivery across the nation.[30] The consumer's desire and need to be forewarned of those substandard practitioners discovered in the course of PSRO review may conflict with the physician's interest in maintaining the secrecy of data showing a pattern of substandard care.[31] The statutory language does little to resolve these tensions; and while regulations and the actual operation of the program will confront some of them, the policy decisions which will resolve most of these conflicts may answer the needs of one PSRO participant at the expense of another. Indeed, such resolution is, in some cases, unavoidable. In other situations, the choice that is made may be directly antithetical to consumer interests, and motivated solely by the desire to accommodate powerful vested interests with easy access to policymakers.[32] In every situation where such choices are made, it is important to recognize which perspective and whose values prevail. Where it can be shown that powerful vested interests were chosen at the expense of consumer interests for no reason other than simple accession to financial power (and therefore political clout), the recognition of that motivation ought to lead to policy changes to achieve a better balance.

Throughout this study the competing values, and the possible policy choices within the statutory structure which reflect them, are elucidated. In each case, the arguments for the consumer interest are presented. Ultimately though, only the actual implementation and operation of the full PSRO program will reveal which values determined each decision. The theme underlying the analysis which follows is that seeking out and responding to consumer input, at the very least as an *equal* consideration in policy determinations, will result in a better, more credible, and, therefore, more effective system in a democratic society. The most direct and effective means for discovering and giving recognition to those interests is the inclusion of consumers themselves in policymaking as members of those bodies whose day to day interpretations of the PSRO statute and regulations will determine the actual functioning of the program.[33] This is not to suggest that PSROs should be consumer controlled. Consumers by definition are incapable of making technical, medical evaluations.[34] But in this or any society with limited resources available to be spent on health care for the poor and aged, many nontechnical choices will be made which must, necessarily, compromise some consumer interests. The negotiation of those compromises, the choices of which sacrifice must be made, should take place in an open, participatory forum where all interests are fairly and equally represented. In the PSRO program to date, those choices have been made in a less than open forum from which consumers have been excluded. The decisions reflecting those choices, then, were not made in an equitable way, and will be replicated throughout the system unless consumers are included in the process which will further implement PSROs.

THE LAW SUMMARIZED

Under the law, the Secretary of HEW, after consultation with national and local health associations, was to designate PSRO areas on a nationwide basis by January 1, 1974.[35] Areas range from part of a city to an entire state depending on the number of physicians in each area. Three hundred physicians was the minimum number required for participation in the creation and operation of PSRO.[36] Although the localism of PSROs was designed to permit active participation by a broad range of physicians, the overall structure of the system calls for a tripartite organization on local, state, and national levels.

Medical societies and medical foundations will be invited to submit plans to establish other entities as the local PSRO for their area.[37] If by 1976 those organizations, or other physician organizations initially approached, fail either to submit a plan or to fulfill a plan to establish a PSRO, then the Secretary can appoint nonpracticing physicians to PSROs and may designate other non-physician-controlled entities to act as PSROs.[38]

Although appointment of non-physician organizations is possible under the law, only physicians may make final determinations in the appraisal process,[39] and only physicians who have staff privileges in PSRO-area hospitals can evaluate hospital care.[40] PSROs are encouraged to achieve for their membership the broadest possible representation of area doctors and to rotate their members on review committees "on an extensive and continuing basis."[41] Doctors "ordinarily should not be responsible for, but may participate in the review of care" in the same hospitals where they have staff privileges.[42] Nor can they review the care they provided their own patients or care provided in an institution in which they have a financial interest.[43]

In performing review, PSRO physicians have the power to examine all relevant provider records and to inspect facilities.[44] The Secretary of HEW is authorized to reimburse the PSRO for the services of specialists and for all other reasonable and necessary expenses.[45] The Secretary may also provide for the coordination of activity between and among PSROs, intermediaries, carriers, and state agencies, including the exchange of data and the use of mechanical and other information gathering equipment and processes.[46] The primary impact of PSROs is created by the provision that no payment can be made by an intermediary, carrier, or state agency if the PSRO makes an adverse determination as to medical necessity or the level of care provided.[47]

In each state served by three or more PSROs, a Statewide Review Council, consisting primarily of physicians, but required to include also four public members "knowledgeable in health care" (at least two of whom are recommended by the governor), will coordinate the activities and review the performance of PSROs.[48] In addition, representatives of health delivery institutions and practitioners other than physicians will comprise Advisory Groups so that their roles and problems as health services providers may be better understood by the Statewide Councils.[49]

The PSRO hierarchy is completed by the National Professional Standards Review Council whose impact will be felt nationwide. This body consists of eleven physicians who are appointed by the Secretary to three year terms,[50] and all of whom are required to have "recognized standing and distinction in the appraisal of medical practice."[51] The Council reports directly to the Assistant Secretary of Health and coordinates efforts of the other government agencies involved in the program (e.g., Medicaid, Bureau of Health Insurance, Bureau of Quality Assurance, Social Security Administration).[52]

Once a PSRO is in full operation, its activity will preempt all utilization and quality review of practitioner and institutional care by inter-mediaries and carriers.[53] The PSRO must, however, "utilize the services of, and accept the findings of" institutional utilization review committees, but only to the extent that the PSRO is satisfied that the institutional committee is acting "effectively and in timely fashion."[54] The statute does not specify how the PSRO is to evaluate the effectiveness of these committees. PSROs will be performing many of the cost and quality control functions previously charged to Medicare institutional utilization review committees and fiscal intermediaries which will no longer review those physician determinations.[55] The law also grants PSROs the authority to determine in advance whether "any elective admission to a hospital or other health care facility, or . . . any other health care services which will consist of extended or costly courses of treatment" would be medically necessary and provided at the proper level of care (in-patient or out-patient, hospital or nursing home).[56]

Three criteria for review determinations are mandated for all decisions which would authorize an individual's admission to an institution or extend his length of stay: the care rendered must be (1) consistent with professionally recognized health care standards; (2) medically necessary; and (3) [in certain cases] impossible to be provided more economically in a different facility.[57]

The law prescribes the methodology for PSRO review. "Each [PSRO] shall apply professionally developed norms of care, diagnosis, and treatment based upon typical patterns of practice in its regions (including typical lengths-of-stay for institutional care by age and diagnosis) as principal points of evaluation and review."[58] Norms, though locally developed, must be approved by the National Council for each region served by a PSRO.[59] If, however, the PSRO determines that the actual norms of care for its area "are significantly different from professionally developed regional norms of care, diagnosis, and treatment approved for comparable conditions," then, with the approval of the National Council, it may apply variant norms.[60] The law also permits a presumption of entitlement to payment for care where prior authorization for care has been granted on the basis of norms, and care is provided in compliance with such guidelines.[61]

Although the statute provides for insulation of the physician from malpractice liability if his practices have conformed to professionally established norms and standards,[62] strict sanctions for continuing violation of treatment guidelines have also been established.[63] Finally, hearings and appeals mechanism is provided for physicians, providers, and consumers who are dissatisfied with a PSRO determination.[64]

WHY EXAMINE PSROs?

The Legislative Context: Other Regulatory Techniques Enacted and Proposed.

The PSRO program has developed in the context of a plethora of related legislative and governmental activity directed at the regulation and delivery of health care. A number of other programs and approaches to cost and quality control were enacted as part of the Social Security Amendments of 1972.[65] Some of these will duplicate or parallel PSRO activities.

Social Security Act Amendments. As part of the Medicare program, in each state there will be Program Review Teams,[66] consisting of physicians, other professional personnel, and consumer representatives, with authority to review individual cases, analyze statistical data, and make recommendations to the Secretary on excessive fees or other charges. The law provides that PSROs may be used instead of Program Review Teams.[67] Advance approvals of care in extended care facilities or of home health services for a limited period of time immediately following hospitalizations are now possible under the Medicare program.[68] PSROs also will review proposed care in extended care facilities.[69] Payments now available for patients suffering from "end-stage renal disease"[70] (advanced kidney disease) will be reviewed by Local Medical Review Boards "which will be an integral part or agent of (PSROs) once they become functional."[71]

Several new sections of the Social Security Act impose requirements for disclosure of information about the quality of health services delivered under Medicare and Medicaid. Disclosure of the pertinent findings in state surveys of health care facilities eligible for reimbursement under Medicare and Medicaid[72] and of information on the performance of carriers, intermediaries, state agencies, and providers of services under those programs is now mandatory.[73] At the same time, PSROs themselves will be developing a wide variety of information relevant to the quality of care delivered across the country.[74] The interaction and comparison of activities between PSROs and other review authorities will be significant for the future evaluation and possible modification both of PSROs and of other programmatic approaches.

Much recent discussion has centered on the relative merits of particular cost control and quality assurance systems. Though of only limited extent before the PSRO law's enactment, the intensity of the debate around other proposed programs was fed by the passage of PSROs. These other proposals would supercede, replace, or absorb entirely the functions of PSROs. To evaluate meaningfully the success of the PSRO program, as well as the validity of those other proposals, it is important to recognize the basic distinctions between these competing (or complementary) approaches and to consider whether and how PSROs work better or are more acceptable than the proposed alternatives.[75] Although various commentators suggest different modifications, three principal proposals form the context of the continuing debate surrounding cost and quality review: (1) Peer Review Organizations (PROs) promoted by the American Medical Association (AMA),[76] (2) the "Health Outcomes Commission" notion sponsored by InterStudy,[77] and (3) the Commission on the Quality of Health Care,[78] an element of "The Health Security Act."[79]

AMA Peer Review Organizations. The essential characteristic of the AMA's Peer Review Organizations is their direct link to and control by state medical societies. It was this proposal which the AMA took to Bennett leading him to create PSROs.[80] Each PRO would have review jurisdiction over the same populations PSROs serve plus those covered by the AMA's Medicredit national health insurance proposal.[81] In each state, this responsibility would be exercised by the state medical society or its designee, or by another organization appointed by the Secretary of HEW to serve as the PRO Commission in that state. An advisory council consisting of representatives of consumers, providers, and carriers would be appointed by the state society and impaneled to serve the commission as appropriate. The Commission would designate geographic areas within the state to be administered by Commission-appointed local review panels and local advisory councils, and would act as a review tribunal where censure or disciplinary matters were involved. Under the proposal, the Commission would itself act as a local panel where none existed. The local panel, for its part, could delegate its review authority for a hospital to that hospital's utilization review committee. Complaints or other reports relating to such issues as the reasonableness of fees charged or the need for and quality of services rendered by a provider in the area could be submitted to the local panel by any interested party. If the panel's initial review were to find that the accusation provided sufficient basis for a hearing, it would offer an opportunity for informal discussion with the provider "with a view toward conformance by [him] with generally acceptable professional practices."[82] Only after such discussion had failed to resolve the dispute satisfactorily would a hearing be held, giving to the provider extensive procedural rights. The Commission would review the panel's evidence, findings, and determinations and could accept, reject, or modify them. The Commission could terminate payment to a provider who it found had, in a substantial number of cases, substantially overcharged, overtreated, or rendered services "of a quality substantially below generally acceptable professional practices."[83] First offenses would be sanctioned by termination of payment for no more than six months. Subsequent offenses would result in termination for as long as the Commission deemed appropriate. The Commission could reinstate payments as it chose. Judicial review of the Commission's findings would be available; but its records and any evidence it had used would be unavailable for use in any other civil or criminal actions. Under the PRO system, it would be the responsibility of the provider against whom disciplinary action had been taken to notify patients that government payments for services rendered by him would no longer be available. Other aspects of the AMA's proposal include a national advisory council, insulation from liability for information generated within the PRO system for its purposes, and reimbursement to PROs by the government for reasonable expenses incurred in the establishment and operation of the system.

The basic differences between the AMA's PRO proposal and PSROs are the following: (1) PROs would not have ongoing case review responsibility;[84] but would merely respond to complaints; (2) PROs would not disallow payment for excessive services in an individual case;[85] (3) PROs would not be required to use norms or other standards of review;[86] (4) PROs, as proposed, give no review authority to the Secretary of HEW;[87] (5) the proposal includes no reporting requirements or other stipulations for "public accountability," let alone consumer accountability;[88] (6) PROs review charges;[89] (7) PROs have no information generating or data processing components;[90] and (8) state medical societies would control the establishment and functioning of the program.[91]

Health Outcomes Commission. The InterStudy Health Outcomes Commission (HOC) proposal presents a vivid contrast with the AMA approach. Although the proposal is aimed at the regulation of health maintenance organizations,[92] it would establish an independent regulatory agency in the executive branch with jurisdiction extending to any provider choosing to submit to it. Federal in scope, the agency would have little local administration. HOC review would concentrate on the clinical outcomes of care (the actual result of treatment to the patient measured against his status prior to care).[93] Local providers would be aided in creating internal quality assurance systems and would be offered direct financial incentives to accept HOC jurisdiction, thereby exempting themselves from other regulatory authorities, including PROs. Research to assess varying modes of quality review; to compare differing techniques of delivering and financing health care services; and to ensure maximal dissemination of information about health care to the public figures prominently in the HOC scheme.

Ongoing HOC quality assessment activities would focus on locally determined high priority disease areas chosen according to their amenability to improved results from care. Review would be financed by the federal government in an amount equal to 2 percent of the provider's total gross revenues. Under the HOC plan, solo practitioners choosing HOC jurisdiction would be required to form groups numbering at least five; each such group would maintain its own internal assessment system. Technical assistance to providers to help them meet minimum requirements for routine screening of cases would be available. The aggregate figures developed through this screening, showing utilization of services by categories (e.g., number of laboratory tests per month, hospital patient days per month, X-rays per month, and out-patient days per month) would be reported to the HOC, but used locally to develop standards, guidelines, and criteria for care. Although the HOC would not establish parameters for measuring care, the "norms" used by internal systems could be changed by the commission if providers, consumers, and others had been given both notice and an opportunity to rebut the commission's decision.

Sanctions for substandard performance would be levied according to results of HOC evaluations of routine screening. A "satisfactory" rating would result in no sanction's being applied. A rating of "provisional in quality assurance" would lead to further in depth examination of the provider's records and procedures, or its voluntary compliance with ongoing monitoring by the HOC. A rating of "probationary" would require notice to the public and the selective temporary removal of exemptions from other regulations with reductions of federal monies given to the provider. An "unsatisfactory" quality assurance rating would result in the termination of federal financial assistance available by virtue of the provider's having accepted HOC jurisdiction, and the repayment, with interest, of whatever federal financial assistance had been given during the two years preceding the unsatisfactory rating. Finally, fines could be imposed for fraud or criminal behavior.

Public disclosure of a variety of information would be required of both the HOC itself and those providers over which it had authority. Providers would be required to maintain internal grievance mechanisms for use in medical injury disputes. The failure of those mechanisms to resolve disputes would lead to binding arbitration, with costs allocated at 75 percent paid by the provider, 25 percent by the consumer.

The HOC approach is distinguished from PSROs by its focus on aggregate rather than case by case review or review of individual services or individual practitioners. This emphasis, excluding any HOC concern with cost control, reflects the belief of its proponents that cost control will be achieved inherently through the HMO delivery mechanism. In addition, the HOC's independent research mandate has no parallel in the PSRO system. The HOC program would operate as a complete, closed system alternative to the PSRO model, avoiding HEW jurisdiction, and also, for the most part, judicial dispute resolution.

Quality of Health Care Commission. The Commission on the Quality of Health Care, as proposed in Title III of S.3, in January 1973,[94] falls somewhere between the AMA and InterStudy models. The Commission, established within HEW, would consist of eleven members, seven representing providers or "non-governmental organizations engaged in developing standards pertaining to the quality of health care," and four consumers.[95] The primary functions of the Commission would be the development of methods for assessing the quality of health care furnished under the Health Security Act national health insurance proposal and development of techniques for utilizing such methods; little review of individual cases is contemplated by this proposal. A systematized nationwide data base would provide the necessary foundation for determining how best to assess the following four aspects of health care delivery: (1) the qualifications of personnel and facilities; (2) patterns of health practice in episodes of care; (3) patterns of utilization of the components of health care systems; and (4) the health of patients "during and at the conclusions of episodes of health care."[96] The statistical norms and ranges (either national or regional in scope as the Commission chose) yielded by such analysis would then be used to set the standards forming the basis for recommendations to both the Secretary and a Health Security Board for control and improvement of quality. (The Health Security Board is the agency proposed to administer national health insurance under S.3.)

A research component, similar to that in the InterStudy model, is proposed. Research would focus on (1) improvement of technology for quality assessment, including input and end results of care; (2) comparison of the quality of care under differing modes of delivery and payment; (3) the effects of consumer health education programs and preventive health care; (4) the effectiveness of different approaches to medical malpractice; and (5) how best to obtain a variety of information relevant to health care delivery. Although neither the research findings nor the standards they would help would be available upon implementation of the program, pending their development the Commission could, nonetheless, advise the Secretary and the Health Security Board.

The Health Security Board itself also would have a role in quality control.[97] It would both issue regulations, and, upon the Commission's recommendation, review them. The Board would regulate the qualifications of health care personnel and establish continuing education requirements for them. Facilities could also be regulated. Major surgery and other specialized services would only be covered under the Health Security Act if performed by specialists. If the Commission on the Quality of Health Care so recommended, the Board would contract with a PSRO (or similar entity) "to monitor the quality of some or all institutional and other services furnished under the Act" and report its findings on the quality of care in those institutions to the Board.[98]

The bill seeks to control costs by virtue of the Board's ability to sanction those practitioners and providers it determines have, in a substantial number of cases, furnished unnecessary, poor quality, or negligent services. Such determinations could result in suspension or termination of participation under the Act, after consultation with "an appropriate professional organization or committee constituted by the Board after consultation with such an organization."[99] Hearings and judicial review would be available to anyone dissatisfied with a Board determination.

The main differences between the Quality Commission in S.3 and the PSRO program is the absence of case by case review under S.3, and the diminished role of PSROs to only secondary monitoring entities. Although the Commission would conduct research and develop data for use in setting norms and standards, no specific methodology for review is mandated. The commission's focus on personnel and facility quality is entirely absent from the PSRO scheme, although it is present in the Social Security Act generally.[100] In most respects the S.3 Commission on the Quality of Health Care model is not as detailed as the program established in the PSRO statute; and its more discretionary approach provides for substantial interpretation through regulations.

Health Maintenance Organization Act. The three quality review models discussed above are essentially alternatives to or parallels of the PSRO program as presently conceived. None of them has been enacted. At least one major piece of legislation was enacted after the PSRO statute, however, and it may have a long range effect on the PSRO program. The "Health Maintenance Organization Act of 1973"[101] authorizes a five year program of financial assistance for the planning, development, expansion, and operation of HMOs.[102] Under this act, an HMO must have an ongoing internal quality assurance program which stresses health outcomes but also provides for review by physicians and other health professionals of the process followed in the provision of health services.[103] Of great implication for PSROs, however, is the research and evaluation program (examining the effectiveness, administration, and enforcement of quality assurance systems) for which federal moneys have been asked in the legislation: $4,000,000 for the fiscal year ending June 30, 1974; $8,000,000 for 1975; $9,000,000 each for 1976 and 1977; and $10,000,000 for the fiscal year ending June 30, 1978.[104] An annual report by the Secretary to the Congress is required; the first report due no later than March 1, 1975. In addition, the Secretary was required to contract with a private organization to undertake an independent analysis of quality in health care developing five specific studies:[105] (1) an analysis of past and present legally required and voluntary mechanisms to assure the quality of health care, especially the strengths and weaknesses of major prototypes and their comparable costs; (2) a set of basic principles for an effective quality assurance system, including scope; methods of assessment; data requirements; development of criteria and standards relating to desired outcomes; and, significantly, mechanisms for assuring responsiveness to the needs and perceptions of consumers; (3) an assessment of programs for improving the performance of practitioners and providers, including the effectiveness of sanctions and educational programs; (4) a definition of the specific needs for a program of research and evaluation of quality assurance systems; and (5) development of methods for assessing the quality of health care from the point of view of consumers. Ten million dollars, with no fiscal year limit, was asked for this study.[106] An interim report was due by June 30, 1974, with the final report to be submitted by January 31, 1976.[107]

Concurrent with submission of the final report will be the Secretary's initial designation of alternative organizations, if any, to serve as PSROs.[108] Because the required quality assurance studies under the HMO Act are not linked exclusively to HMOs, PSROs will no doubt be examined as part of the study.[109] Assessment of them in a comprehensive, systematic comparison of quality review systems will be significant for future legislative activity.

National Health Insurance Proposals. Other legislative activity may also affect PSROs. National health insurance proposals have received serious congressional consideration during the last several years. Three of the four major bills recently under consideration would rely on PSROs for cost and quality control.[110] The Health Security Act, originally sponsored by Senator Kennedy and Representative Griffiths,[111] would employ the InterStudy Outcomes Commission approach relabeled as the "Commission on Quality Health Care Assurance." At least five other national health insurance proposals contain some quality review and cost control mechanisms.[112] Of the major bills, only the "Medicredit" proposal sponsored by the AMA[113] gives the government no role in cost and quality review, nor for that matter does it include PROs, the AMA's own proposal which was the original impetus behind PSROs.[114]

In reviewing the legislative context in which the PSRO program was developed and will be implemented, it is evident that PSROs represent a first major step by government into the regulation of health care generally, and the control of costs and quality specifically.[115] Analysis of the issues presented by PSROs, if sensitive to the needs of consumers, will shed considerable light on the many other options now before Congress.

The Potential Impact of PSROs

PSROs are the first major intrusion of government into the private delivery of health care, and an outgrowth of the increasing concern in many quarters regarding cost control and quality assurance in the provision of medical services: their development will be the basic test for both government and the private sector in this type of activity. Acknowledging that problems will undoubtedly arise in attempting so massive an undertaking, the Senate Finance Committee said:

> It should be emphasized that in recommending operational, rather than experimental authority, it is recognized that the successful development of (PSROs) can encompass a variety of prototypes and that changes in technology can be expected to result in continued modifications in procedures, and that much remains to be done in the area of the development and refinement of professional norms. It is believed, though, that the proposal can be implemented within an overall framework of innovation and flexibility. The committee believes further, that only a full implementation effort will provide the impetus needed to establish effective and equitable comprehensive professional review throughout the Nation.[116]

Successful implementation is by no means certain. Dependence on acceptance by physician groups has seriously hampered the program. Although a year and a half after the law's enactment a variety of organizations had applied for PSRO planning grants, conditional PSRO status, and designation as Statewide Support Centers,[117] at least 18 state medical societies had declared their intention to seek repeal of the PSRO statute.[118] Attempts by other health care–related organizations—Blue Cross, Blue Shield,[119] the American Hospital Association,[120] the American Association of Foundations for Medical Care[121]—to win control of various aspects of the program further complicate implementation.

Administrative struggles within the HEW bureaucracy, initially brought to light with the resignation of the program's first director after only six months in office,[122] have seriously impeded the effective development of PSROs from the government's end.[123] HEW's delays in beginning implementation, in part, led to major cuts in the PSRO appropriations asked for fiscal 1975. The House initially reduced the $57 million requested by $7 million. The Senate Appropriations Subcommittee on Health slashed that figure further to $27 million.[124] Whether PSROs survive will also depend on the balance between the costs of operating the program and the costs saved through review. The government is now spending $25 billion annually on Medicare and Medicaid.[125] HEW projected costs for the PSRO program when fully implemented have ranged from $60 million[126] annually to $100 million.[127] Estimates vary on potential savings that could accrue with a cost control program. One estimate (not specifically related to PSROs) projects the following reductions across the population, if not offset by the cost of substitute services: (1) $1.3 billion would be saved by a 5 percent reduction in the number of people "in any population group" who are hospitalized; (2) $3 billion would be saved by a one day reduction in the average length of stay for hospitalized patients (now 7.6 days); and (3) $0.7 billion would be saved by reducing in-patient services by 5 percent. Taken together, a savings of $5 billion would be realized by reductions as indicated.[128] Although those figures are claimed to apply to all population groups, and PSROs, at first, will serve a specified minority, reductions like those indicated would be significant.

While the government undoubtedly would view such cost savings as a demonstration of PSRO success, consumers' satisfaction will turn on different factors; and their satisfaction should be considered important by those policymakers and analysts who seek more than lip service to notions of consumer accountability in this pluralistic society. PSROs have the potential to yield beneficial results which can meet previously elusive consumer needs and goals. These needs are common to all health care consumers and fulfillment of them will be critical to an effective national health insurance program as well.

This study examines the program's potential positive and negative effects on consumers. The most important potentially beneficial effect would be improved quality of care. Through scrutiny of medical services on an objective basis, the worst health care practitioners may be improved. Continuing education for physicians through PSRO participation also may contribute to generally improved care. The information developed by PSROs, if widely disseminated, would contribute to consumer education and better informed consumption of health care generally. The use of norms to review care may result in the elimination of "artificial benefits packages" (limitations on coverage provided by governmental programs based on fiscal needs with little considera- tion for medical necessity), particularly for Medicaid patients, thereby giving these consumers greater access to care than they have had previously.[129] The use of variant norms can statistically identify medically underserved areas, and, if channeled into planning and development activities, could improve overall health care delivery. Possible revitalization of hospital utilization review committees may result in local institutions which are more responsive to the needs of the patients they serve. The local orientation of the PSRO program may provide easier consumer access to it in contrast to preexisting statewide or national efforts. The use of advance determinations and concurrent review may eliminate harsh, retroactive denials of benefits to consumers. Hearings and review under this program may give better procedural rights to Medicare beneficiaries.

But many detrimental and even pernicious effects may come from PSROs. The general lack of consumer accountability in the operation of PSROs may result in continual disregard of consumer interests. Use of advance determinations may deny consumers access to health institutions and services. Norms may stifle innovative medical practice. The authority given to PSROs to delegate review responsibility to institutional utilization review committees may only serve to replicate the problems of the preexisting systems. While the hearings and review scheme may grant more rights to Medicare beneficiaries, it may deny presently well-established rights to Medicaid recipients.

The policy choices which will dictate the balance between the PSRO program's contrasting effects will have immediate and direct impact on the Medicare and Medicaid populations. Although the program's scope was initially limited to services rendered to the poor and aged, it is now clear that PSROs (or a similar program) ultimately will monitor the medical services delivered to most of the American population. The fate of Medicare and Medicaid patients now, at the hands of the PSRO program, will directly affect the fate of larger groups under a national health insurance plan enacted in the future. Recognition of the legitimate interests of consumers in the continuing development of PSROs is, then, a vital issue for everyone concerned about delivery of medical services in this country.

Notes for Chapter One

1. §249F, P.L. 92–603, the Social Security Amendments of 1972, Title XI–B, the Social Security Act, §§1151 *et seq.*; 42 USC §1320c *et seq.*

    The citations in this book will be given with the section from the Social Security Act first, followed by the section from the United States Code, unless otherwise indicated.

2. "Medicare" is the popular name for Title XVIII of the Social Security Act, §§1801–1879; 42 USC §§1395–1395pp. Patients receiving Medicare benefits are referred to as "beneficiaries."

    "Medicaid" is the popular name for Title XIX of the Social Security Act, §§1901–1910; 42 USC §§1396–1396i. Patients receiving Medicaid benefits are referred to as "recipients."

    Sections 501–515; 42 USC §§701–715 provide Maternal and Child Health and Crippled Children's Services. Primary attention in this book has been given to the Medicare and Medicaid programs because they involve many more patients and the laws governing their operations contain more specific cost and quality control provisions. The words "consumers" and "patients," used throughout this book, are meant to include Title V patients unless otherwise indicated.

    It is not the purpose of this study to summarize the coverage, operation, or financing of any of these programs. Throughout the book, explanations of the differences among the programs are presented, where relevant. For other summaries and basic information about each of the programs and their differences the following works are useful:

    1974 Social Security and Medicare Explained – Including Medicaid, (Chicago: Commerce Clearing House, Inc., 1974). Health Law Project, "A Poor Children's Health Crisis," *Clearinghouse Review*

(May 1973), at 5–13 (Title V). Health Law Project, "Medicare Level-of-Care Determinations," VI *Clearinghouse Review* 234–253 August-September 1972). Butler, "The Medicaid Program: Current Statutory Requirements and Judicial Interpretations," 8 *Clearinghouse Review* 7–18 (May, 1974).

3. See this chapter at 8 *infra* for a summary of the law.

4. See this chapter at 16 *infra* for a discussion of these proposals.

5. 116 *Cong. Rec.* S22475 (July 1, 1970).

6. Other proponents include, among others, representatives of the Utah Professional Review Organization, the Colorado Foundation for Medical Care, the Pennsylvania Medical Care Foundation, and the New Mexico Foundation for Medical Care. See "Implementation of PSRO Legislation," *Hearings Before the Subcommittee on Health*, Committee on Finance, U.S. Sen. (93d Cong., 2d sess.), May 8–9, 1974 [hereinafter cited as *PSRO Oversight Hearings*] at 355, 402, 209, and 473.

7. Examples include the American Society of Internal Medicine, the American Osteopathic Association, and the American College of Physicians. See *PSRO Oversight Hearings* at 83, 90, and 52.

8. Included among them are Rep. Rarick (D–La.) sponsoring H.R. 9375, H.R. 11444; Rep. Ashbrook (R–Ohio) sponsoring H.R. 11394; and Rep. Harsha (R–Ohio) sponsoring H.R. 12879, all bills 93d Cong., 2d sess. (1974).

9. See, for example, "Thunder from Medicine's Right Wing," *Medical World News*, June 21, 1974; *PSRO Oversight Hearings* at 250–345; and Thomas, "You'll Work with Big Brother Watching," 11 *Physician's Management* 21 (September 1974).

10. For the only published work existing at the time of this writing which examines some of the implications of the PSRO program for consumers, see Lander, "PSROs," 59 *Health-PAC Bulletin* 1–19 (July-August 1974).

11. §1156; 42 USC §1320c–5.

12. §§1861(e) (6), (j) (8), (k), 1903 (i) (4); 42 USC §§1395x(e) (6), (j) (8), (k), 1396b(i) (4). This is only one of many "conditions of participation" which institutions must meet in order to be eligible for government reimbursement for their services to eligible patients.

13. §1155(e); 42 USC §1320c–4(e).

14. Although authorities differ on the definition of "health maintenance organizations," generally HMOs are groups of physicians in public or private organizations which provide medical services to member patients who have enrolled by paying a single annual prepaid fee.

15. §1816, 1842; 42 USC §§1395h, 1395u.

16. §1159; 42 USC §1320c–8.

17. For example: "It is interesting to note that even the PSRO program is essentially a consumer initiative," Walter J. McNerney, President, Blue Cross Association, in "Medicine Faces the Consumer Movement," *Prism* (September 1973) at 13, 15. "I see [PSRO] as part of a trend toward consumerism that's affected nearly every pro-

fession." Morris Fishbein, M.D., in "PSRO: promise and perils as seen by MWN's advisory board," *Medical World News*, May 3, 1974, at 23.

18. Although Senator Bennett made it clear several times that "the genesis of the amendment was the professional review organization proposal of the American Medical Association" which would have had minimal implications for cost control (See this chapter at 11 *infra*) his changes in their proposal firmly established the cost control purpose. 116 *Cong. Rec.* S17865 (October 13, 1970).

19. 116 *Cong. Rec.* S22475 (July 1, 1970).

20. 116 *Cong. Rec.* S29604 (August 20, 1970).

21. 116 *Cong. Rec.* S17865 (October 13, 1970).

21. 118 *Cong. Rec.* S418 (January 25, 1972).

23. *Id.*

24. Overutilization may also include the use of incorrect services in the absence of correct services. Underutilization, where insufficient services are rendered, also undermines quality. All these terms are, however, relative and measurement of overutilization or under-utilization of medical services depends on comparison of the services rendered with an established concept of good quality, acceptable, or optimal care.

   It is beyond the scope of this discussion to attempt to define "quality" in health care. There is an enormous body of literature discussing that definition. As this book will demonstrate, a determination of quality may depend on the particular requirements of a specific situation and may vary in different contexts. We are assuming that PSRO standards will entail at least the most minimal quality levels. Whether optimal levels are ever achieved will depend to a large extent on the relative weight accorded cost control needs.

25. Dr. William Bauer, former Director of HEW's Office of Professional Standards Review (OPSR), quoted in Reynolds, "National Peer Review—how tough and how soon," *Medical Economics*, June 11, 1973, at 4.

26. In health care politics there is no such thing as a monolithic public interest. Every actor can have a different interest at different times. For a more extensive discussion of this theory see Chapter Six, at 174 *infra*.

27. PSROs have specific authority to review some in-patient care on a prospective basis to determine whether it could "consistent with the provisions of appropriate medical care, be effectively provided on an out-patient basis or more economically in an in-patient health care facility of a different type." §1155(a) (1)(C); 42 USC §1320c–4(a) (1) (C).

28. See Chapter Two at 32 *infra*.

29. The Secretary of HEW has the authority to review PSROs, compare them, and withdraw contracts for unsatisfactory performance. §§1152(d), 1162(c); 42 USC §§1320c–1(d), 1320c–11(c).

30. The statute grants a right to confidentiality in §1166; 42 USC

§1320c–15 with penalties for its violation. It also gives to the PSRO the responsibility to develop profiles of patients, practitioners, and providers [§1155(a) (4); 42 USC §1320c–4(a) (4)] and gives PSROs the right to "examine pertinent records of any practitioner or provider" [§1155(b) (3); 42 USC §1320c–4(b) (3)]. For a detailed discussion of these problems see Chapter Six at xxx *infra*.

31. Each PSRO has the authority and responsibility to discipline chronic violators of its standards for care, and through that discipline and the profiles will identify poor performers [§1160(b); 42 USC §1320c–9(b)]. See Chapter Seven at 231 *infra*. An example of one attempt by a vocal physician group to shield such data is the following amendment to the PSRO statute proposed by the American Medical Association:

> Section 1167 should be amended to provide that the written records of Professional Standards Review Organizations, Statewide Professional Standards Review Councils, and the National Professional Standards Review Council shall not be subject to subpoena or discovery proceedings in any civil action; nor shall the identity of any member, employee, or person providing information, counsel, or services be subject to subpoena or discovery proceedings; nor shall the discussion or deliberations of any organization, council member, employee or person by [sic] subject to subpoena or discovery proceedings in any civil action.

PSRO Oversight Hearings at 76.

32. See n. 48, *infra*.
33. Chapter Six expands on this concept. See also Tancredi and Barsky, "Technology and Health Care Decision Making—Conceptualizing the Process for Societal Informed Consent," XII *Medical Care* 845 (October 1974).
34. See Chapter Two at 32 *infra*.
35. §1152(a) (1); 42 USC §1320c–1(a) (1). There are 203 areas, each of which will have one PSRO serving it. 39 *Fed. Reg.* 10204, March 18, 1974.
36. *Report of the Senate Finance Committee to accompany H.R. 1,* Social Security Amendments of 1972, (Rpt. No. 92–1230, 92d Cong., 2d sess.) [hereinafter cited as *Sen. Fin. Comm. Rpt.*] at 259.
37. Medical societies cannot qualify directly as PSROs because of their dues-paying requirements. §1152(b) (1) (A); 42 USC §1320c–1(b) (1) (A).
38. §1152(c) (1); 42 USC §1320c–1(c) (1). State or local health agencies may be designated at that time. See Chapter Six at 206 *infra*.
39. §1155(c); 42 USC §1320c–4 (c).
40. §1155(a) (5); 42 USC §1320c–4(a) (5).
41. §1155(d) (2); 42USC §1320c–4(d) (2). See Chapter Seven at 238 *infra*.

42. §1155(c); 42 USC §1320c–4(c).
43. §1155(a) (6); 42 USC §1320c–4(a) (6).
44. §1155(b) (3) and (4); 42 USC §1320c–4(b) (3) and (4).
45. §1155(b) (1) and (f) (2); 42 USC §1320c–4(b) (1) and (f) (2).
46. §1165, 42 USC §1320c–14. See Chapter Four at 124 *infra* on data activities.
47. §1158; 42 USC §1320c–7.
48. §1162; 42 USC §1320c–11. See Chapter Six, at 203 *infra* on consumer participation. Although there is no specific authority for them under the statute, the Secretary has also created Statewide Support Centers to give state medical societies a role in the PSRO system. The battle of statewide versus local control of the program was waged by state societies. The Social Security Amendments of 1973, H.R. 3153 (93d Cong., 2d sess.) technical and conforming amendments contained a proposal that §1152 be amended so that creation of a statewide PSRO could not be refused solely because of the number of physicians which would be included in its area (H.R. 3153, §188). A third amendment would establish Statewide Councils in every state with at least one PSRO, and would alter the membership require-ments to give the PSROs in the state more representatives (H.R. 3153, §189). These proposals were not enacted during the 93d Congress. See Chapter Six at 180 *infra* for a history of the development of Statewide Support Centers.
49. §1162(e) (1); 42 USC §1320c–11(e) (1).
50. §1163(a); 42 USC §1320c–12 (a).
51. §1163(b); 42 USC §1320c–12(b). The Council has been named and is operating. See Chapter Six at 201 *infra.*
52. There have been many administrative problems in coordinating the activities of other agencies which deal with matters related to PSROs and establishing administrative authority for the program. Some of the HEW offices involved include Office of Professional Standards Review (OPSR), Bureau of Quality Assurance (BQA), Bureau of Health Insurance (BHI), Social and Rehabilitative Services (SRS), Bureau of Hearings and Appeals (BHA), and the Social Security Administration (SSA) generally. For a discussion of some of these difficulties, see Turner, "Health Report/HEW Begins Medical Review, AMA, hospitals mount opposition," *National Journal Reports,* January 19, 1974, at 90. A "Memorandum of Under-standing" clarifying interagency relationships and responsibilities has been reported. See *PSRO Letter* (semimonthly McGraw-Hill publica-tion) [hereinafter cited as *PSRO Letter*] (no. 18), May 1, 1974, at 3, and (no. 20), June 1, 1974, at 2. For information on the development of relationships among the administrative agencies within HEW see the following editions of the *PSRO Letter:* (no. 1), August 15, 1973, at 2–4; (no. 2), September 1, 1973, at 3; (no. 3), September 15, 1973, at 7; (no. 4), October 1, 1973, at 3,5,8; (no. 5), October 15, 1973, at 4,8; (no. 6), November 1, 1973, at 1; (no. 10),

January 1, 1974, at 4; (no. 11), January 11, 1974, at 3; (no. 13), February 15, 1974, at 3; (no. 14), March 1, 1974, at 2,4; (no. 15), March 14, 1974, at 7; (no. 16), April 1, 1974, at 1; and (no. 26), September 1, 1974, at 2.

53. §1155(a) (1); 42 USC §1320c–4(a) (1). See Chapter Four at 121 *infra* for a summary of the activities which will be preempted.
54. §1155(e) (1); 42 USC §1320c–4(e) (1). See Chapter Three at 71 *infra.*
55. See Chapter Four at 109 *infra.*
56. §1155(a) (2) 42 USC §1320c–4(a) (2).
57. §1160 (a) (2); 42 USC §1320c–9(a) (2).
58. §1156(a); 42 USC §1320c–5(a). See Chapter Two 29 *infra.*
59. §1156(c) (1); 42 USC §1320c–5(c) (1). See Chapter Two at 34 *infra.*
60. §1156(a); 42 USC §1320c–5(c) (1). See Chapter Two at 47 *infra.*
61. See Chapter Two at 44 *infra.*
62. §1167(c); 42 USC §1320c–16(c). See Chapter Seven at 232 *infra.*
63. §1160(b); 42 USC §1320c–9(b). See Chapter Seven at 235 *infra.*
64. §1159; 42 USC §1320c–8. See Chapter Five at 137 *infra.*
65. P.L. 92–603.
66. §229, P.L. 92–603; §§1862(d) (4); 1866(b) (2) (F); 42 USC §§1395y(d) (4), 1395cc(b) (2) (F).
67. §1157; 42 USC §1320c–6. See Chapter Six at 207 *infra* for a more detailed discussion.
68. §228, P.L. 92–603; §1814(h), (i); 42 USC §1395f(h), (i).
69. §1155(a) (2) (B); 42 USC §1320c–4(a) (2) (B). See Chapter Five at 149 *infra* for more discussion of this type of PSRO approval.
70. §229I, P.L. 92–603, §§226(e)–(g); 42 USC §§426(e)–(g).
71. "Final Policies, P.L. 92–603, Section 299I, End-Stage Renal Disease Program of Medicare," April 1974, Office of Policy Development and Planning, Office of Assistant Secretary for Health, DHEW, at 5; *PSRO Letter* (no. 18), May 1, 1974, at 4–5.
72. §299D(a), P.L. 92–603; §1864(a); 42 USC §1395aa(a); 299D(b), §1902(a), 42 USC §1396a(a).
73. §249, P.L. 92–603; §1106(d), (e); 42 USC §1306(d),(e).
74. For a discussion of PSRO information policies and potentials see Chapter Six at 182 *infra.* Other proposals which were not enacted include §216, H.R. 1 establishing an "Inspector General for Health Administration" in the Department of Health, Education and Welfare, independent of subagency control, answerable only to the Secretary, with oversight authority for Titles XVIII and XIX and any other federal health care programs. See *Sen. Fin. Comm. Rpt.* at 57.
75. This study does not consider proposals to continue the previously existing utilization review system. For a summary of the quality and cost control programs in effect before PSROs, see Chapter Three at 67 *infra;* and Chapter Four at 112 *infra.*
76. S. 1898 (92d Cong., 1st sess., 1971) (Sen. Fulton); H.R. 8684 (92d Cong., 1st sess., 1971) (Rep. Broyhill).

77. See Ellwood, et al., *Assuring the Quality of Health Care,* (Minneapolis, Minn.: InterStudy, 1973), at 89–125, and Appendix II at 1–26.

78. Title III, S. 3 (93d Cong., 1st sess., 1973) (Sen. Kennedy) is identical to H.R. 22 (Rep. Griffiths). These bills, in substantially the same form but without the quality commission title, had been introduced in 1971. See S. 3, (92d Cong., 1st sess., 1971); H.R. 22 (92d Cong., 1st sess., 1971). After their initial reintroduction in 1973, the provisions on the quality assurance commission were substantially revised as part of the Kennedy HMO Act Proposal—so that the quality assurance commission in S. 3 represented essentially Ellwood's health outcomes commission approach. See Title II, S. 3 (93d Cong., 1st sess., 1973), 119 *Cong. Rec.* S9137 (May 15, 1973).

79. See this chapter at 16 *infra* on PSROs and national health insurance proposals.

80. See n. 18 *supra.*

81. See n. 113 *infra* on "Medicredit."

82. S. 1898 (92d Cong., 1st sess., 1971) at §2102(c).

83. *Id.* at §2103.

84. The PSRO authority exists in §1155, 42 USC §1320c–4.

85. PSRO authority is given in §§1151, 1158; 42 USC §§1320c, 1320c–7.

86. §1156; 42 USC §1320c–5. Norms are prescribed for PSRO use.

87. See n. 29 *supra.*

88. See Chapter Six at 174 *infra* for a discussion of program elements necessary to consumer accountability.

89. PSROs are forbidden to review costs. See Chapter Six at 208 *infra.*

90. See Chapter Six at 184 *infra.*

91. See n. 37 *supra.*

92. See Ellwood et al., *supra* n. 77, generally. The discussion in the text which follows is based on InterStudy's book. InterStudy defines an HMO this way: "An HMO is a public or private organization which provides, either directly or through arrangement with others, health services including, at a minimum, hospital and physician services, to enrollees on a per capita, prepayment basis." *Id.* at 19. According to InterStudy's theory, HMO quality assurance is maintained through free market competition. "Such organizations will be responsible for the quality and availability of their services and are expected to compete for voluntarily enrolled consumers with other providers including other HMOs." *Id.* For other discussion of PSROs and HMOs see Chapter Three.

93. Review of quality usually focuses on three aspects of care: (1) input, (2) process, and (3) outcomes. Inputs are those aspects of quality which affect personnel and facilities qualifications such as personnel licensure and approval by the Joint Commission on Accreditation of Hospitals (JCAH). Process review examines the actual treatment rendered and the manner in which it was delivered—for example, whether the treatment was appropriate to the diagnosis. Outcomes or end result review examines the result of medical services to the

patient. For a more detailed discussion, see Chapter Two at 30 *infra*.

94. See n. 78 *supra*.
95. S. 3 at §1202(b).
96. *Id.* at §1202(a) (1).
97. *Id.* at §141.
98. *Id.* at §145.
99. *Id.* at §132(c).
100. Conditions of participation for providers under Medicare impose some quality standards, such as approval by the Joint Commission on Accreditation of Hospitals, §§1861(e), 1865; 42 USC §§1395x(e), 1395bb. Under Medicaid, other types of programs assuring the standards of institutions are required. §§1902(a) (22) (B), 1902(a) (26), 1902(a) (31); 42 USC §§1396a(a) (22) (B), 1396a(a) (26), 1396a(a) (31).
101. P.L. 93–222 (93d Cong., 2d sess., 1973).
102. The definition of an HMO under the Act is different from the InterStudy definition, *supra* n. 92. There are at least 11 separate requirements to qualify as an HMO under the act. §1301(c) (1–11). See "Joint Explanatory Statement of the Committee of Conference," in *Health Maintenance Organization Act of 1973, S. 14* (Comm. Print., 1974) prepared for the Senate Subcommittee on Health of the Commission on Labor and Public Welfare, February 1974, at 41.
103. P.L. 93–222, §1301(c) (8).
104. P.L. 93–222, §399c. The general HMO budget for fiscal year 1975, was drastically cut by the House from $58 million requested to $18 million approved. See *Health Systems* (Washington, D.C.: Morris Associates Report, July 30, 1974); "The HMO bandwagon traveling at slower pace," *American Medical News,* October 14, 1974, at 1; and "HMOs," *Medical World News,* January 27, 1975, at 53.
105. P.L. 93–222, §4. The conferees specifically indicated that the Institute of Medicine of the National Academy of Sciences be included among those given the opportunity to conduct the study. See *Joint Explanatory Statement, supra* n. 102, at 72.
106. P.L. 93–222, §4(d).
107. P.L. 93–222, §4(c).
108. §1152(b) (2) and (c); 42 USC §1320c–1(b) (2) and (c). See this chapter at 8 *supra* and Chapter Six at 206 *infra*.
109. Although the law requires the study to examine some aspects of quality assessment from the consumer point of view, there is no requirement that consumers participate in or consult on those sections of the study.
110. "Comprehensive Health Insurance Act of 1974," S. 2970, H.R. 12684 (93d Cong., 2d sess.) (Mills-Packwood), the administration's proposal; "Comprehensive National Health Insurance Act of 1974," S. 3286, H.R. 13870 (Kennedy-Mills); and "The Catastrophic Health Insurance Act," S. 2153 (Long-Ribicoff). Other bills that include PSROs are the "Health Rights Act of 1973," S. 2756 (Scott-Percy),

which would rely on PSROs with some additional features; and the "National Health Insurance Partnership Act of 1971," H.R. 2618 (Railsback).

111. See n. 78 *supra.*

112. "National Health Care Services Reorganization and Financing Act," H.R. 1 (Ullman); "National Health Care Act of 1973," H.R. 5200, S. 1100 (Burleson-McIntyre); "National Health Care Act of 1973," H.R. 559 (Fuqua); "National Health Insurance and Health Services Improvement Act of 1973," S. 915 (Javits); "National Comprehensive Health Benefits Act of 1973," H.R. 11345 (Staggers); and "National Health Insurance Act," H.R. 33 (Dingell).

113. "Health Insurance Act of 1973," S. 444, H.R. 222 (Fulton-Broyhill); H.R. 288 (Ashbrook).

114. See n. 18 *supra.*

115. For a discussion of recent trends and issues in health regulation, see Iglehart, "Health Report/Executive-congressional coalition seeks tighter regulation for medical services industry," *National Journal Reports,* November 19, 1973, at 1684. For an examination of PSROs and other traditional methods of government regulation, see Cohen, "Manpower and Social Controls," 48 *Hospitals, JAHA* 105 (April 1, 1974); and Cohen, "Regulatory Politics: The Case of Medical Care Review and Public Law 92–603" Paper delivered at American Political Science Association Meeting, New Orleans, September 5, 1973, on file with the author.) For another examination of regulatory trends, see Havighurst, "Regulation in the Health Care System," 48 *Hospitals, JAHA* 65 (June 16, 1974), which is a summary of Havighurst's longer piece, "Regulation of Health Facilities and Services by 'certificate of need'," 59 *Va. L. Rev.* 1149 (October 1973).

116. *Sen. Fin. Comm. Rpt.* at 259.

117. "Background Material Relating to Professional Standards Review Organizations (PSROs)," *Sen. Fin. Comm.* (Comm. Print, May 8, 1974), at 11.

118. See *American Medical News* of the following dates: April 10, 1973; May 7, 1973; May 21, 1973; May 28, 1973; June 4, 1973; September 10, 1973; September 17, 1973; October 29, 1973; November 26, 1973; January 1, 1974; April 22, 1974; May 20, 1974; May 27, 1974.

A law suit was filed challenging the constitutionality of the PSRO law. At this writing the opinion in the case was expected shortly. *Association of American Physicians and Surgeons, et al. v. Weinberger,* No. 73 C 1653, (N.D. Ill., filed June 26, 1973.) The Texas State Medical Society initially planned to sue to overturn the area designation for Texas, but the suit was never filed. See *American Medical News,* April 15, 1974, at 3.

One physician reportedly retired rather than "tolerate" PSROs. See "PSRO prompts surgeon to retire," *American Medical News,* January 14, 1974, at 5.

It was not until the last week of June 1974 that the AMA, internally shaken by dissent over PSROs, cautiously agreed to cooperate. See "Showdown at the AMA: Delegates Take Over," *Medical World News*, July 19, 1974, at 15; and "Peer Review: The AMA Says Yes," *The New York Times*, June 30, 1974, at 9E.

119. See Chapter Four at 124 *infra.*

120. Although PSROs will only review services ordered by physicians, PSRO review will directly affect hospital budgets. The American Hospital Association reports that 80 to 85 percent of costs in a hospital's budget are generated by physician orders. "Quality Assurance Program: AHA's attempt to keep the medical review functions in the hospital," *Modern Hospital*, March 1973, at 40.

121. See "Organizations Vie for PSRO Power," *American Medical News*, May 14, 1973, at 14.

122. See "Dr. Bauer quits as head of federal PSRO agency," *American Medical News*, September 24, 1973, at 1.

123. See Constantine, "On the Other Hand," *Medical World News*, September 24, 1973, at 1.

124. See *PSRO Letter* (no. 26), September 1, 1974.

125. "Background Material," *supra* n. 117, at 23.

126. See testimony of Henry Simmons, Director, OPSR, *PSRO Oversight Hearings* at 26.

127. See Turner, *supra* n. 52, at 98, quoting Simmons.
One operating PSRO analyzes its costs per admission review at $13 to $14 and that figure is expected to double in the near future. Another PSRO estimates a $9 cost per admission review. "PSROs: How the first ones are working," *Medical World News*, October 25, 1974, at 56, 59.

128. 1 Q 74, *Perspective* (Blue Cross Association), at 7.

129. See Chapter Two at 44 *infra.*

Chapter Two

Norms[1]

If PSROs are to yield beneficial effects through improved quality of care, and consequently improved health status among patients,[2] those results will depend on the norms that are selected and their application. The keystone to the PSRO program, and the major determinant of its success as a cost control and quality assurance system, is the development and use of norms as the "principal points of evaluation and review"[3] of the medical care rendered to Medicare and Medicaid patients. "[N]orms of care, diagnosis and treatment ... including lengths-of-stay for institutional care"[4] by age and diagnosis are the basic standards for all review of the medical necessity, appropriateness, and quality of care.[5] The concept of norms (described more fully below) has been the most controversial element of the PSRO program, presenting the greatest obstacle to the program's acceptance by physicians.[6] Physician opponents have asserted that this direct intrusion by government into the delivery of care will, at best, lead to standardized care and stifled innovative practices; at worst, they claim it will alter radically the basic practice of medicine.[7] Control of the norms-setting process is of major concern also to those physicians who are not intransigently opposed to a peer review system which uses some sort of objective standards.[8]

For consumers, as well as other analysts of PSROs, the basic programmatic tension between cost and quality is epitomized in the norms-setting and application processes.[9] At every point that a decision is made to limit the range of covered services by establishing norms, the problem of domination of cost or quality factors is present. Because, for example, the law requires that norms for each condition must consider which facility is "the type in which health care services which are medically appropriate ... can be most economically provided,"[10] cost considerations are built into the choice of norms. The relative weight given to cost elements can alter standards significantly. The following extreme example highlights how this can work. In deciding whether a patient who has had a heart attack needs the level of care available in a sophisticated coronary care unit, that choice must be evaluated against the risks of treating him at home. Obviously, the care available in a coronary unit will be more expensive than care in the patient's home with physician backup services only in case of an emergency. If norms were to carry cost consciousness to an absurd point they would approve no care: the least costly care is no care at all—a choice that is politically, realistically, and humanistically unacceptable. We must assume good faith on the part of both the designers of the PSRO program and its physician implementers. In establishing norms, physicians, then, must strike a balance between cost and quality; to do so, they must have some notion of what "quality" is and how to evaluate it. The parameters which PSROs apply will, in essence, embody the PSRO program's resolution of this crucial, though elusive, definition.

How physicians strike that balance depends on the methodology and focus of review. Quality assessment generally focuses on three aspects of care:[11] (1) *structure* or *input*—the context in which actual services are delivered, including the physical environment, the qualifications of personnel, and the organizational structure of the institution;[12] (2) *process*—how care is delivered, including technical competence and the appropriateness of the services to the condition;[13] and (3) *outcomes* or *end results*—what happened to the patient as a result of care, i.e., improvement, deterioration, no change.[14]

PSRO review based on norms is maladapted to an input review program. Nowhere does the statute mention personnel or facilities licensure; and, in fact, these elements of care are ordinarily the subject of other types of laws.[15] The PSRO approach puts the major emphasis on the process of care through its requirement of review of the discrete services rendered to patients. The review of the process of care is more amenable to serving the two different PSRO interests, cost control and quality assurance. In review of process each service can be quantified as a separate cost factor. As each service is approved or disapproved for coverage it can also be reviewed for quality—whether it is appropriate to the patient's condition. For example, in evaluating the appropriateness of and necessity for a hysterectomy, physicians would not approve the procedure as the treatment of choice for a patient with an inflamed appendix, although similar symptoms might dictate a hysterectomy or appendectomy in certain cases. If through review the services are deemed medically appropriate, their scope can be examined. For example, although a drug to control joint inflammation may be correct treatment for a patient suffering from arthritis, certain medications should be given for only short periods of time; prolonged use of such drugs can be ineffective or harmful. At each point where it is determined that a service is not within the established parameters of care, that individual service can be disapproved and simultaneously costs will thereby be cut. Review of process, using these separate steps, is better adapted to a single review for both cost and quality factors than are other methods.

In contrast, end result review looks at the totality of the patient's condition as a result of care.[16] Generally, however, this type of review is aimed at "maximizing desired outcomes over a population and not necessarily for each patient";[17] and, therefore, a determination as a result of outcomes review that an individual patient's condition had worsened or was unimproved would not necessarily imply a decision that care was not of high quality. Also, because outcomes review examines patterns of care, as a methodology it is not easily linked to specific measures for cost control in individual cases, such as those sought in the PSRO program.[18] PSRO process review, as established by the statute, also is essentially oriented toward a fee for service delivery mechanism—the patient (or the government on his behalf) pays a fee for each service to him—in contrast with end result review which is most often associated with prepaid financing mechanisms.[19] In addition, although process review can be done prospectively to avoid unnecessary services and costs, end result review must, by definition, take place after care has been delivered.

Despite the utility of process review for cost control, consumers (and others) will be concerned about whether the use of norms as objective standards for evaluating care will change the quality of care rendered to Medicare and Medicaid patients.[20] The PSRO statute creates systemic incentives for practitioners to both apply and adhere to the PSRO's norms.[21] If norms are set with concern for high quality care, as a result of those incentives, depending on their effectiveness, practitioners and providers whose patterns of practice fall below PSRO standards may be forced to upgrade their practices. Conversely, if norms are oriented primarily toward cost control at the expense of quality, incentives to adhere to norms will result in lower quality care. Improved care as a result of using norms may also result from the educational value to physicians of establishing and applying a detailed quality assessment system—a method which also has been cited as an effective technique to improve quality without sanctions and penalties.[22]

The development and use of norms as the program's foundation most significantly brand PSROs as peer review entities. The Senate Finance Committee specifically chose the peer review course: "The Committee believes that the review process should be based upon the premise that only physicians are, in general, qualified to judge whether services ordered by other physicians are necessary."[23] In addition to the choice of peer review for the future, the Committee's decision to use physician-established norms anticipated the inclusion of past physician review experiences.[24] As this chapter will suggest, other choices were and are available. The decision to create a total physician-oriented program was motivated by the Senate Finance Committee's "aware[ness] of increasing instances of criticism directed at the use of insurance company personnel and government employees in reviewing the medical necessity of services."[25] At least three separate situations will arise in the course of establishing and applying norms where consumer input will be appropriate and probably beneficial.

1. There are many areas of medicine where the choice of treatment is controversial. Tonsillectomies, circumcisions, breast cancer, and stomach ulcers have recently been citied.[26] One reason for such disputes is a lack of quantifiable and conclusive evidence indicating which treatment should be preferred. If peer review has any validity, it lies in the expertise of physicians in technical medical matters. Unless a clear technical consideration is the basis of a physician's preference for treatment, he has no expertise by virture of his profession to make the choice. Medical decisions where there is no overriding technical factor mandating a specific choice are not, in fact, medically determined decisions; they may, instead be guided by psychological, financial, or social factors. Physicians have no monopoly on the ability to make nonmedical determinations. Where controversial procedures are the subject of norms, consumer input will be no less valid than "peer" dialogue in making some determinations.

2. Many aspects of the quality of care involve socioeconomic factors affecting the patient's condition. An example would be an elderly widower living alone on the top floor of a three story, walk-up apartment building who falls and breaks a hip. Although his immediate needs might extend only to having the fracture set and convalescing until ambulatory, PSRO norms of care must have the ability to confront the fact that at the time when strictly technical medical concerns might dictate his discharge, the patient will be unable to climb the three flights of stairs in his building or care for himself. To discharge that man from an institution might represent poor quality care because of the potential risks to him of reinjury and complications. In setting standards which accommodate socioeconomic factors, consumers, again, have valid insights to offer.[27]

3. The third situation involves nontechnical elements of care which can directly affect the results of treatment. Doctor-patient communication, for example, is a major factor in the delivery of medical care. With good communication the patient will be more likely to follow his physician's instructions and contribute psychologically to his own recovery; poor communication can be directly inimical to good treatment results.[28] If PSROs are a quality review system, these factors will have to be recognized by and incorporated into the standards PSROs set. Consumers' inclusion in the establishment, if not the evaluation, process will help ensure that a quality-oriented program is created.

Norms can benefit consumers or be detrimental to their interests depending on how they are used. If norms help generate improvement in the quality of medical care by forcing bad practitioners to meet higher standards of practice, they will help consumers. If the standards applied are widely disseminated to consumers, they will contribute to health education and give consumers the ability to take a more active role in their health care.[29] If norms include nontechnical elements of care, including elements in patients' "Bills of Rights,"[30] and socioeconomic aspects of care, by drawing attention to the patient's total needs the program will have wide-ranging positive effects. With review for medical necessity based on accepted professional standards, the result may be expanded Medicare and Medicaid coverage, severing these programs from the artificial benefits packages now used to control costs.[31] Because of the PSRO system's ability to use norms to pinpoint underserved areas,[32] norms can form the basis for improved health facilities and manpower planning and funding.[33]

Norms also have the potential to mold all other PSRO processes to work against consumers' interests. If norms cover only the most minimal levels of care, PSRO authority to review care prospectively in order to certify proposed treatment for payment can deny consumers access to institutions.[34] Because of the PSRO statute's malpractice exemption for physicians who comply with PSRO norms, if a physician's practice, though in accord with PSRO norms, nonetheless injures a patient, the patient may have no way to sue the physician and recover damages.[35] If, where there is significant medical controversy, physicians choose norms solely on the basis of cost considerations, and without input from consumers, consumers will suffer doubly: not only will they have been unable to influence the choices of standards, but their options for medical care will have been limited by the choice. Because norms will form the basis for establishing physician, provider, and patient profiles,[36] their being skewed to control costs will bias the result of all other evaluations based on them. Profiles attempting to show patterns of practice will not be valid indices of the quality of care delivered in this country if norms are set so low that physicians must abide by them or suffer financially unabsorbable expenses of noncoverage.[37] Under those circumstances, profiles will show only compliance with norms, and their value as documentation of medical care will be decreased.[38] Finally, if norms are rigidly applied, despite an orientation toward quality, they will hamper physicians' abilities to respond to aberrant medical problems. Strictly standardized care, even if high quality, can lead to inappropriate care for patients whose conditions present an unusual course of disease. If norms do not strike an acceptable balance between costs and quality standardization will affect more patients. Because in the PSRO system there is great potential for manipulation of the processes by which norms will be set and applied, the range of possible effects from their use is also wide. It is unlikely that all the negative effects just described will occur. But the PSRO statute's definite emphasis on cost control makes it just as unlikely that review will yield uniformly beneficial results. The real effects of this form of objectified review will, in the end, be determined by the discretion given to each PSRO and its use of that authority. The statute itself only begins to define the parameters of responsibility for setting norms and applying them.

STATUTORY REQUIREMENTS

Norms are not defined in either the statute or the legislative history; they are characterized. Their functions are stated; their scope is indicated. Norms are to be used as "principal points of evaluation and review."[39] They will be "professionally developed,"[40] "based on typical patterns of practice,"[41] and will extend to care, diagnosis, and treatment.[42] Lengths of stay for institutional care by age and diagnosis will be included in them. Under the law, norms will consider the types and extent of services appropriate to particular illnesses or conditions "taking into account differing modes of treatment."[43] Norms will be used to evaluate the appropriateness of the particular health care facility in which treatment is rendered with regard to its being the most economical but still medically acceptable approach.[44]

The statute mandates several uses for norms. They provide the basis for all review of the medical necessity and quality of care as well as the appropriateness of the delivery facility to the treatment.[45] They may be applied retrospectively, after care has been delivered, or prospectively when elective (nonemergency) admissions or other services "which will consist of extended or costly courses of treatment" have been proposed.[46] Norms will form the basis for the PSRO to establish those points in time after admission when the physician will be required to certify the medical necessity of the patient's continued stay.[47] Finally, by implication, norms will provide the foundation for the physician, provider, and patient profiles which are used to evaluate patterns of medical practice.[48]

The statutory provisions on establishing norms are ambiguous. It is clear norms are to be "professionally developed."[49] Each PSRO has the responsibility to "apply" and "utilize" norms based on typical patterns of practice "in its regions."[50] The National Professional Standards Review Council "shall provide for the preparation and distribution ... [to each PSRO] ... of appropriate materials indicating the *regional norms to be utilized.*"[51] The statute also provides for the National Council to approve the use of norms other than those generally applicable to the region in areas "where the *actual norms* in a (PSRO) area are significantly different."[52] These provisions, taken together, make it appear that the National Council will establish the norms to be applied by each PSRO; and, in fact, that apparent authority has been the subject of serious controversy.[53] Many physicans have claimed that these provisions constitute a specific call for nationwide, uniform standards of care.[54] The confusion is aggravated by distinct references to PSRO "areas" elsewhere in the statute;[55] "regions" are mentioned only in the norms section.[56]

The first guidelines issued under the statute are contained in the *PSRO Program Manual*[57] and attempt to define norms and to clarify the allocation of responsibility for establishing them. The *Manual's* provisions, though, are only guidelines; since they are not regulations, modifications without procedural formalities are possible and contemplated.[58] The *Manual* provides that "[m]edical care appraisal norms [be] numerical or statistical measures of usual observed performance."[59] Under this definition norms can only apply to elements of care which are susceptible to quantification (e.g., average lengths of stay, or ranges of normal values for laboratory studies). They are to be "derived from aggregate information related to health care provided to a large number of patients over time."[60] Because quantifiable care factors alone are insufficient for evaluating the quality of services delivered to patients, the *Manual* creates two other parametric categories: "*Standards* ... professionally developed expressions of the range of acceptable variation from a norm or criterion...," and "*Criteria* ... predetermined elements against which aspects of the quality of medical service may be compared."[61]

For their development, criteria will rely heavily on professional expertise and professional literature and each will catalogue those services which should be rendered to treat a patient with a specific condition. In treating a patient with a myocardial infarction (heart attack), the following elements, among others, might be included among the criteria for care: a medical history, electrocardiograms, chest X-rays, complete bed rest, myriad laboratory studies, and a variety of drugs. This partial listing indicates the diversity of elements which can be subsumed under the label "criteria." "Standards" will indicate how often each of those elements should be present in a course of treatment. For example, a medical history should always be taken. Electrocardiograms might be required daily or more often initially, but less frequently toward the end of hospitalization. A single chest X-ray during the patient's length of stay might be indicated according to standards, but performing an X-ray daily or not at all would be unacceptable variations. Whether norms, as the statute discusses them, are applied flexibly or rigidly is a function of the "standards" for each condition. In other words, the narrower the range of acceptable deviation, the stricter the standard. Establishing the ranges will be the most critical factor in determining whether cost or quality interests dominate in PSRO review.

Clarifying the statutory ambiguity, the *Manual* requires that each local PSRO establish and apply its own norms.

> The PSRO is responsible for the development and ongoing modifica-
> tion of the criteria and standards and the selection of the norms to
> be used in its area. While PSROs may structure themselves in many
> ways to perform these duties, the overall responsibility for the
> development, modification and content of norms, criteria and
> standards rests with the PSRO.[62]

The National Council is to furnish each PSRO with sample sets of norms and criteria.[63] PSROs may then adopt or adapt the sample sets or develop their own variables,[64] subject to ultimate National Council approval. Because the process of selecting and establishing parameters for review will take time, the *Manual* specifies considerations for assigning priorities among the conditions to be evaluated: the frequency with which a condition or problem is seen in hospitalized patients; the degree to which health can be improved by identifying and treating particular problems; and the degree to which subjective or objective evidence indicates inappropriate utilization or substandard quality.[65]

PSROs will also be responsible for developing norms, criteria, and standards for use in developing profiles of physicians, providers, and patients.[66] Dissemination of norms, criteria, and standards will be directed primarily at physicians and providers;[67] and modifications are expected.[68] Although physicians have the ultimate responsibility for review, the *Manual* specifically requires that PSROs enlist nonphysician health care practitioners[69] to participate in establishing, modifying, and applying the norms, criteria, and standards relevant to their respective disciplines.[70]

SELECTING AND APPLYING NORMS

The statute's reference only to "norms" (not standards and criteria) creates an ambiguity. Will the hallmark of norms be their reflection of the highest quality care or mere codifications of existing practice? The *Manual*'s use of "standards" and "criteria" is an attempt to achieve some balance between quality and actual practice. "Norms," as the *Manual* and statute define them, are statements of existing typical patterns of practice. Criteria represent optimal levels of care as established by experts. Standards determine the balance by delimiting the acceptable range of deviation from norms and criteria.[71] But the choice of criteria can directly shift the standards. Many specialty societies have established criteria for various diagnoses of concern to them.[72] One analyst has estimated that there were at least 50 different criteria sets in existence before the implementation of PSROs had even begun.[73] Those in existence, as well as those any individual PSRO might develop, may be biased according to which specialists collaborated in their creation. If, for example, surgeons develop a set of criteria for hypertension (high blood pressure), that set might include surgical intervention as the treatment of choice, whereas a set developed by internists might not ordinarily suggest surgery. On the other hand, standards mitigate those biases depending on the influences exerted at the standards-setting level. If surgeons dominate the criteria selection process, but internists dominate the standards committee, the internists may seek to vitiate the effect of the surgical prejudice. Although there is no necessary correlation between consensus selection of standards among specialties and improved quality of care, a consensus approach will guarantee that no single specialty group dominates, and will, thereby, widen the range of options for medical care for consumers.[74]

In establishing norms, problems may arise from reliance on

particular data sources. If, for example, data developed by Medicaid state agencies[75] is the source for establishing norms, the patterns of practice reflected in Medicaid claims forms will undoubtedly reflect the limitations on coverage imposed by the state's Medicaid plan. For example, in one state, Medicaid state agency data may identify hospital stays totaling less than 30 days per years as a typical practice for all Medicaid patients in that state, regardless of their conditions, because the state plan covers only 30 days of hospitalization. In that case, the data may demonstrate only that the physicians treating Medicaid patients do not order services exceeding coverage because of the risk of nonpayment. Exclusive reliance on state agency data would prejudice the PSRO's norms against Medicare patients whose coverage may be more liberal. If it is true that poor people and old people have utilization rates different from the general population, it is critical to recognize that fact in the development of norms. Beyond this though, reliance on information developed from claims forms data will almost certainly prejudice norms in favor of cost control.[76]

Whether cost or quality concerns prevail will be reflected in the scope of norms, criteria, and standards. If these variables confront only coverage issues (i.e., which benefits can be approved and what services Medicare and Medicaid will not pay for), other factors which can affect the quality of care will be ignored. Socioeconomic considerations such as diet and living environment, can prolong, aggravate, or cause recurrence of a condition. One of the difficulties in including these factors in a quantified approach to care is that they are not easily reduced to checklists or numerical variables and are even more difficult to evaluate comparatively. That socioeconomic factors do affect the patient's condition is indisputable; that physicians include them in selecting treatment has been demonstrated in studies.[77] It is critical that PSROs develop the technology and analytic capability to permit the inclusion of these factors in medical care evaluation.

Other nontechnical aspects in the delivery of care affect its quality. Informed patient consent to procedures is now widely accepted as an element in the proper delivery of care. Good physician-patient communication is also vital to good care because without it treatment often cannot proceed. In reviewing these aspects of care, consumer involvement will be essential both to meaningful analysis of the problem and development of corrective programs. Physicians cannot effect better relations with patients if their existing failure to do so rests on misunderstanding or ignorance of patients' needs. Patients themselves are best able to explain why they were unable to understand their physician's instructions. The involvement of nonphysician professionals, such as social workers, whose training may specifically orient them toward confronting socioeconomic and other nontechnical aspects of care, also would contribute to the general quality assessment activities of PSROs.[78]

For these kinds of quality assessment issues, end result review may be more useful for discovering and correcting poor practices. Part of an end result or outcomes-oriented approach is a focus on consumer responses to physician treatment:

> "...[T]he outcomes definition of quality implies a little recognized responsibility of the health care system: the responsibility for patient compliance. If the quality of health care lies in maximizing the outcomes for patients, then it is not enough just to diagnose, treat and prescribe."[79]

In relating actual results of care to expected outcomes, end result review contemplates analysis of the reasons why poor results exceed preestablished estimates. For example, if the estimated outcome for treatment of venereal disease in a particular institution was a rate of 95 percent controlled conditions after administration of antibiotics, but review revealed that 20 percent of the patients evaluated were still infected, physicians using end result review would analyze why results fell below their estimates. Such analysis might discover that patients failed to take medication because they did not understand the relationship between the medication and their condition, or that patients failed to return for follow-up care.[80] These types of quality "failures" are not the result of technical incompetence. They do, however, implicate physician attention to nontechnical aspects of care.

Although PSROs are directed toward process evaluation, there is nothing which precludes inclusion of outcomes review techniques in some review and the *Manual* permits outcomes review in individual institutions.[81] The most effective quality review would combine elements from both approaches.[82] Because the outcomes review notion entails a consensus on anticipated treatment results among the physicians in an institution, an individual PSRO may not be the appropriate entity to establish estimates of outcomes for its constituent institutions. A PSRO could, however, require each institution over which it has jurisdiction to review nontechnical aspects of care (through outcomes review) and to submit its outcomes estimates to the PSRO for its own review of practitioners and providers.[83]

THE PROCESS OF REVIEW

Whichever norms, criteria, and standards the PSRO chooses, they will be used in four different types of medical review: (1) preadmission review; (2) concurrent admission certification; (3) continued stay review; and (4) retrospective review.[84] This listing follows a time continuum from preadmission review, before any services have been delivered, through retrospective review, which is performed after the patient has been discharged. To examine briefly the types of review which a PSRO can perform, the following discussion considers the steps in review of a hypothetical elective (nonemergency) hospital admission for a hysterectomy.[85]

If the PSRO, at its discretion, has included elective hysterectomies among the procedures it reviews prior to admission,[86] the physician would first present to it his reasons for seeking the admission. The PSRO would then compare the data supplied by the physician with its norms, criteria, and standards for hysterectomies. Among the issues for the PSRO would be the indications that the hysterectomy was necessary; for example, whether for a 45 year old woman with recurrent mid-menstrual cycle bleeding the PSRO's criteria included hysterectomy as an approved procedure. Relevant laboratory studies (e.g., results of a recent Pap smear) would be presented if the criteria required them. Whether the proposed treatment would be an abdominal or a vaginal hysterectomy, and total (removal of the uterus, cervix, and both ovaries) or partial (removal only of the uterus and cervix) would be considered by the PSRO in determining the appropriate length of stay. The specificity of PSRO-required information will depend on the scope of its norms, criteria, and standards as well as the individual PSRO's implementation of preadmission review. Obviously, the PSRO's ability to assess the proposed admission is contingent on its having complete information, but, beyond that, it will be necessary for physicians to cooperate in supplying the required data.[87] Past experience suggests that both the accuracy and completeness of medical records will be a recurring problem at every level of PSRO review.[88] Approval would also be affected by the flexibility provided by standards—i.e., how many criteria must be met for approval to be granted. PSRO approval of the admission would, according to the Senate Finance Committee, "provide the basis for a presumption of medical necessity for purposes of Medicare and Medicaid."[89] Appeal would be possible where the PSRO had disapproved an admission.[90]

If the admission were approved, the physician and patient would arrange for hospital accommodations. The *Manual* stipulates that all in-patient cases will be subject to admission certification. At least initially, "concurrent certification of elective admission will be performed on *all* elective admissions unless the PSRO can clearly identify in their [sic] review plan diagnoses (or problems) or physicians which do not require such review."[91] Notwithstanding a PSRO's choice to review elective hysterectomies on a preadmission basis, generally the same information required in such review would be considered by the PSRO within one working day following admission[92] in assigning an appropriate length of stay (based on norms and standards) and assuring that an appropriate level of care would be provided.[93] The hysterectomy patient might be assigned a seven day length of stay.

On the seventh day or before, the patient's case would be reassessed.[94] Such continued stay review is used to evaluate "the medical necessity of a patient's need for continued confinement at a hospital level-of-care and may also include a detailed assessment of the quality of care being provided."[95] Whether a case is subject to continued stay review depends on the PSRO's criteria on (1) the types of services which can be provided only in a hospital and (2) the indications for discharge.[96] Had the hysterectomy patient developed a stitch abcess or a postoperative phlebitis (blood clot), for example, a continued stay would probably be approved. A new certification point for another review would be assigned at that time, giving, for example, a four day extension.[97] A PSRO could also choose at this point to perform an in depth quality assessment of the care rendered so far based on criteria "specifying the critical indicated and contraindicated diagnostic and therapeutic services (including their frequency, timing and quality)."[98] It would be at this point in review that the physician's choice of a total or partial hysterectomy could be thoroughly evaluated, as might his postoperative routine use of antibiotics without evidence of infection.

If, after consultation with the attending physician, the PSRO did not approve a continued stay, notice of that disapproval would be given to the hospital, the attending physician, the patient, and, in the case of a Medicaid patient, the Medicaid state agency.[99] An appeal of the disapproval would, ordinarily, be possible.[100]

The three types of review just discussed (together with medical evaluation studies)[101] are intended to meet the needs of the PSRO program. But PSROs are also authorized to perform retrospective review,[102] the type of review which had predominated under the old utilization review system. The Senate Finance Committee has recognized, by implication, at least one situation in the PSRO process when retrospective review will be appropriate:

> ...[I]t is recognized that there are situations in which stays for certain diagnoses may be quite short in duration. In such situations the PSRO might decide against requiring certification at or before expiration of the period of usual length of stay on the grounds that the certification would be unproductive: for example, when the usual duration of stay is two days or less.[103]

In addition, at least where preadmission certification (prior approval) has been given, some retrospective review will be required. Because "advance approval of institutional admission would not preclude a *retroactive finding* that ancillary services (not specifically approved in advance) provided during the covered stay were excessive,"[104] some mechanism for making that retroactive finding is contemplated.[105] Despite the fact that preadmission review may be implemented immediately, the *Manual* indicates that "[r]etrospective review of individual hospital claims is not an initially required PSRO review mechanism ... [and] ... will be used only when required forms of review have not been implemented, or where implemented, have not been performed effectively."[106] The implication is that the *Manual* provides no mechanism to determine whether, for example, private duty nurses, not contemplated by the PSRO norms, were assigned to the case during the hysterectomy patient's recovery from a stitch abcess. Without retrospective review, admission review (prior and concurrent) and continued stay review will be the only procedures required of the PSRO for its determinations to be binding (subject to subsequent appeals).[107]

Once reviewed by the PSRO, services rendered will be reimbursed according to the PSRO's determinations based on its norms, criteria, and standards. The use of those variables is, as this section suggests, the foundation of the PSRO system and determinative of every other aspect of the PSRO scheme. Despite the enormous impact of these variables, the PSRO process does include a mechanism for screening by nonphysician coordinators, usually trained nurses.

The Senate Finance Committee specifically suggests the use of nonphysicians.[108] However, the statutory requirement that none but physicians render final determinations[109] means that all review by nonphysicians (trained nurses or others) will have to be strictly conditioned.[110] Most suggestions for employing nonphysicians to perform review recommend that they "screen" cases.[111] On screening, the *Manual* says only that, based on norms, criteria, and standards "from a number of cases, those requiring more in-depth review"[112] will be sifted. The National Council, however, considered the definition of screening at some length. Although the Council's members initially had agreed to define screening as "a process in which norms, criteria and standards are used to analyze large numbers of items, activities, or transactions in order to select a smaller sample for study in greater depth...,"[113] later deliberations led the Council's Subcommittee on Data and Norms to adopt an altered definition: "Screening is a process in which norms, criteria or standards are used *to analyze large numbers of cases in order to select those cases not meeting these norms, criteria or standards.*"[114] The second definition makes clearer which cases will be subject to further review; that is, only those cases which do not match established patterns. The clarification indicates that physicians can delegate to nurses the responsibility for preliminary determinations. But such delegations will be efficient only if the standards and criteria are so clearly stated that a nonphysician will be able to determine if the case under review falls within those parameters. Criteria conditioned by such phrases as "when indicated" or "under certain circumstances" vitiate whatever advantages derive from delegating initial review.[115]

Nurses or other nonphysician reviewers will need training in applying norms, criteria, and standards if the pitfalls of the old utilization review system are to be avoided.[116] So will most physicians whose experience with such techniques of assessment is, at best, minimal.[117] In addition, questions about applying norms, criteria, and standards to the care rendered by interns and residents have been raised,[118] recognizing that the care delivered by those who are learning may not conform with established patterns of practice. The *Manual* does not confront this problem at all. But unless specific attention is devoted to applying parameters to physicians who provide care as part of their education, patients will suffer doubly when care does not match established patterns: (1) the quality of care they receive will be inferior if they are rendered unnecessary or inappropriate services; and (2) they will be forced to bear the financial burden of any PSRO-disapproved services rendered to them by interns and residents. [119]

Finally, issues in the case of *Bell* v. *Heim* [120] portend problems in selecting and applying norms, criteria, and standards which may arise during the later implementation of PSRO review. The New Mexico Foundation for Medical Care had, prior to the PSRO program's enactment, developed norms and guidelines for nursing home care which redefined the levels of care appropriate for specific conditions and specific kinds of facilities. The foundation then contracted with the state to use those guidelines to review the care rendered to Medicaid patients. Many of the Medicaid recipients who had been in skilled nursing facilities were reclassified as being eligible only for boarding home care, in accordance with the foundation's guidelines. [121] The plaintiffs, Medicaid patients, sought an injunction against the state's reduction in the levels of care for nursing home patients (based on the foundation's guidelines and application of them by the state) without providing those patients with a hearing prior to either declassification or transfer. This denial of any means to challenge the propriety of the changes was a violation of federal regulations, the patients asserted. [122] The complaint was amended later when the plaintiffs learned that the effect of the redefinitions would be the virtual elimination of skilled nursing home care for Medicaid patients in New Mexico. The case was finally resolved by a stipulated order (order approved by the court which the defendant and plaintiff agreed to) which set definitions of levels of care to reinstate skilled nursing home care as a service which would be available generally to Medicaid patients requiring it. In addition, because the court recognized the patients' legal right to the services by virtue of their Medicaid status, the state was permanently enjoined from terminating or reducing the level of care given to nursing home patients until specific procedural requirements had been met. [123]

The lesson of *Bell* v. *Heim* is that, in selecting and applying norms, criteria, and standards, PSRO actions may be subject to judicial override if they will adversely affect patients, as they would tend to do if a cost control orientation predominated. Delegation of definitional chores and the responsibility for establishing guidelines for review from the state (or the federal government) to a PSRO does not necessarily insulate either entity from specific legal requirements. [124] *Bell* v. *Heim* holds an additional hopeful note for consumers, because the court was unwilling to approve cost control at the expense of individual patients' needs and rights.

INCENTIVES TO USE NORMS

Because the use of norms, criteria, and standards is central and fundamental to the program, the PSRO system is forced to provide incentives to physicians to adopt the new techniques of review in order to ensure its own viability. Those incentives exist in three primary forms, all essentially financial in nature: (1) the PSRO's direct authority to deny approval and therefore payment for services; (2) the malpractice exemption; and (3) specific legal obligations to comply with norms.

The major weight of a PSRO's authority lies in its ability to disallow payment for services it disapproves (subject to appeal). Physicians and providers who fail to comply with norms, criteria, and standards will not be reimbursed. A financial incentive is thereby created because the physician (or provider) will seek to prevent the financial loss to himself which will result if he is forced to suffer no payment for his services. Because he is usually reimbursed for each service he renders, though, the same incentive which will prevent his exceeding established levels of care may equally well encourage him to provide as many services as he can within approved levels. That financial incentive to render services up to the limit of approval is what creates much of the overutilization problem which Senator Bennett cited. [125] While the use of norms, criteria, and standards may help to control overutilization, their use will not necessarily affect the incentive to utilize services maximally within the established ranges. [126] Because physicians subject to these financial incentives will establish the parameters, their interest in maximizing reimbursement can affect the norms-setting process. [127]

The malpractice exemption creates an incentive to comply with norms, criteria, and standards by protecting those physicians who rely on them. Under the statutory provision, no physician (or provider) "shall be civilly liable to any person ... on account of any action taken by him in compliance with or reliance upon professionally developed norms of care and treatment applied by a [PSRO]..." [128] The Senate Finance Committee expressly intended that the provision "remove any inhibition to proper exercise of PSRO functions, or the following by practitioners and providers of standards and norms recommended by the review organization." [129] Under the law, the physician who is not negligent and does conform with PSRO norms is, despite any injury to the patient, absolved of liability if he otherwise exercised due care in his behavior. Because physicians are so wary of malpractice charges and litigation, this incentive appears to be a strong one. [130]

Finally, the statute provides specific legal obligations to comply with norms. These obligations are imposed on individual practitioners (or providers) [131] and require them, in part, "to exercise ... professional responsibility" to assure that any care they order for their patients but do not themselves provide will, nonetheless, "be of a quality which meets professionally recognized standards of health care"[132] (i.e., norms, criteria, and standards). Continued violation of obligations to comply with norms and assure compliance by others will provide the basis for imposition of sanctions,[133] among which are exclusion from the right to be reimbursed by Medicare and Medicaid altogether or fines in the amount of the services whose provision violates the obligations, up to $5000.[134] This incentive is also essentially a financial one and will work only if physicians are sufficiently interested in the potential income from serving Medicare and Medicaid patients that they will seek to avoid exclusion from these programs.[135] The schedule of fines is merely an aggregation of individual case by case PSRO disapprovals. In the final analysis, then, not only are norms, criteria, and standards used to control overutilization and therefore costs, but the systemic incentives to use them also rely on the financial interests of the overutilizers.

SYSTEMIC IMPLICATIONS OF 'STANDARDIZED' REVIEW

Expansion of Coverage

As the opening discussion in this chapter suggested, review based on norms, criteria, and standards can create beneficial or harmful effects for consumers, or both, because of the more objective, quantified, and delimited nature of the parameters. Depending on the degree of review standardization, the PSRO system may be able to permit the state and federal governments to provide better coverage benefits to consumers, if those governments' previously existing fears that physicians and providers will abuse the benefits for financial gain are proved (by effective review) to be groundless. Consumers would benefit if elimination of governmental fears resulted in (1) the creation of broader entitlements to care and (2) the elimination of artificial Medicare and Medicaid benefits packages presently limited by government commitment to cost control.[136]

Governmental reliance on PSRO review for determinations of medical necessity is the key to both of those possibilities. In giving PSROs the authority to review medical necessity, the Senate Finance Committee precluded to them "questions concerning reasonableness of charges or costs or methods of payment ... [and] ... internal questions relating to matters of managerial efficiency in hospitals or nursing homes..,"[137] The report emphasizes that "[t]he PSRO's responsibilities are confined to evaluating the appropriateness of medical determinations so that medicare and medicaid payments will be made *only for medically necessary services* which are provided in accordance with professional standards of care."[138] The system uses norms, criteria, and standards as the basis for such medical determinations.[139] The Committee also cites the PSRO's authority "to approve the medical necessity of all elective hospital admissions in advance—solely for the purpose of determining whether Medicare and Medicaid will pay for the care" [140] as another means by which PSROs will monitor services for medical necessity. Although these passages underscore the Committee's intention to have approved only those services which are, in fact, medically necessary, by implication *any* services which are medically necessary should be approved. If this emphasis on medical necessity gives impetus to administrative practices truly aimed at ensuring that Medicare and Medicaid patients get any and all care which they need, the established parameters for determining their need will themselves provide the basis for expanding coverage of services rendered to individuals in the two ways described below.

The creation of broader entitlements to care—that is, more legal rights extending to more people to receive services—may be possible in the context of preadmission review. The Senate Finance Committee explicitly stated:

> [w]here advance approval by the review organizations for institutional admission was required and provision of the services was approved ... such approval would provide the basis for a presumption of medical necessity for purposes of Medicare and Medicaid benefit payments.[141]

Without such a presumption, advance approvals would be subject to complete review on a retrospective basis, and therefore meaningless.

The presumption will entitle an individual patient with a specific condition to any of the services which would be covered according to the appropriate norms, criteria, and standards applied to his or her case. For example, if the previously discussed hypothetical hysterectomy case were approved by the PSRO prior to admission to the hospital, it might be assigned a seven day length of stay. The patient and physician could then assume that during the seven day period coverage would extend to the approved operation, the laboratory studies which should precede it, the nursing care and medication which should follow the procedure, and any physical therapy the criteria might contemplate.[142] If review revealed that some of the services which the PSRO had approved for the case had not been rendered,[143] the right to services arising from the presumption of coverage could provide a basis for the PSRO to approve the omitted services at no cost to the patient, under appropriate circumstances. However, full and conscientious use of concurrent review[144] would probably lessen, if not obviate, the need for such a mechanism. Had the same hysterectomy patient not received physical therapy despite its inclusion as a covered element of treatment, concurrent review would uncover the omission before the patient's discharge, thereby providing an opportunity to assure the delivery of physical therapy services during the initial approved period or on the basis of an approved extension for that purpose.

There will be circumstances, however, when other services (e.g., indicated X-rays, diagnostic procedures, or sufficient antibiotics) will not have been prescribed, nor their administration begun, before the patient's discharge, despite both their established medical necessity and the presumption of coverage resulting from advance approval. If providing those services, even though the patient has been discharged, would contribute to improving the patient's health by upgrading the quality of care rendered to her or him, at best the PSRO should affirmatively seek to ensure the provision of those services; at the least, a patient seeking those services (or a physician seeking to provide them) should be entitled to expedited approval and coverage for them. [145] In that way, the PSRO could extend its approval to those services which, though medically necessary, might not otherwise be provided to the patient.

Medical necessity is also the key to elimination of artificial benefits packages limited according to fiscal necessity, particularly in Medicaid programs. Because Medicaid is administered locally by each state, using combined state and federal moneys, and each state determines the details of the plan it offers its eligible citizens (subject to certain federal requirements), Medicaid benefits vary from state to state. [146] An artificial benefits package is one whose coverage is limited for fiscal purposes, regardless of actual medical need for the services for which a claim is presented. Examples include limitations on hospital stays to a total of 45 days a year, on out-patient hospital visits (clinics) to 30 in any one year, and on drugs to $20 a month. [147] If norms, criteria, and standards reflect professional determinations of medical needs, then logic and justice dictate that all services which a PSRO approves as medically necessary should be covered irrespective of the peculiarities of state plans. Otherwise, there would be no use for PSROs: their existence would merely duplicate the fiscal management efforts of the state agency. If local norms, criteria, and standards are linked to and based on restrictive state plans, they will not meet the program's professed goal of approving for payment all services which are medically necessary. The Senate Finance Committee stated the principle underlying their grant to PSRO's of authority to review all Medicare and Medicaid services in their areas: "to establish a unified review mechanism for all health care services under the aegis of the principal element in the health care equation, the physician." [148] Clearly, the intent was to create a review system for all services using the same norms, criteria, and standards regardless of the specific financing program—Medicare or Medicaid—or their differing benefits packages. [149] Medical necessity (with concern for quality), then, was to be the sole dictate of approval for payment. [150]

Unfortunately, the political realities of the Medicaid program are such that restrictive coverage designed solely to meet fiscal needs will probably be eliminated only if PSROs do yield controlled costs. For example, the

Medicaid agency in New Mexico agreed to accept PSRO-type review in place of its own restricted benefits because the reviewing group had succeeded in reducing costs to the state. [151] Without a demonstrable cost control result, states seem to have no incentive to substitute PSRO review (or other review aimed at assuring quality) in place of their own fiscally determined artificial coverage. For consumers, however, a state's requirement that a PSRO show cost control success (which often will be the factor determining a state's acceptance of PSRO review) would eliminate the beneficial potential of the tendency toward elimination of artificially restricted coverage. The result might be programs insignificantly different from fiscally predetermined packages.

The potential for a state government's resistance to PSRO review dependent on cost control success is real. [152] The realization of that contingency ultimately could deprive consumers of vital medical benefits. The only sure technique for overcoming the political pressures dictating state government retention of artificial benefits packages is sufficient opposing political pressure. Although PSROs can affect health care delivery to consumers undesirably, the expansion of benefits through creation of broader entitlements and elimination of artificial benefits packages would be important beneficial effects of the PSRO system. These goals merit active consumer attention because the factors militating against their achievement are political, and potentially vulnerable to countervailing political activity.

Improved Planning Capabilities

From a long range perspective, the use of variant norms may benefit consumers of health care services. The statute provides that,

> [w]here *actual* norms of care, diagnosis and treatment in a [PSRO] area are significantly different from professionally developed regional norms of care, diagnosis and treatment approved for comparable conditions, the [PSRO] concerned shall be so informed, and in the event that appropriate consultation and discussion indicate reasonable basis for *usage of other norms* in the area concerned...[153]

the PSRO may apply its "actual" norms if they are approved by the National Council. These norms, varying from "regional" norms, would be keyed to the actual practice in a PSRO area and would reflect differing capabilities of practitioners and institutions in that area. [154] If the actual norms indicate that lesser quality care is being delivered in a medically underserved area, the use of variant norms, although grounded in reality, would effectively approve poor quality care. Patients obtaining services in a PSRO area using variant norms, would, in effect, be penalized with regard to medical care, in comparison with similar patients in a neighboring area where "regional" norms were applied.

If the PSRO system is committed to improved quality in medical care delivery, the recognition that variant norms are needed because of deficient medical services (e.g., insufficient numbers of practitioners, too few hospitals, poorly equipped facilities) must be channeled into facility and manpower planning and funding programs. Because each approved variation in a norm or standard would identify specific deficiencies (further corroborated by provider and practitioner profiles [155]), the actual needs in a PSRO area will be statistically demonstrated, thereby facilitating planning and funding. [156] If variant norms are applied in a PSRO area with a surplus of superspecialized medical facilities (Houston, Boston, and New York are examples), the patients of other lesser institutions in that area would suffer if the parameters were geared only to the most specialized care. [157] Expanding the range of variables so that care in either type of institution could be approved might, however, result in the elimination of incentives to improve deficient facilities. Whatever orientation is selected, though, the benefit of variant norms lies in their ability to identify specific needs for improved manpower and facilities.[158]

Inability to Affect Underutilization

While the above-stated potential benefits are important and wide-ranging, other possible effects of standardized review may be detrimental to consumer interests. Because in case by case review the most immediate feedback lies in disapproval of inappropriate services, there is some question about a PSRO's ability to rectify underutilization and so improve quality.[159]

Underutilization (like overutilization) is a relative concept based on comparison of the services rendered against norms, criteria, and standards. It occurs primarily where too few of the appropriate services are provided, but may also occur when inappropriate services are rendered in the absence of proper care. If standards called for X-rays to determine changes in heart size during a 21 day hospital stay for a myocardial infarction (heart attack) and no X-ray was taken, underutilization would have occurred. Underutilization would also be present if a patient complaining of heartburn and chest pains were diagnosed as having a peptic ulcer and treated with a special diet, mild sedatives, and bed rest, but was not given the electrocardiogram called for by criteria to rule out a heart attack. In this example, the underutilization would go unrecognized unless it were somehow discovered that the patient had actually suffered a heart attack; at that point, depending on the injury suffered by the patient as a result of the misdiagnosis, a malpractice suit might be in order.

Because the PSRO will usually approve payment when too few, but still appropriate, services are rendered, there is no mechanism that can immediately affect the physician's techniques of delivery in cases of underutilization. Where inappropriate services are rendered in the absence of appropriate care and the differences are sufficiently great that the PSRO does not approve payment, there is no immediate means of assuring delivery of the needed services.[160] In instances where two different conditions with similar symptoms require different treatment, services will likely be approved unless it is demonstrated that the wrong diagnosis was made.[161] Although profiles have the capacity to uncover patterns of underutilization, PSRO review is not designed to detect and remedy underutilization in individual cases.[162]

Denial of Access to Institutions

An additional negative effect from the use of norms, criteria, and standards can arise through patients being denied access to institutions on the basis of advance determinations of lack of medical necessity. If, in reviewing care prior to admission, the PSRO disapproves the proposed admission, the hospital or nursing home may choose to refuse the admission sought by the patient and his physician rather than risk relying on the patient's ability to pay. If in the appeals process[163] the PSRO's disapproval is upheld, the patient will have but two options: (1) to wait until the condition degenerates to a level at which the proposed procedure can no longer be considered "elective"; or (2) to accept legal responsibility for the hospital bill. The Senate Finance Committee has said that a "denial of certification for admission would not bar admission of any patient to an institution if his physician desires to admit him and if the institution accepts the admission."[164] Whether a patient can overcome the PSRO's denial in order to gain admission may rest on the relationship between his physician and the institution, and his physician's authority and credibility there. The committee report adds, "In this regard medicare [*sic*] parallels private health insurance where a private policy might determine that care proposed or rendered was not reimbursable under the terms of the policy."[165]

Implications for Hospital Financing

Utilizing standardized review can have serious consequences for hospital financing. PSROs are required by law to consider economic factors in the review process.[166] Because of unrealistic out-patient reimbursement rates, particularly in Medicaid,[167] almost every procedure which, from a technical perspective, can be performed on an out-patient basis or in facilities other than a hospital would be more economically performed without the hospital admission. Issues arising from the relative weight given to economic considerations in establishing parameters for review have already been discussed here. The balance achieved between the established ranges and the additional economic considerations required by the statute will also have consequences for hospital finances in general if so much emphasis is placed on lowering costs that PSROs consistently approve only care provided on an out-patient basis or in less expensive facilities. Most hospitals can ill afford the shift of their patient load to their clinics (or out of the hospital altogether to nursing homes). Health delivery finances may respond in several ways: (1) In-patient hospital costs might soar to make up revenues lost as a result of the interaction between PSRO review and Medicaid out-patient reimbursements. (2) Hospitals might have to close down beds (eliminate patient usable space) or other in-patient services wholly or in part. (3) Clinics, unable to bear the increased patient load, might be forced to deny services to patients despite PSRO approval of clinic care. Similar results could arise from shifts to nursing homes unable to absorb the increased demand.

Such drastic developments are unlikely. The financial incentive to physicians to develop guidelines which approve in-patient hospital care (generally reimbursed at higher levels) would restrain a tendency toward sudden and enormous utilization shifts as described. In addition, the statute tempers the consideration of economy (and a preference for out-patient care) with the conditions of medical propriety and effectiveness.[168] The strict application of the provision to assure that services are provided economically will undoubtedly result in some significant changes in hospital utilization rates and, therefore, hospital finances. In fact, the basic thrust toward cost control is intended to change some utilization and, therefore, financing patterns.

Finally, if, in fact, there is validity to the notion of local norms in that patterns of practice across the country do differ, it will be important to assure that norms reflect a local orientation if it serves to improve quality. Where practice differs but is of poor quality,[169] the local orientation should ultimately be abandoned to provide incentives to improve care (although the "typical" practice and "actual" practice requirements would have to be overcome). Because the National Council will issue sample sets of norms, there is the possibility that PSROs will adopt those sets in toto without consideration for local peculiarities.[170] Although the statute and legislative history are vague on the use and significance of "regional norms"[171] it would seem that norms, criteria, and standards developed to reflect regional differences could provide a basis for comparison to flag inappropriate, nonspecific norms which might be indiscriminately accepted or promulgated by a PSRO.[172] In sections of the country where particular conditions occur more frequently for environmental, economic, dietary, or other reasons, the parameters of review should recognize the local differences. Increased incidence of intestinal parasites in southern rural areas would be an example. Without a technique to assure that significant local differences are considered in reviewing care, the national norms, uniformity of review, and rigidly standardized care that would result would be to consumers' disadvantage.

Notes for Chapter Two

1. Setting and applying norms present the most difficult technical medical problems in the PSRO system. It is beyond the scope of this study to consider technical considerations in the methodology of selecting norms. This chapter analyzes the broad systemic implications to consumers of norms and their applications.

2. Whether PSROs can begin to achieve such positive results through the use

of norms is itself a speculative matter. Inexperience with a methodology seeking three principal ends—cost control, improved quality of care, *and* improved health—will present problems in the system. For a particularly incisive analysis of these issues, see Brook, "A Skeptic Looks at Peer Review," *Prism,* October 1974, at 29.

3. §1156(a); 42 USC §1320c–5(a).

4. *Id.*

5. §1155(a) (1); 42 USC §1320c–4(a).

6. See, for example, *PSRO Oversight Hearings* at 71, 97, 250–345, and 482. See also "PSRO Issues: 'quality' norms, jurisdiction," *American Medical News,* April 23, 1973, at 6; and "Interpreting PSRO 'norms of care'..." *American Medical News,* May 20, 1974, at 19.

7. See, for example, "You'll work with Big Brother watching," 11 *Physician's Management* 21 (September 1974).

8. See, for example, testimony of American College of Physicians, American Society of Internal Medicine, American College of Surgeons, and Pennsylvania Medical Care Foundation, *PSRO Oversight Hearings* at 53, 84, 161, and 212.

   The Senate Finance Committee chose to institute norms as the basis for review because without them,

   [t]he present review process ... becomes a long series of episodic case-by-case analyses on a subjective basis which fail to take into account in a systematic fashion the experience gained through past reviews or to sufficiently emphasize general findings about the pattern of care provided. The committee believes that the goals of the review process can be better achieved through the use of norms which reflect prior review experience.

   Sen. Fin. Comm. Rpt. at 257.

9. See Caper, "The Meaning of Quality in Medical Care," 291 *NEJM* 1136 (November 21, 1974); and Chapter One at 4 *supra.*

10. §1156(b) (2); 42 USC §1320c–5(b) (2).

11. For some short surveys of different quality assessment approaches, see Donabedian, "Evaluating the Quality of Medical Care," XLIV *Milbank Memorial Fund Quarterly* 166 (July 1966); Lewis, "The State of the Art of Quality Assessment, 1973," XII *Medical Care* 799 (October 1974); Brook and Appel, "Quality of Care Assessment: Choosing a Method for Peer Review," 288 *NEJM* 1323 (June 21, 1973); and Brook, "Assessing the Quality of Care: The Role of Teachers of Preventive Medicine" (Paper presented at American Public Health Association Meeting, San Francisco, November 1973).

12. See, for example, Worthington and Silver, "Regulation of Quality of Care in Hospitals: The Need for Change," XXXV *Law and Contemporary Problems* 305 (Spring 1970).

13. See Donabedian, *supra* n. 11; and "Promoting Quality Through Evaluating the Process of Patient Care," VI *Medical Care* 181 (May-June 1968).

14. See Ellwood, "Quantitative Measurement of Patient Care Quality," pt. I, 40 *Hospitals JAHA* 42 (December 1, 1966); pt. II, 40 *Hospitals JAHA* 59 (December 16, 1966).

15. See n. 12 *supra*.

16. The proponents of end result review do recognize review of "intermediate outcomes," points in the process of care when an evaluation of the patient's status may be made. See n. 14 *supra*.

17. Ellwood et al., *Assuring the Quality of Health Care,* (Minneapolis, Minn.: InterStudy, 1973), at 27.

18. This is not to say there is no place for end result review in the PSRO process. Some of its principles can be more "consumer-oriented" than process review. See this chapter at 38 *infra*. Neither process nor outcomes review, used singly, will adequately serve the patients' best interests.

    Assessment of quality of care on the basis of physician performance [i.e., process] may be inappropriate because many physicians' activities have not been proved to relate to improved health. However, assessment of quality of care on the basis of the results of care may be similarly inappropriate since the results of care depend not only on the medical care received, but also on the demographic, social and economic characteristics of the patient population.

    Brook and Appel, *supra* n. 11.

19. See Chapter Three at 89 *infra* for a discussion of tensions between PSROs and health maintenance organizations created by this orientation.

20. One study of a 20 year old program using norms in a peer review process found that while "statistically significant" alterations in practice patterns occurred after review, these changes could not be attributed exclusively to review. Public pressures, publicity, and other factors could have influenced physician behavior as well. See Buck and White, "Peer Review: Impact of a System Based on Billing Claims," 291 *NEJM* 877 (October 24, 1974).

21. See this chapter at 73 *infra*.

22. See Chapter Seven at 246 *infra*.

23. *Sen. Fin. Comm. Rpt.* at 256.

24. *Id.*

25. *Id.* Some quality assessment systems have focused on consumer evaluations of care. For a survey of some of these studies, see Lebow, "Consumer Assessments of the Quality of Medical Care," XII *Medical Care* 328 (April 1974). See also "The Role of the Consumer in Assuring Quality Health Care" (June 1973), New Mexico Regional Medical Programs (270 Frontier N.E., Alburquerque, New Mexico); and Mitchell, "Quality of Medical Care—Mutual Responsibility of Consumers and Providers," *Quality Assurance of Medical Care Monograph,* HEW (February 1973), at 83.

26. See Caper, *supra* n. 9.

27. One might argue that poor people and old people are in some instances *better* able to isolate the social and economic factors contributing to and aggravating their conditions than their physicians.

    The problem of accommodating the patient whose needs no longer dictate an acute level of care available in a hospital has plagued the Medicare utilization review process for years. Many of the court cases appealing fiscal intermediary decisions have focused on the needed level of care vs. available facilities dilemma. See Chapter Five at *xx infra*. It would be unfair for the PSRO's profile of a hospital to include the extended stay as part of the hospital's typical practice in treating an elderly patient with a fractured hip, if the hospital recognizes that the level of care required in fact is *not* acute hospital care. But the PSRO must allow flexibility of norms to permit accommodation of the patient for whom socioeconomic factors dictate an extended stay because of the lack of available facilities (e.g., nursing homes). The obvious implication of the PSRO's recognition through approval of the services is the need for governmental and societal recognition of the need for more long term care facilities. PSRO data development could demonstrate statistically the extent of this need. See Chapter Six at 184 *infra*.

28. One aspect of doctor-patient communication (the obverse of "patient compliance") is patient education based on information supplied by the doctor. Compliance is a passive process of following instructions. Education entails an active give and take between the physician and patient so that the patient is capable of making some decisions about his own care according to information supplied by the physician. Recent discussions have called for increased attention to those issues. For some short practical discussions, see Werner and Schneider, "Teaching Medical Students Interactional Skills," 290 *NEJM* 1232 (1974); and Brady, "Teaching Students How to Talk and Act with Patients," 291 *NEJM* 367 (1974).

29. In considering whether PSRO norms should be publicized, Dr. Henry Simmons, Director of the Office of Professional Standards Review, is reported to have said, "I would like to see a situation where a patient tells a doctor he has a cold, the doctor begins writing a prescription for an antibiotic, and the patient interrupts with, but doctor, you haven't taken a throat culture yet." *PSRO Letter* (no. 15), March 15, 1974, at 4.

30. See American Hospital Association's Patients' Bill of Rights, November 17, 1972; Joint Commission on the Accreditation of Hospitals (JCAH) Preamble, 1971; and, generally, Health Law Project Materials on Health Law, vol. 8, *Individual Patients' Rights*, rev. ed., 1972.

31. It makes little sense to implement a government-mandated review system unless the government will abide by the system's determinations. See this chapter at 44 *infra*.

32. See this chapter at 47 *infra*.

33. See this chapter at 48 *infra*.

34. §1155(a)(2); 42 USC §1320c–4(a)(2). See this chapter at 49 *infra*.
35. §1167(c); 42 USC §1320c–16(c). See Chapter Seven at 235 *infra* for a full discussion of the malpractice exemption.
36. See Chapter Six at 185 *infra*.
37. Obviously there is minimal possibility of such low cost–oriented norms because the physicians establishing norms have a financial incentive to extend Medicare and Medicaid coverage to as many services as possible. See Chapter Seven at 246 *infra*.
38. See Chapter Six at 185 *infra* for a discussion of potential benefits from profiles and their dissemination.
39. §1156(a); 42 USC §1320c–5(a).
40. *Id.*
41. *Id.*
42. *Id.*
43. §1156(b)(1); 42 USC §1320c–5(b)(1).
44. §1156(b)(2); 42 USC §1320c–5(b)(2).
45. §1155(a)(1); 42 USC §1320c–4(a)(1).
46. §1155(a)(2); 42 USC §1320c–4(a)(2).
47. §1156(d); 42 USC §1320c–5(d). See Chapter Three at 74 *infra* for a discussion of this process.
48. §1155(a)(4); 42 USC §1320c–4(a)(4). See Chapter Six at 185 *infra* for a discussion of profiles' significance to consumers.
49. §1156(a); 42 USC §1320c–5(a).
50. §1156(a), (c); 42 USC §1320c–5(a),(c).
51. (Emphasis added.) §1156(c)(1); 42 USC §1320c–5(c)(1).
52. (Emphasis added.) §1156(a); 42 USC §1320c–5(a).
53. Senator Carl Curtis (R–Neb.), a member of the Senate Finance Committee, asserts that the law gives the Secretary all power to apply and set norms. See *PSRO Oversight Hearings* at 21 and 39, for example.
54. *Id.* at 101, for example; and "Interpreting PSRO 'norms of care'–Cookbook medicine or textbook medicine?" *American Medical News,* May 20, 1974, at 21.
55. §§1152, 1153, 1154, 1155, 1162; 42 USC §§1320c–1, –2, –3, –4, –11.
56. The Senate Finance Committee Report repeats the confusion, consistently referring to "areas" except in discussing "regional norms." *Sen. Fin. Comm. Rpt.* at 257, 258, 259, 263.
57. Distributed by the Office of Professional Standards Review (OPSR), HEW, issued March 15, 1974. (Hereinafter cited as *Program Manual.*)
58. "The manual is subject to revision based upon the experience of organizations participating in the PSRO program and the comments of concerned organizations and individuals. As experience is gained, portions of the material contained in the manual will be issued as proposed regulations." Foreword, *Program Manual.*
59. *Program Manual,* Chapter VII, §709 at 16.
60. *Id.* at 17.
61. *Id.* at 16. For background information on the development of these definitions, see Farrell, "Norms/Criteria/Standards," remarks before

the National Professional Standards Review Council, July 9, 1973 (available from OPSR), and *PSRO Letter* (no. 8), December 1, 1973, at 6.

62. *Program Manual,* Chapter VII, §702.2, at 4. Secretary Weinberger cited this section of the *Manual* specifically in his testimony before the Subcommittee on Health of the Senate Finance Committee, to indicate that he did not want the authority to set norms for PSROs and if he had such authority he would support a change in the statute to remove it. *PSRO Oversight Hearings* at 17.

63. *Program Manual,* Chapter VII, §709.11 at 17.

64. *Id.* §709.12 at 17.

65. *Id.* §709.13 at 17. Because of differences in approach among physician specialties and types of institutions, the last factor may cause some dispute among physicians selecting priority conditions. There are some objective sources of data which can indicate quality or utilization problems. See Chapter Six at 184 *infra.*

   One commentator has suggested that priorities be selected differently.

   My proposed system overcomes this difficulty ... [the insurmountable difficulty of establishing objective criteria for the measurement of increasing gradations of positive health] ... by identifying those health events that should not occur and are easy to measure in the form of unnecessary disease, unnecessary disability, and unnecessary untimely death.

   Rutstein, "New Incentives for Quality Care," *Prism,* September 1974, at 3.

66. *Program Manual,* Chapter VII, §709.16 at 19. See Chapter Six at 185 *infra.*

67. *Program Manual,* Chapter VII, §709.2 at 19–20.

68. *Id.* §709.3 at 20.

69.   Non-physician health care practitioners are those health professionals which (a) do not hold a Doctor of Medicine or Doctor of Osteopathy degree, (b) are qualified by education, experience and/or licensure to practice their profession, and (c) are involved in the delivery of direct patient care or services which are directly or indirectly reimbursed by the Medicare, Medicaid or Maternal and Child Health programs.

   Id. §730.2 at 31. See Chapter Six at 203 *infra.*

70. *Program Manual,* Chapter VII, §730 at 31–33.

71. There has been some experience with different models of setting norms, criteria, and standards. Beginning in 1970, the federal government financed 10 experimental medical care review organizations (EMCROs) to develop working models to test the feasibility of conducting systematic and ongoing reviews of medical care in a manner which would be acceptable to professionals, the public, the

government, and third party payers. Various approaches were tried. The grantee in Georgia concentrated on nursing home care. The Oregon EMCRO assayed ambulatory care of physicians who volunteered for the program.

In choosing methodologies, the Utah EMCRO (later the first PSRO) settled on criteria with "high discriminatory value" which represent "a crystalization of factors which are truly *essential* to *ideal* care of a particular problem or diagnosis." Nelson, "The EMCRO Project and the Utah Professional Review Organization," *Quality Assurance of Medical Care,* monograph (Washington, D.C.: Department of Health, Education and Welfare, Regional Medical Programs Service, Health Services and Mental Health Administration, February 1973), at 265. The Sacramento, California, program worked on developing entirely normative criteria, seeking to document actual practice only. In Charlottesville, Virginia, the EMCRO undertook lengthy documentation of criteria, relying on extensive surveys of professional literature. As of this writing, no final reports on these experiments had been published. For information on the EMCRO program, see Nelson, *supra;* A. D. Little, Inc., *Experimental Medical Care Review Organization (EMCRO) Programs,* (Washington, D.C.: Department of Health, Education and Welfare, Publication No. (HSM) 73–3017, National Center for Health Services Research and Development, March 1973); and Sanazaro et al., "Research and Development in Quality Assurance," 287 *NEJM* 1125 (November 30, 1972). (This last study was also published in 44 *Medical Record News* 47 [April 1973].) The Charlottesville experience, although recognized as atypical, has been specially singled out for praise. See Brook, "A Skeptic Looks at Peer Review," *Prism,* October 1974 at 32.

72. For example, the American College of Physicians, the American Society of Internal Medicine, and the American College of Surgeons presented testimony to the Subcommittee on Health of the Senate Finance Committee on their work in developing criteria. *PSRO Oversight Hearings* at 52, 83, and 159.

Under the PSRO program, almost $1.5 million in contracts have been awarded to different groups for the development of norms, criteria, and standards. The AMA has a contract to develop model sets of criteria to cover those diagnoses, problems and procedures that account for approximately 75 percent of short stay hospital admissions in each specialty area. The AMA has further subcontracted with other groups such as the American Academy of Pediatrics. See 25 *News + Comment* (Amer. Academy of Ped.) 5 (October 1974). The American Nurses Association will develop model criteria for use in reviewing nursing care. Podiatric care criteria will be developed by the American Podiatry Association; and the American College of Physicians has a contract to develop criteria on antibiotic use. *HEW News Release,* July 19, 1974 (HEW–E31); and *PSRO Letter* (no. 22), July 1, 1974, at 5.

73. Brook, "Assessing the Quality of Care: The Role of Teachers of Preventive Medicine" (Paper presented at the American Public Health Association Meeting, San Francisco, November 1973).

74. For a study which involved consensus selection of standards within specialties, see Brook and Appel, "Quality of Care Assessment: Choosing a Method for Peer Review," 288 *NEJM* 1323 (June 21, 1973). Consensual norms have been criticized because they lack a demonstrable, empirical base, and in particular, consensually established lengths of stay have been criticized because they often adopt unexplained number preferences (particularly multiples of seven). See Donabedian, "The Numerology of Utilization Control," XI *Inquiry* 229 (September 1974).

75. See Chapter Three at 94 *infra* for a discussion of PSROs and Medicaid state agencies.

76. In some contexts it may be difficult to find *any* competent data source to rely on other than claims forms. For example, there may be no national data available to demonstrate "typical" practice in nursing homes. See Chapter Six at 184 *infra*. Availability of data is only one problem in the assessment of ambulatory care. See Hare and Barnoon, *Medical Care Appraisal and Quality Assurance in the Office Practice of Internal Medicine* (Department of Health, Education and Welfare [Contract HSM 110–70–420], National Center for Health Services Research and Development, July 1973). San Francisco, Calif.: American Society of Internal Medicine, July 1973. Developing criteria (and review in general) for psychiatric conditions may prove equally elusive. For consideration of general issues in review of psychiatric care, see "Psychiatric Utilization Review: Principles and Objectives," American Psychiatric Association, June 1968.

77. One study has found that out of 252 patients admitted to a municipal hospital, extramedical factors contributed to the decision to admit 21 percent (54) of the patients. Eight percent (20) would not have required hospitalization if the extramedical factors were not present. Inability of the patient to understand directions, no one at home to assume responsibility for the patient's care, and lack of alternative facilities for care were the primary factors cited. Mushlin and Appel, "Extramedical Factors in the Decision to Hospitalize Medical Patients" (Available from Mushlin at Columbia Medical Plan, Columbia, Maryland 21044), 1973. See also, *American Medical News,* November 26, 1973, at 15.

78. See Chapter Six at 200 *infra* on nonphysician participation in PSROs generally.

79. Ellwood et al., *supra* n. 17, at 27.

80. This is an area of demonstrated problems in quality assurance. See, for example, Brook et al., "Effectiveness of Inpatient Follow-up Care," 285 *NEJM* 1509 (December 30, 1971); and Sanazaro and Williamson, "Physician Performance and its Effects on Patients," VII *Medical Care* 299 (July–August 1970).

81. *Program Manual,* Chapter VII, §705.35(d) at 15.
82. See n. 18 *supra.* See also, Williamson, "Evaluating Quality of Patient Care: A Strategy Relating Outcome and Process Assessment," 218 *JAMA* 564 (October 1971).
83. See Chapter Three, at 87 *infra.*
84. Medical care evaluation studies will be performed by PSROs and hospitals to which they have delegated review authority. These studies, which examine problem areas in medical care delivery rather than individual cases, will not use PSRO norms, criteria, and standards employed in the other forms of review, and will not, therefore, be considered here. See *Program Manual,* Chapter VII, §705.35 at 15.

    The process of each PSRO's review is similar to, but conceptually different from, case by case review in hospitals over which PSROs have authority. For a full discussion of these issues, see Chapter Three.
85. The *Manual* gives special consideration to emergency cases. They will be subject to norms, criteria, and standards but not to all of the levels of review indicated here. See *Program Manual,* Chapter VII, §705.15 at 7–8.
86. Preadmission review is considered optional in the *Manual* and the statute. *Program Manual,* Chapter VII, §705.14(b) at 7. The statute provides that each PSRO "shall have the authority to determine in advance, in the case of ... elective admissions ... or other health care services which will consist of extended or costly courses of treatment" whether the services were medically necessary and proposed to be performed in an appropriate facility. §1155(a)(2); 42 USC §1320c–4(a)(2).
87. Pro forma compliance with the system (i.e., filling out forms only to meet the requirements of the program for payment without real cooperation with it) was a recurring problem cited by the staff of the Senate Finance Committee in its extensive report on Medicare and Medicaid. See *Medicare and Medicaid: Problems, Issues and Alternatives,* Report of the Staff to the Committee on Finance, U.S. Senate (91st Cong. 2d sess.), February 9, 1970 (hereinafter cited as *Medicare and Medicaid 1970*), at 105–112. Physicians will always have the option of writing records to meet payment demands only rather than with regard primarily for quality. If the PSRO program is oriented toward cost control alone, that incentive will inhibit some quality-oriented record keeping efforts. Where physicians demonstrate poor record keeping practices, adherence to PSRO program demands will create at least a minimal quality level.
88. One recent study has demonstrated a correlation between good medical record practices and good medical care performance. Lyons and Payne, "The Relationship of Physicians' Medical Recording Performance to Their Medical Care Performance," XII *Medical Care* 714 (August 1974). For a study of five different medical record formats

and their utility for rapid, accurate retrieval of information, see Fries, "Alternatives in Medical Record Formats," XII *Medical Care* 871 (October 1974).

89. *Sen. Fin. Comm. Rpt.* at 263. See this chapter at 45 *infra* for further discussion of the systemic implications of such a presumption.

90. See Chapter Five, at 144 *infra* for an extensive discussion of the PSRO appeal process.

91. *Program Manual,* Chapter VII, §705.14(a) at 7. Presumably preadmission and initial admission certifications would not be performed on the same case because they are duplicative processes.

92. *Id.* §705.13 at 6–7. See *Id.* §705.18 at 8–9 for a list of data needs for admission certification.

93. *Id.* §705.12 at 5.

94. *Id.* §705.24 at 11.

95. *Id.* §705.21 at 10.

96. *Id.* §705.25 at 11.

97. This point would be the 75th percentile of the average length of stay for patients with the same diagnosis and same age grouping—that is, the point at which 75 percent of those patients will have been discharged. *Id.* §705.26 at 11–12. Initial certifications will be established generally at the 50th percentile of lengths of stay. §1156(d)(2); 42 USC §1320c–5(d)(2); *Sen. Fin. Comm. Rpt.* at 263. See Chapter Three at 74 *infra.*

98. *Program Manual,* Chapter VII, §705.25(c) at 11.

99. *Id.* §705.24 at 11.

100. See Chapter Five, at 144 *infra.*

101. See n. 84 *supra.*

102. §1155(a)(1); 42 USC §1320c–4(a)(1).

103. *Sen. Fin. Comm. Rpt.* at 263.

104. *Id.*

105. See Chapter Seven, at 249 *infra* for a discussion of the need for retrospective review of preadmission determinations in some situations.

106. *Program Manual,* Chapter VII, §707(b) at 16.

107. See Chapter Five, at 144 *infra.* Other types of retrospective review in addition to medical care evaluation studies include medical audit, which also measures services rendered against criteria. For a discussion of some medical audit issues, see Trustee, Physician, Administrator (TAP) Institutes, "Procedure for Retrospective Medical Care Audit in Hospitals," Joint Commission on Accreditation of Hospitals, 1973; and Richardson, "Methodological Development of a System of Medical Audit," X *Medical Care* 29 (January-February 1971).

108. "Another way to conserve physician time would be through the use of other qualified personnel such as registered nurses who could, under the direction and control of PSRO physicians, aid in assuring

effective and timely review." *Sen. Fin. Comm. Rpt.* at 264.

109. §1155(c); 42 USC §1320c–4(c); *Program Manual,* Chapter VII, §730.55 at 32.

110. See Chapter Four at 112 *infra.*

111. See, for example, "Interpreting PSRO 'norms of care'–cookbook medicine or textbook medicine?", *American Medical News,* May 20, 1974, at 21.

112. *Program Manual,* Chapter VII, §701 at 2.

113. *PSRO Letter* (no. 8), December 1, 1973, at 6.

114. (Emphasis added.) *PSRO Letter* (no. 11), January 15, 1974, at 7.

115. See comments of Alan R. Nelson, M.D., reported in *American Medical News,* May 20, 1974, at 21.

116. See Chapter Three at 70 *infra* and Chapter Four at 112 *infra.*

117. If the program finally is implemented fully, techniques of PSRO review perhaps should be taught in medical schools. See Brook, "Assessing the Quality of Care: The Role of Teachers of Preventive Medicine" (Paper presented at the American Public Health Association meeting, San Francisco, November 1973).

118. See, "PSRO issues: 'quality' norms, jurisdiction," *American Medical News,* April 23, 1973, at 6.

119. The 1972 Social Security Amendments amended the Medicare provisions to confront the problem of Medicare reimbursement for in-patient care rendered to nonprivate patients (i.e., ward patients) by interns, residents, and supervising physicians in teaching hospitals. §227, P.L. 92–603; amending §§1861, 1814, 1832, 1835, and 1842; 42 USC §§1395x, 1395f, 1395k, 1395n, and 1395u. See, *Sen. Fin. Comm. Rpt.* at 194–198.

Under §227, whether payment would be made to the supervising physician on the basis of costs or charges (essentially comparable to the difference between wholesale and retail hospital costs) would be determined in part by the nature and extent of his supervisory duties. A portion of interns' and residents' salaries is reimbursed to the Medicare participating hospital under §§1835(e), 1861(b)(4); 42 USC §§1395n(e), 1395x(b)(4). For an analysis of reasonable cost reimbursement to hospitals generally under the Medicare program, see Law, *Blue Cross: What Went Wrong?* (New Haven: Yale University Press, 1974).

Although no comparable provision exists under the Medicaid program, the Senate Finance Committee report does provide that "[w]here States elect to compensate for services of supervisory physicians under medicaid, Federal matching should be limited to reimbursement not in excess of that allowable under medicare." *Sen. Fin. Comm. Rpt.* at 198. Implementation of the new Medicare provision was postponed until June 1976 by P.L. 93–368 (H.R. 8217, 93d Cong., 2d sess., 1974), an unrelated trade bill.

The activities of teaching hospitals in the PSRO system are problematic in general. Higher costs, higher utilization rates, research activities, educational functions, and generally larger size are all factors which have been cited as presenting difficulties in the application of PSRO norms, criteria, and standards. Kavet and Luft, "The Implications of the PSRO Legislation for the Teaching Hospital Sector," Health Care Policy Discussion paper Number 12, Harvard Center for Community Health and Medical Care, Boston, August 1973. If teaching institutions are to continue their activities which distinguish them from ordinary community hospitals, they will necessarily assume active roles in the norms setting process. See Chapter Seven at 243 *infra*.

120. No. 9189 Civil, (D.C. N. Mex., 1971). Reported at ¶15,275 *CCH Poverty Law Reporter* (Chicago, Ill.: Commerce Clearinghouse).

121. Before the reclassification, 500 patients were receiving skilled nursing care. Applying the new definitions, only 25 patients would have been eligible for skilled nursing care. Amended Complaint, *Bell v. Heim*, No. 9189 Civil, (D.C. N. Mex., 1971). Reported at ¶15,275 *CCH Poverty Law Reporter* (Chicago, Ill.: Commerce Clearinghouse) (hereinafter cited as *CCH Pov. L. Rpt.*).

122. See Chapter Five, at 150 *infra*.

123. The state was required to provide to each patient, at least 15 days prior to any termination or reduction, individual written notice stating fully (a) the proposed termination or reduction, (b) the reasons therefore, (c) the right to request a fair hearing regarding the termination or reduction, (d) the method by which a hearing could be obtained, and (e) all information concerning the recipient's rights. Stipulated Judgment, *Bell v. Heim*, No. 9189 Civil (D.C. N. Mex., 1971). Reported at ¶15,275 *CCH Pov. L. Rpt.*

   Recent changes in the federal regulations might affect the outcome of the case if it were brought today. Under new regulations, the state need not provide notice 10 days before reductions in care or transfers become effective when the recipient has been placed in skilled nursing care, intermediate care, or long term hospitalization, or when a change in level of care is prescribed by the recipient-patient's physician. 45 CFR §205.10(a)(4)(ii)(D),(H). See Chapter Five at 151 *infra*.

124. See n. 113 Chapter Five, *infra* for a discussion of PSROs as state (government) action. See Chapter Three at 94 *infra* for a discussion of tensions between PSROs and Medicaid state agencies created by their dual responsibilities in these activities.

125. See Chapter One at 4 *supra*.

126. Contrast this incentive with the incentive to low utilization which exists in HMOs. See Chapter Three at 90 *infra*.

127. It should be noted that the financial incentives considered here do not operate without constraints. Most physicians acting in good faith are motivated to render quality care consistent with the needs of their patients.

128. §1167(c); 42 USC §1320c-16(c). See Chapter Seven at 235 *infra* for a complete discussion of this provision.

129. *Sen. Fin. Comm. Rpt.* at 267.

130. But see Chapter Seven at 235 *infra* for a discussion of the real impact of this apparently powerful incentive.
131. §1160(a); 42 USC §1320c–9(a).
132. §1160(a)(1)(E); 42 USC §1320c–9(a)(1)(E).
133. See Chapter Seven at 231 *infra*.
134. §1160(b); 42 USC §1320c–9(b).
135. See Chapter Seven at 246 *infra* for a discussion of whether the financial weight of the program is sufficient to generate physician compliance.
136. The discussion of potential "entitlements" to specific services is applicable to individual patients. The elimination of artificial benefits packages (see text below) will have similar effects, but will apply to classes of patients rather than individuals.
137. *Sen. Fin. Comm. Rpt.* at 261.
138. (Emphasis added.) *Id.* at 261–2.
139. §1156; 42 USC §1320c–5.
140. *Sen. Fin. Comm. Rpt.* at 262.
141. *Id.* at 263.
142. "However, advance approval of institutional admission would not preclude a retroactive finding that ancillary services (not specifically approved in advance) provided during the covered stay were excessive." *Id.*
143. See Chapter Seven at 249 *infra* for consideration of the need for some retrospective review of advance approvals.
144. See this chapter at 38 *supra*.
145. In order for the patient to give force to the presumption in this way, he must have access to the norms, criteria, and standards applied to his case. See Chapter Six at 189 *infra*.
     See this chapter at *xx infra* for a discussion of PSROs' abilities to remedy underutilization generally.
146. See Chapter Three at 94 *infra*.
147. For a survey of benefits packages available in each state see, "Characteristics of State Medical Assistance Programs Under Title XIX of the Social Security Act," HEW, Public Assistance Series Number 49, 1970 ed. For updated material, see also *CCH Medicare and Medicaid Guide* ¶¶ 15,550–660.
148. *Sen. Fin. Comm. Rpt.* at 262.
149. Unified review using identical standards for all patients is the first step on the road to a national health insurance program with universal entitlement to care and broad coverage. See Chapter One at 16 *supra*.
150. Medical necessity has been used increasingly as the lever to extend Medicare coverage in level of care determination appeals. See n. 83 *infra*, Chapter Five.
151. When review by the New Mexico Foundation for Medical Care for the New Mexico Health and Social Services Department began, the state Medicaid program was reported to be bankrupt. The legislature had threatened to jail the state health and welfare director for exceeding

his budget. Two years later, accepting PSRO-type review, state officials claimed savings of $85,000 a year on physician bills and $500,000 a year from reducing the average length of hospital stays by one day. Auerbach, "New Mexico: Self-Reform by Doctors," *Washington Post,* May 7, 1973, at 1, col. 5. See *PSRO Oversight Hearings* at 474. The President of the New Mexico Medical Society reported further:

Parenthetically, because of these [cost and quality] results, we have been able to have removed arbitrary restrictions on patient benefits, such as the limit of 30 days hospitalization per year, limiting visits to physicians to 12 visits per year, and limitations on necessary hospital consultations. We have also been able to increase reimbursement to physicians from the 50th percentile of a 1968 base to the 75th percentile of 1970. This has increased physician willingness to cooperate and participate.

Statement of Armin Keil, President, New Mexico Medical Society, *PSRO Oversight Hearings* at 474.

152. See Chapter Three at 185 *infra.*
153. (Emphasis added.) §1156(a); 42 USC §1320c–5(a). There is no legislative history on this provision.
154. According to the statutory language, the determination that actual practice differs from regional norms would be made by the National Council or some other entity. The PSRO only "shall be ... informed" that actual practice varies from norms. §1156(a); 42 USC §1320c–5(a). This provision is ambiguous in light of the apparent locally controlled norms-setting process. See this chapter at 34 *supra.*
155. See Chapter Six at 185 *infra.*
156. The use of variant norms appears to apply only between PSRO areas. But norms applied within an area necessarily will include institutions with varying degrees of specialized services, sophistication of equipment, and funding available to maintain their services. If norms, criteria, and standards for a specific condition were to require particular equipment for proper, efficient treatment of the condition, and a hospital did not have such equipment, depending on the flexibility in applying the established variables, three results would be possible: (1) care without the indicated equipment would be approved; (2) care without the indicated equipment would not be approved but the patient would choose to stay in that hospital anyway absorbing the cost of the disapproved services; or (3) the patient would go to an institution which could provide the services in the prescribed manner. One physician who has worked extensively with the Charlottesville, Virginia EMCRO (see n. 70 *supra*) has stated his belief that if norms, criteria, and standards were established to require specific equipment, the law would require the

transfer of a patient in a deficient hospital to one which had the capability to perform according to the guidelines. Comments of James Respess, M.D., Professor of Internal Medicine at the University of Virginia, Federal Bar Association meeting, June 8, 1973, Washington, D.C. The use of such explicitly predetermined criteria has been criticized as leading to stifled innovation, increased costs, increased demand for scarce manpower resources, and increased risk of harm to the patient from the care itself. See Institute of Medicine, *Advancing the Quality of Health Care* (Washington, D.C.: National Academy of Sciences, August, 1974), at 21.

157. Because of the cost control orientation of the program, it is unlikely that variant norms will be applied in areas where superspecialists practice in great numbers. Because, in general, norms are to reflect "typical patterns of practice" [§1156(a); 42 USC §1320c–5(a)] which, by definition, are not unusually specialized or sophisticated, without variant norms there is the possibility that medical practice innovators and researchers will find their work curtailed by the scope of norms. The possibility of stifling innovation and extraordinary procedures will also rest on the flexibility of the applied parameters. It would be possible for a PSRO to approve unusual care not specifically included in norms, criteria, and standards if the variables are used *only* as principal or initial points of evaluation. To standardize care to the point of requiring uniformity would not benefit consumers because it would deny them flexibility in approach to and options among treatment and individualized care. See also n. 119 *supra* and accompanying text.

158. For an example of the use of PSRO-type information for planning purposes, see Wennberg and Gittelsohn, "Small Area Variations in Health Care Delivery," 182 *Science* 1102 (December 14, 1973); and Bloom and Peterson, "End Results, Cost and Productivity of Coronary Care Units," 288 *NEJM* 72 (January 11, 1973).

There are organized entities required by federal law to manage and scrutinize health planning throughout the country. Originally these entities were comprehensive health planning councils which advised state agencies on planning matters. Under the law state agencies must approve expansion, reduction, or new construction of health facilities which receive federal moneys before that money can be committed to such facilities. Data developed by PSROs would be important to these agencies. The American Association of Comprehensive Health Planners has called for state and areawide planning agencies to be given review and comment responsibility in PSRO applications and overall implementation of the program. *PSRO Letter* (no. 1), August 15, 1973, at 7. Other local agencies and councils are reported to be involved in the formation of PSROs and nominations to Statewide Councils. *Consumer Clearinghouse for PSRO Action* (no. 2), August 8, 1973, at 3. For a summary of the review authority of comprehensive health planning agencies, see

"The Review and Comment Responsibilities of State and Areawide Comprehensive Health Planning Services," DHEW, No. (HSM) 73–14,003 Rev. February 1973; and Corbett, "Health Planning: Some Legal and Political Implications of Comprehensive Health Planning," 64 *Amer. J. of Pub. Health* 136 (February 1974). The law establishing these entities, and mandating 51 percent consumer membership on them, was P.L. 89–719 (89th Cong., November 3, 1966), "Comprehensive Health Planning and Public Health Services Amendments of 1966," of which §3 amended §314 of the Public Health Service Act (42 USC §246) authorizing grants to states for comprehensive health planning.

There has been significant criticism of these agencies, and new legislation requires the establishment of health services agencies which would combine the functions of comprehensive health planning agencies with several other planning and development functions. These entities will need and use PSRO generated data. See the National Health Planning and Resources Development Act of 1974, P.L. 93–641 (93d Cong., 2d sess., 1974).

159. See Chapter Six at 190 *infra*.
160. If, in the course of concurrent review, an affirmative effort is made to assure delivery of appropriate services (see this chapter at 39 *supra*), underutilization could, in some instances, be corrected.
161. This is not to imply that a determination after the fact that the diagnosis was incorrect should result in disapproval for payment purposes. Rather, in those circumstances, medical care evaluation studies and medical audit techniques ought to be used in creating physician education programs. See Chapter Three at 73 *infra*.
162. This deficiency is particularly important in review of HMO care. See Chapter Three at 89 *infra*.
163. See Chapter Five at 137 *infra*.
164. *Sen. Fin. Comm. Rpt.* at 263.
165. *Id.*
166. "...[I]n case such services or items are proposed to be provided in a hospital or other health care facility on an in-patient basis, such services and items could consistent with the provision of appropriate medical care, be effectively provided on an out-patient basis or more economically in an in-patient health care facility of a different type." §1155(a)(1)(C); 42 USC §1320c–4(a)(1)(C).
167. In Pennsylvania, for example, all out-patient visits are reimbursed at a flat rate of $6, regardless of the services provided or treatment performed. The $6 fee was raised in 1973 from $4. *Medical Assistance Memo No. 4*, Commonwealth of Pennsylvania, Harrisburg, January 15, 1973. It was recently recommended to raise the flat rate reimbursement to $9 a visit. This rate does not compare favorably with in-patient reimbursement on a reasonable cost basis (the reimbursement formula prescribed by law for Medicaid in-patient services). For a discussion of reasonable cost reimbursement

under Medicaid, see Law, *Blue Cross: What Went Wrong?* (New Haven: Yale University Press, 1974), at 102–104. Nursing home reimbursement under Medicaid is also less favorable financially. See also Chapter Seven at 246 *infra.*

168. §1155(a)(1)(C); 42 USC §1320c–4(a)(1)(C).

169. See "Health Care in the South: A Statistical Profile," (Atlanta: Southern Regional Council, 1974); and "Southern health care lags behind others study says," *American Medical News,* September 9, 1974, at 3.

170. One neurosurgeon has reported that neurosurgical specialty societies decided against development of national treatment guidelines as part of the AMA's Advisory Committee on PSROs which is developing model treatment criteria. "Once things get written down in a book 600 pages long, people might say, 'Why should we do any work? It's all written down right here.' " Comments of Russel H. Patterson, M.D., reported in "Interpreting PSRO 'norms of care'—cookbook medicine or textbook medicine?" *American Medical News,* May 20, 1974, at 20. At this writing those sample sets had not been issued.

171. See This chapter at 34 *supra.*

172. Apparently, regional norms would encompass areas larger than PSRO 'areas' but would be more particularistic than national norms or model sets.

Chapter Three

PSROs and Institutional Review

The previous chapter demonstrated that the use of norms, criteria, and standards will fundamentally alter the practice of medicine by practitioners as well as in institutions. Of primary concern to health care institutions—hospitals and nursing facilities—is the fact that the PSRO system changes the basic roles of those institutions in cost control and quality assurance. Prior to the PSRO law's enactment, the essential activities for cost control and quality review were located in those institutions. Hospitals and nursing homes participating in Medicare and Medicaid were required, as conditions of their participation in those programs, to have operational "utilization review committees." These committees, composed of members of the staff of each institution, were charged with the responsibility of reviewing care in individual cases. Their function was established by law. An institution's utilization review plan was considered sufficient, if it required

> ... review on a sample or other basis of admissions to the institution, the duration of stays therein, and the professional services (including drugs and biologicals) furnished, (A) with respect to the medical necessity of the services and (B) for the purpose of promoting the most efficient use of available health facilities and services.[1]

The goals of the institutional review program were "high quality care and an increase in effective utilization of hospital services to be achieved through an educational approach involving study of patterns of care, and the encouragement of proper utilization."[2] As this chapter will discuss, the program failed for a variety of reasons, but its failure was the principal impetus behind the creation of PSROs. The function of these institutional "utilization review committees" (sometimes labeled differently in individual institutions) was very similar to the responsibilities now charged to PSROs. Because those functions now lie with PSROs, conceptually the role of institutional review, if it is to exist, must be quite different. Otherwise it would simply duplicate PSRO efforts. Institutional review does have a place within the PSRO scheme; essentially, institutions are to augment the PSROs' review capabilities by concentrating on the development of their own techniques to improve their health care delivery. As a practical matter, PSROs may have to rely heavily on institutional review committees to perform case by case review because of the many other responsibilities the law gives to PSROs (e.g., development of norms, hearings, data development, and analysis of profiles of care).

How utilization review committees fulfill their roles within the PSRO program is important to consumers for several reasons. First, utilization review committees represent the most local element in the PSRO review system. Because of their particularized focus, they have the potential to be the element in the system best able to respond to community needs and consumer interests. The political power of community pressure on a local service institution can be more effective where it is more concentrated because of a specific focus. Significantly for consumers, there are no exclusionary restrictions imposed on utilization review committee membership. The regulations establish minimal standards for staff participation, but unlike the PSRO statute, they do not prohibit consumer participation in committee processes. In fact, nonphysicians who enjoy no "professional" role in the delivery of care in some cases have already been included on utilization review committees as a result of pressures from private insurers.[3] Because the PSRO law gives each PSRO the authority to delegate case by case review to institutional committees,[4] a committee's effectiveness will determine whether the PSRO exercises that authority.

Second, as this chapter explores, the differences in case by case review as practiced by an institutional committee compared with the PSRO performing the same duties may be significant to consumers. Before the promulgation of new regulations governing utilization review, the law made it clear that an institutional committee, unlike a PSRO, was bound to rely primarily on the attending physician's judgment in approving or disapproving services.[5] That provision was particulary important to patients seeking coverage of services subsequently disapproved by a paying agent.[6] The revisions in the utilization review system, conforming it to the needs and dictates of PSROs, eliminated the provision mandating reliance on the attending physician's judgment. Now lost to consumers is the right to place primary faith in their physician's opinion alone. Norms have been substituted for his judgment, and patients may find the change significant in practical terms of realizing their expectations of reimbursement.

In other ways, too, the proficiency of utilization review by an institutional committee can be important to a consumer seeking review of PSRO-disapproved services which he had no notice would not be covered. Under the "waiver of liability" provisions (or "hold harmless" provisions as they are also called)[7] the patient will not be held responsible for otherwise noncovered services if he had no notice they would not be covered. The provider-institution would then be liable unless, it, too, had no notice the services would not be paid for by the government. The provider will not be held liable for the disapproved services (and the government will therefore absorb the costs) if, among other criteria, it has an effective utilization review program operating. If its program is effective, "[i]n general, there will be a presumption in favor of the provider that [it] did not have knowledge, actual, or imputed, that such items or services are excluded from coverage."[8] One standard which has been used for determining effectiveness is a demonstrated rate of 5 percent or fewer denials of coverage on bills submitted by the provider for payment.[9] When a provider is entitled to the presumption of coverage, it will have less incentive to transfer liability for uncovered services back to the patient by showing that the patient *did* have notice that services would not be covered.

Finally, consumers may also benefit as a general matter from the incentives which the PSRO law creates in institutional committees to actively cooperate with and support the PSRO, because those incentives may serve to revitalize utilization review committees. With the new mission to work effectively within the PSRO system, these institutional committees, if they accept a positive role in the PSRO program, may take on unique functions which go beyond the basic statutory requirements given them. For example, it would be appropriate (and beneficial to the PSRO system, as well as to consumer-patients) for a utilization review committee to examine the psychosocial factors in medical care, the amenities of care, and the socioeconomic factors relevant to individual cases, whether or not the PSRO itself reviews such elements. "Utilization" of an institution and its facilities entails more than the length of stay, symptomatology, and diagnosis of individual patients. It can, for example, include the efficiency of the institution, as demonstrated by patients' waiting times between procedures, itself affected by the availability of equipment within the institution. It can include the ability of the institution to reach out into its community as a health service center providing its resources for more than technical problems of hospitalization or other confinement. The work of social service departments, common in most urban hospitals, has expanded as they confront problems of financing care through public programs, follow-up on care delivered in the institution, patient health education, and other aspects of health care delivery not immediately included in the medical process of diagnosis, prescription, and treatment. The participation and cooperation by other health care practitioners in the effective management of those nontechnical aspects of care, as part of the revitalization of institutional review processes, would contribute to the welfare of patients along with the increased efficiency and usefulness of the institution as a unique community resource. Because the costs of utilization review to meet the demands of the PSRO system will be borne by the government,[10] consumers and institutions which recognize the legitimacy of these broadened review activities should seek to obtain PSRO recognition of them as well.

Whether any revitalization will succeed, either minimally to satisfy basic PSRO requirements or broadly as the fulcrum to fundamental change in the roles of health care institutions in their communities, will depend on the ability of the PSRO mechanism to overcome the deficiencies of the previously existing utilization review system. The failures of utilization review as the primary method of cost and quality control for Medicare and Medicaid, in part, were inherent in the creation of those institutional committes, but they were especially aggravated by poor performance. The Senate Finance Committee, in its work in developing PSROs, analyzed at least four inherent deficiencies: (1) lack of coordination between the Medicare and Medicaid review systems; (2) lack of integrated review for all services, institutional and noninstitutional, available to or prescribed for a patient; (3) lack of adequately developed norms of care; and (4) lack of sufficient support and involvement from physicians.[11] In designing the PSRO system, the Committee attempted to meet each of these criticisms. Medicare and Medicaid services will now be reviewed by a single entity, the PSRO.[12] Eventually, PSROs will review care in hospitals and nursing facilities and, if they choose, will monitor ambulatory care as well.[13] Professionally developed norms will be applied to all review,[14] and the program has been made entirely dependent for its operation and success on physicians' support and involvement.[15]

Although the inherent deficiencies in the system's design which the Senate Finance Committee confronted may have been met, the poor performance of the various entities responsible for utilization review presents a greater challenge. Voluntary acceptance of the PSRO program by physicians and institutions and enforcement of the system are not made achieveable simply by writing laws requiring compliance,[16] particularly since the law has faced serious opposition from those on whom its success depends. The two most critical failures of the utilization review program were (1) a pervasive derogation by the committees of their statutory responsibilities, and (2) their acquiescence in the usurpation of activities they were intended to perform themselves by fiscal intermediaries (the private agencies charged with the responsibility of actually paying the government's money to beneficiaries for services the public programs cover).[17]

The Senate Finance Committee characterized the utilization review committees' performances as "of a token nature and ineffective as a curb to unnecessary use of institutional care and services,"[18] and noted that their failure had in itself contributed to upward spiraling medical costs. A 1968 sampling of the nation's hospitals by the Social Security Administration found that 10 percent of the hospitals performed no review of extended care cases; 47 percent were not reviewing admissions; and 42 percent failed to maintain at least abstracts of medical records or other form of summary for review purposes.[19] The 1970 report of the staff of the Senate Finance Committee on Medicare and

Medicaid called attention also to the Social Security Administration's (SSA) own dereliction of its obligations in administering the utilization review program. SSA's failures were evident in three major areas: (1) lack of adequate regulations; (2) lack of administrative direction and follow-through to ascertain that the various participants performed according to their contracts and statutory requirements; and (3) failure to produce and furnish fiscal agents and providers with data useful to effective utilization review.[20] Not only did the Social Security Administration fail to provide the relevant data, but the staff noted that initially SSA had discouraged the development and dissemination of data by intermediaries themselves, but had changed its position in 1970.[21] Contributing to the general collapse of the utilization review program, the Committee found, was that the little review paying agents did perform stifled minimal institutional utilization review committee activities and led to physicians' "resentment that their medical determinations [were being] challenged by insurance company personnel."[22]

At the bottom of this flimsy hierarchy of review was the patient, who, unfortunately, suffered the impact of the ineffectiveness of the system. Indiscriminate approvals of coverage by pro forma committees, established solely to meet the conditions of participation but never truly functional, often resulted in retroactive denials of coverage by fiscal intermediaries. Patients who had consented to the "disputed" procedures, presuming that Medicare or Medicaid would pay, found that utilization review committee approval of their care, if the committee functioned at all, could still be overruled by the paying agent, with little opportunity to challenge the denial. The patient would then be required to pay for the desired services himself or was sued by the hospital for failure to pay. Where patients were so poor that a hospital could not recover the cost of services from them, the hospital itself was forced to absorb the loss. This could in turn lead the hospital to recover these "bad debts," created by their own negligence, by clever accounting techniques, or charging the loss to other public programs under which they were required to render a certain amount of free services to poor people.[23] With their quotas of free service met through accounting manipulation, patients legitimately eligible for free care under the law could not get it.

The PSRO law was written to overcome those failures. This chapter examines the relationships which the law creates between PSROs and institutions, in light of the previous system's collapse, and analyzes the factors that will structure their interaction and the possible implications for the viability of the PSRO system and its potential for consumer service.

DELEGATING CASE BY CASE REVIEW

The provision governing the relationship between PSROs and institutional utilization review committees is set forth among the duties and functions of PSROs:[24] "Each [PSRO] shall utilize the services of, and accept the findings of, the review committees of a hospital or other operating health care facility or organization located in the area served by [it] .... ."[25] The operation of the provision is specifically conditioned. Approval and acceptance of committee review is to occur "only when and only to the extent and only for such time that such committees have demonstrated to the satisfaction of [the PSRO] their capacity to review activities. .... ."[26] The selection of criteria for evaluating committee performance is not, however, exclusively discretionary with the PSRO. Approval will be governed by any regulations the Secretary may issue to carry out the provisions of the PSRO statute relating to institutional committees.[27] Once criteria have been established, the PSRO's application of them will be subject to review in two ways: (1) the Secretary may for good cause disapprove any PSRO's acceptance of a utilization review committee's activities[28] and (2) PSROs themselves may be reviewed by the Secretary on a comparative basis. Improvident PSRO acceptance of committee activities would result in the Secretary's giving the PSRO an unfavorable rating. The Senate Finance Committee has cautioned PSROs to "use this authority carefully ... [as] ... indiscriminate acceptance of hospital and other review activities would undoubtedly be reflected in an overall poor performance rating when a PSRO was measured against other PSROs operating in careful fashion."[29]

Subject to these conditions, utilization review committees must satisfy the PSRO for their area that they are capable of timely and effective performance of their responsibilities. There are, however, no specific statutory requirements or standards for PSRO approval or evaluation of institutional committees.[30] The Senate Finance Committee has indicated only one prerequisite to acceptance of committee activity; no institutional committee will be accepted which does not participate in PSRO review activities.[31] The Committee does expect the Secretary to create a reasonable mechanism for institutional committees to appeal any unfavorable PSRO determinations about their effectiveness.[32] This mechanism would counteract any bias or "nonprofessional" prejudice on the part of the PSRO.[33]

Direct regulatory interpretation of the provisions discussed above determines three separate aspects of the PSRO–institutional committee relationship: (1) the responsibilities allocable to each entity; (2) the criteria for approving in-house committees; and (3) the process by which the committees will be monitored, and with what effect. The PSRO-committee relationship in the law, as further detailed by regulations, creates various incentives to delegate review to committees as well as to withhold approval. The following discussion elaborates on the interpretations given the statute in the *PSRO Program Manual* and guidelines, and considers the various incentives created in the two groups of entities—PSROs and in-house committees.

Allocated Responsibilities
Practically all PSROs will approve some committees to perform case by case review:

> The PSRO would ... be required to acknowledge and accept, in
> whole or in part, an individual hospital's own review of admissions
> and need for continued care, on a hospital-by-hospital basis, where it
> has determined that a hospital's in-house review is effective. It is
> expected that where such in-house review is effective this authority
> would be exercised.[34]

The *PSRO Program Manual*, at least initially, carries that authority further
through its requirement that both planning contractees and conditional PSROs
present "a timetable for phasing-in review in those hospitals not performing
review under an authorization from the PSRO,"[35] implying that eventually all
committes will be approved.[36] However, there is no legislative history supporting
an intent to approve all committees. Later transmittals from the Bureau of
Quality Assurance, issuing further guidelines on the delegation of review to
hospitals, held out the possibility that some hospitals might not be approved in
the delegation process. Among the steps in that process is "PSRO evaluation of
hospital plan and determination of review functions, *if any*, which shall be
delegated."[37] There has been no further clarification on whether all hospitals
should eventually be approved.

In all cases, the PSRO is itself responsible for all case by case review:

> PSROs ... will assume full responsibility for all decisions having to
> do with quality, appropriateness and necessity of services[38] ... [and
> will be] ... responsible for assuring the effectiveness of all medical
> care review which [they] are authorized to perform. Thus while a
> PSRO may delegate review functions to effective institutional review
> committees, it retains responsibility for assuring the continued
> effectiveness of that review.[39]

A PSRO need accept only that part of a hospital's review which it finds
satisfactory, but does so knowing that any review activities it does not accept it
must perform itself.[40] The *Program Manual* permits hospitals to perform three
kinds of review for the PSRO:[41] (1) *admission certification* a "form of medical
care review in which an assessment is made of the medical necessity of a
patient's admission to a hospital";[42] (2) *continued stay review*, "a form of
medical care review which occurs during a patient's hospitalization and consists
of an assessment of the medical necessity of a patient's need for continued
confinement at a hospital level of care and may also include a detailed
assessment of the quality of care being provided";[43] and (3) *medical care
evaluation studies*, "a type of retrospective medical care review in which
in-depth assessment of the quality and/or the nature of the utilization of health
care services is made."[44] These types of review are the basic review responsibilities of the PSRO, and the requirements imposed on the PSRO for each type
of review apply equally to the hospital seeking approval of its committee.[45]

The requirements for approval by a PSRO are slightly different from those which institutional review committees are required to perform as a condition of their institution's participation in Medicare and Medicaid. (The differences are explained further in the next section of this chapter.) When hospital activities in review are approved, in whole or in part, review may be performed by the hospital's personnel alone or in combination with PSRO personnel.[46]

Where the PSRO has *not* approved a committee and is therefore responsible for performing those activities itself, the law establishes the PSRO processes. The PSRO must specify appropriate points in time after admission when the attending physician must certify "that further in-patient care in such institutions [e.g., hospitals and nursing facilities] will be medically necessary effectively to meet the health care needs of such patient."[47] The certification by the physician must include "such information as may be necessary to enable [the PSRO] properly to evaluate the medical necessity of the further institutional health care recommended by the physician."[48] The times when certification must be performed are to be based on norms and should be "usually not later than the 50th percentile of lengths of stay for patients in similar age groups with similar diagnosis."[49] The Senate Finance Committee would allow the PSRO to choose not to require certification in those cases where the 50th percentile for length of stay is quite short, of one or two days duration. The PSRO is thereby offered greater flexibility than review committees under the old system. Were the PSRO required to establish and apply certification points for every admission, the result would be time-wasting, unwieldy bureaucratic procedures for no purpose. However, unless the discretion to forego certification in short stays is strictly supervised, the potential does exist for PSRO reliance on retrospective review with resulting retroactive denials of coverage to patients who assumed services would be reimbursed. It is not yet clear whether an institutional committee's adherence to PSRO certification points (as distinct from norms) is to be used as a criterion for evaluating its performance for delegation purposes.

Requirements for Utilization
Review by Institutions
Whether or not a PSRO even exists in every area of the country, hospitals and nursing facilities are required to perform utilization review if they expect to be reimbursed for services they render to Medicare and Medicaid patients. Conceptually and practically, utilization review in institutions is an activity distinct from utilization review as performed by a hospital to whom a PSRO delegates review responsibility. The legally established process of review in those institutions is different from the requirements imposed under the law before the creation of PSROs, because institutional committees had failed on their own and PSROs are now intended to remedy their failures. But as PSROs around the country are only becoming operational, institutions seeking

reimbursement under Medicare and Medicaid are required to perform utilization review, consonant with the aims and functions of PSROs.

To revitalize the old system's moribund committees, the Senate Finance Committee left the system essentially intact but changed some of the authority for review. Under the preexisting system in the absence of PSROs, utilization review was created initially in the Medicare program, with specific and detailed criteria for the process of review, the composition of the committees, and their goals.[50] The Medicaid program, however, made no specific demands for utilization review and mandated only that state plans provide generally for methods and procedures "relating to the utilization of . . . care and services available under the plan as may be necessary to safeguard against unnecessary utilization. . . ."[51] Principal review authority was vested in the state agency administering the Medicaid program in each state, while those agencies were also encouraged, by regulations, to delegate review to committees performing review for Medicare purposes.[52] These agencies also had the right to delegate responsibility for monitoring review to fiscal intermediaries performing those functions under the Medicare laws.[53] As a result, the responsibility to safeguard against unnecessary utilization of Medicaid services was contingent on a functional Medicare program. With the failure of Medicare utilization review there was nothing to support Medicaid review activities and the structure collapsed.

The 1972 Social Security Amendments confronted the failure in three ways:[54] (1) Medicaid state plans were specifically required to provide for utilization review; (2) that review was to be coordinated with Medicare review, and, if efficient, performed by the same groups or committees;[55] and (3) where Medicare procedures were not being used or were otherwise ineffective, the Secretary was given authority to waive the Medicare requirements in favor of more stringent and effective Medicaid requirements.[56] At the same time, if states had effective alternate utilization review programs, other than those methods specified by the Secretary, the Senate Finance Committee intended them to be used, in the hope of eventually achieving a functional program to monitor costs and quality, regardless of its sponsorship.[57]

Hospital Responsibilities. Regulations governing hospital utilization review under the 1972 Amendments were among the most hotly contested regulations ever issued by HEW. The usual thirty day comment period was extended for another thirty days during which time more than 4700 comments were received about the new Medicaid requirements and more than 1000 comments were received on the Medicare regulations.[58] The principal provision feeding the controversy was one requiring preadmission review of all non-emergency admissions under Medicare and Medicaid. The provision was deleted in the final regulations in response to criticism that it would be "cumbersome, expensive, and a poor use of limited physician resources."[59] There was almost a year between the issuance of proposed regulations (January 9, 1974) and the promulgation of final regulations (November 29, 1974).

Under the new laws and regulations, hospitals must at least meet the Medicare requirements for utilization review. Each hospital must establish and put into effect a written plan providing for

> "at least the timely review of the medical necessity of admissions, extended duration stays and professional services rendered, and [have] as its objectives both high quality patient care and effective and efficient utilization of available health facilities and services.[60]

The plan, when submitted to the Secretary, must be accompanied by a certification that it is actually in effect.[61] The plan must specify the organization, composition, and frequency of meetings of the committee, as well as the types of records it will keep.[62] These regulations are not substantially different from those which applied before PSROs. In addition, however, the committee must describe the method it will use in performing "medical care evaluation studies" (described more fully below), and the methods and criteria, including norms, where available, that will be used in assigning initial extended stay review dates.[63]

The committee's membership can be constituted in any of three ways: (1) two or more physicians from the staff of the hospital with participation of other professional personnel; (2) a group outside the hospital which is similarly composed and is established by local medical or osteopathic society; and (3) a group, otherwise set up, which has been approved by the Secretary and is capable of performing utilization review.[64] The last option paves the way for a PSRO to perform institutional review in place of a staff committee. Conflict of interest provisions exclude from review activities anyone financially interested in any hospital or any person who was professionally involved in the care of the patient whose case is being reviewed.[65] These regulations are stronger than previously existing ones.[66] Although the regulations specify that utilization review is "the responsibility of the medical profession,"[67] they do not say that, in exercising that responsibility, a hospital committee may not choose to include nonprofessionals.[68]

The details of the process of review are specified in the regulations. In place of the previous standard of primary reliance on the attending physician's opinion,[69] the new regulations require only that the attending physician be given an opportunity to discuss the reasons for his opinion. If the committee's final determination disagrees with him, it must be concurred in by at least two physicians, unless, when offered an opportunity to discuss his reasons, the attending physician does not respond.[70] In that case, a final determination may be made by one physician.[71] In making their determinations, the committee must use written criteria and standards. These regulations use the terms "criteria," "norms," and "standards" as they are used in the *Program Manual*.[72] Recognizing that, at least initially, hospitals will have difficulty complying with the requirement to select and develop norms, the regulations authorize the Secretary to extend the time period for compliance beyond February 1, 1975 if the committee has made a good faith effort to comply, is currently making progress, and establishes a timetable for achieving the requirements.[73]

Each committee is required to perform three types of review: (1) admission review, (2) extended stay review, and (3) medical care evaluation studies. Admission review is performed by a physician member of the committee, or an appropriately trained nonprofessional.[74] Within one working day of elective and emergency admissions, the patient is assigned an extended stay review date based on the criteria selected by the committee. In order to determine whether the case falls within the medical care criteria and represents a condition which "is not associated with unnecessary admissions or frequent furnishing of unnecessary services"[75] the regulations require that the determination be based on specific information:

(i) Identification of the individual (patient) by appropriate means to assure confidentiality, and identification of the attending physician

(ii) The date of admission. . . (and where necessary the date of application for Medicare benefits)

(iii) The diagnosis or symptoms indicating the need for admission

(iv) The physician's plan of treatment

(v) Where appropriate, date of operating room reservation

(vi) Other supporting material (e.g., recent test findings, recent case history, schedule of tests planned) as the committee may require

(vii) In the case of emergency admissions, the justification for such admission[76]

In assigning an extended care review date, the committee is expected to apply norms otherwise in use in the region. The initial date assigned is to be based on the 50th percentile of these norms.[77] This process of review is similar to that established in the *Program Manual* for the PSRO itself.[78] The process does permit modification in the initially approved length of stay because of a change in patient's condition or in the treatment schedule.[79]

Extended stay review must take place prior to or on the date assigned initially. The process is similar to admissions review, and the determination is to be based on the reasons for continued stay and the physician's plan for treatment during that period.[80] Like admissions review, and the processes of review performed by the PSRO itself,[81] notice of determinations contrary to the physician's must be given in writing to the hospital, the attending physician(s), and the patient not later than two days after the determination is made, and in no case later than two working days after the end of the certified period.[82]

The use of norms and the specifications for the informational base on which determinations must be made are the most significant changes in the review process, distinguishing it from the system before PSROs.

An additional significant difference is the requirement that hospitals perform medical care evaluation studies.[83] These studies are in depth analyses of specific problems within hospitals. They are supposed "to further the basic goals of utilization review by emphasizing identification and analysis of patterns of patient care and ... [suggesting] possible changes for maintaining consistently high quality patient care and effective and efficient use of services."[84] Studies are conducted on a sample (or other) basis and must include, but are not limited to: "admissions, durations of stay, ancillary services furnished (including drugs and biologicals), and professional services performed on the hospital premises."[85] The regulations require that at least one study must be in progress at any given time and at least one must be completed each year. The emphasis in them may be on substantive medical problems or administrative problems affecting the hospital's efficiency. By analyzing data obtained from a variety of sources—medical records in the hospital itself, hospital profiles compiled by an external organization, PSROs, fiscal intermediaries, or other providers of services—the hospital is expected to document its analysis and the way in which the results of any such study have been used to "institute changes to improve the quality of care and promote more effective and efficient use of facilities and services."[86]

Although the essential focus of medical care evaluation studies appears initially to be high quality care, the results of them will also be used to achieve cost control. By regulation, the results are directly channeled into cost control efforts in admissions review. The admissions review mechanism "provides for closer professional scrutiny ... of cases involving diagnosis of treatments that are associated with unusually high cost or the frequent furnishing of excessive services ... such cases being identified as a result of medical care evaluation study."[87] These studies are the core of the educational value in the PSRO program, because they require institutions to undergo self-evaluation, monitored by outside agencies—the Secretary and the PSRO.

Should the Secretary find that utilization review procedures established by the State for Medicaid are superior in their effectiveness to the methods described above, hospitals in that state will have to meet the Medicaid requirements.[88]

Primary responsibility for assuring that utilization review is done under the Medicaid program is given to the individual states. Institutions have responsibility for "utilization *review*"; the states provide "utilization *control*."[89] Should states fail effectively to establish and monitor institutional review, they will be penalized by a reduction in the federal share of payments for the Medicaid program in that state.[90] The state agency responsible for utilization control has two other monitoring duties with regard to in-patient hospital services, which may be seen as inherently creating a stricter program for preventing unnecessary costs. In addition to the continuous program of review of utilization similar to Medicare requirements, the agency itself must provide in its plan for other elements of review: "the on-going evaluation, on a sample basis, of the necessity, quality and timeliness of the services provided to eligible individuals";[91] and the establishment and periodic review of detailed written plans of care for each Medicaid in-patient in any Medicaid facility. This review creates a monitoring function that provides an intermediate point for determining whether the program is working, at the same time evaluating actual medical care delivered. If this mechanism operates effectively it may prevent unnoticed poor performance of the system, like that which crippled the previously existing utilization review system, and will better guarantee the provision of good quality care. With states reviewing necessity, quality, and timeliness of services, and the Secretary then reviewing the states' performance, an earlier fail-safe point is established at which time corrective measures would presumably be taken.

The Medicaid program requires an additional cost control device in the "post-payment review process" imposed on states participating in the program.[92] Apparently as a technique for spotting chronic abusers of the system, malingerers, or defrauders, the state must establish a process that "allows for the development and review of *recipient* utilization profiles, provider services profiles, and exceptions criteria; and that identifies exceptions in order to rectify misutilization practices of recipients, providers and institutions."[93] Note that the onus for improper utilization is placed in part on the recipient in these profiles. It is unlikely that the assumption is valid for most patients, considering that services must be ordered for them by a physician before payment can be made. Most patients do not specify to their physician the services they require; and the policy of focusing on the patient and expecting him or her to bear the consequences of the physician's decision to prescribe is a questionable one at best. Admittedly, the regulations mandate scrutiny of providers as well as the establishment of exceptions criteria, but nowhere in the regulations or their prefatory comments is there an indication of the intended use for such profiles. Their compilation as well as their subsequent use should be strictly supervised and conditioned by the Secretary. Consumers will be especially concerned about the uses of these profiles in order to prevent the states' penalizing patients for whom physicians prescribe unnecessary services in anticipation of easy reimbursement by Medicaid, but for whom the state agency unfairly establishes a profile as an abuser of the Medicaid program.

The process of review in hospitals under the Medicaid program is otherwise essentially the same as that for Medicare. The requirements for a written plan are the same;[94] the organization, function, and composition of the committees are the same.[95] Admissions review, continued stay review, and medical care evaluation studies are to be done in the same manner. Where determinations are contrary to the attending physician's opinion, the program adds the requirement that notice be sent to the single state agency administering the Medicaid program, in addition to the administrator, attending physician, and individual, and, in slight variance from Medicare, states that notice of adverse final determinations should also be sent "where possible" to the next of kin.[96] (Medicare requires only that next of kin or sponsor be notified "where appropriate.")

Responsibilities of Long Term Care Facilities. Skilled nursing care is available as a Medicare benefit; and skilled nursing facilities providing those services must have a utilization review plan in effect, also as a condition of their participation in the Medicare program.[97] The process of review is to be conducted similarly to that in a hospital.[98] The organization, structure, and function of the committee is to be the same. Written plans must be submitted to the Secretary. Unlike hospitals, however, in skilled nursing facilities under the Medicare regulations only two types of review are conducted: (1) medical care evaluation studies and (2) extended stay review.[99] Utilization review in skilled nursing facilities under Medicare dispenses with admissions review. Where PSROs are operating, they have the responsibility to approve services and items "proposed to be provided in a hospital or other health care facility on an in-patient basis."[100] And that authority will usually be used to scrutinize nursing home admissions. In addition, if the PSRO chooses it may determine "in advance, in the case of any . . . health care service which will consist of extended or costly courses of treatment"[101] whether it is medically necessary and appropriately performed in the proposed facility. The skilled nursing facility must provide in its plan for periodic review of each current in-patient beneficiary case of continuous extended duration.[102] The plan itself must specify when such periods occur. Different lengths of stay may be assigned to patients with different conditions, or the same length of stay for review may be assigned to every case. In no case may the initial period before any review is performed exceed 30 days, unless the committee can present evidence that the average or median of current length of stay for a specific diagnostic category would exceed 30 days. Unlike hospital review under Medicare, the regulations do not require the use of preestablished regional norms, criteria, and standards for such review. Screening of cases is based on criteria established by the physician members of the utilization review committee.[103] Review is based on "the attending physician's reasons for and plan for continued stay and any other documentation the committee or group deems appropriate."[104]

When the committee determines that further in-patient skilled nursing care is necessary, it must approve the case for another period it deems appropriate, but in any case review must be made at least every 30 days for the first 90 days and thereafter at least every 90 days.[105] A final determination that further stay is not medically necessary is made by at least two physician members of the committee (unless the attending physician does not present his reasons for his decision to extend the stay). Written notification is given to the facility, the attending physician, and the patient (and where appropriate his next of kin) no later than two days after the determination is made, and in no event later than three working days after the end of the previously approved period of time.[106] Finally, Medicare requirements may be ignored in favor of the Medicaid provisions if the Secretary determines that the utilization review procedures established by a state for its Medicaid program are superior in their effectiveness to the Medicare requirements.[107]

The Medicaid requirements for skilled nursing facilities differ from the Medicare requirements. The basic process of utilization review by the institution itself is the same. Medical care evaluation studies and extended stay review are to be performed by the same type of committees using the same procedures that would be appropriate to the Medicare program.[108] The essential differences lie in the additional responsibilities charged to the institutions and to the state as its part of Medicaid utilization control.

Medicaid requires that "discharge planning" be performed for each individual patient. Each patient must have "a planned program of post-facility continuing care which takes into account such eligible individual's post-discharge needs."[109] Each skilled nursing facility must have a written plan setting forth the procedures by which this requirement will be met. Included in the plan must be a description of the staff which will have operational responsibility for the planning, the manner and methods by which the planning will be performed, and the time period in which each patient's need for discharge planning will be determined (in any case no later than seven days after admission to the facility). Time periods for reevaluation, the local resources available to the facility, the patient, and the attending physician for assistance in developing and implementing the individual's plan, and provisions for periodic review of the facility's own discharge planning program must also be described in the written plan submitted to the single state agency administering the Medicaid program.[110] When the patient is discharged, the facility is required to provide to those people responsible for the patient's post—discharge care that information which will ensure "optimal continuity of care," such as current information about his or her diagnoses, prior treatment, rehabilitation potential, physician advice concerning immediate care, and pertinent social information.[111]

Other elements are required in the state's total utilization review program in skilled nursing facilities under Medicaid. The state must assure that a physician certifies the admission of the patient as medically necessary and appropriately given in a skilled nursing facility, and recertifies the admission at least every 60 days.[112] "A program of medical review (including medical evaluation and *on-site inspection* of the care of patients in ... skilled nursing facilities)"[113] must be part of the written plan which the state submits to the Secretary. This review is to be independent of utilization review; it is a medical evaluation, examining the need for and plan of care for the patient.[114] The requirements for medical evaluations are quite detailed and exceed in specificity the Medicare requirements.

Because Medicaid, unlike Medicare, also provides services in intermediate care facilities, they too are required to perform utilization review. The state plan may, however, provide either for review by the facility, or directly by the state agency or people under contract to it.[115] Each intermediate care facility must, in any event, have on file with the state a plan for review of services rendered to patients. At least one or more physicians and other professional personnel must review the necessity for continued stay at least every six months. Independent professional reviews, which are required in intermediate care facilities as well as in skilled nursing facilities, may be used to meet the basic review requirement in intermediate care facilities.[116] The committee or group performing review must base its determination of the necessity for continued stay on written criteria which it establishes. Final determinations in individual cases and notification of them are made in the same manner as in a skilled nursing facility.

Waivers.   Generally speaking, the requirements for utilization review and control under Medicaid now are more specific than those set forth in the Medicare regulations. If they are fully implemented, they may inherently create a program superior in effectiveness to any Medicare program in operation in each state. If that proves to be the case, or if the state has established some alternate system of its own, the law provides that the Secretary may waive the specified requirements in favor of the more effective mechanism, whatever it is.

Criteria for applying the waiver provision will be established by the Secretary. The regulations permit waiver projects to be evaluated between one and two years after February 1, 1975, and reviewed thereafter periodically. A state may apply for a waiver at any time when it believes it has superior procedures in operation, whether on a demonstration basis or otherwise. Waivers may be granted for as much of a utilization review program as the Secretary is satisfied with, and any institution participating in Medicaid which is not covered by a waiver must continue to meet the requirements which the regulations set forth.[117]

Criteria for PSRO Delegation

The requirements for utilization review as conditions of participation are different from the criteria used by the PSRO in determining whether to delegate case by case review authority to an individual hospital (and presumably, later, to nursing homes). Adherence to, and full implementation of, the utilization review requirements are, however, the basic criteria PSROs will use.

In the preparation of guidelines for the exercise of the delegation authority, many different criteria were considered. An early HEW staff paper suggested the following: "(1) whether a hospital utilization review committee has a truly active Utilization Review program; (2) whether the committee participates in an active program of physician education; and (3) whether the committee makes and follows-up on recommendations for improved hospital policies or procedures flowing from their evaluation of patterns of patient care and utilization of beds and services."[118] The AMA suggested three similar, but somewhat more lenient, standards: (1) that the committee review process is actually being followed; (2) that PSRO-approved criteria are being met or progress toward meeting them is evident; and (3) that a program exists for continuing education based on problems identified in review.[119]

The *PSRO Program Manual* has expanded on the general criteria HEW initially considered, and the *Manual* has been further supplemented with a *PSRO Transmittal Letter* setting forth additional guidelines. Several basic principles are to govern the PSRO's exercise of the delegation authority:

1. The PSRO may delegate one or more of its review functions to a hospital, but it must conduct profile analysis for comparing area hospitals and monitoring individual hospital performance.
2. When the PSRO does delegate review activities, it must do so to the whole hospital; individual departments within a hospital may not be delegated review.
3. The PSRO must communicate its review findings, in those institutions for which review has not been delegated, in writing to the medical staff, administration, and board of trustees.
4. The PSRO must accept and consider in good faith any application by a hospital to receive delegated review authority.
5. A process must be established by which a PSRO's determination against delegation may be appealed by the hospital.
6. The Secretary may for good cause disapprove the PSRO's determination, whatever it is.[120]

Nine minimum criteria for delegation are suggested. (1) Concurrent admission certification, continued stay review, and medical care evaluation studies must be performed by the hospital.[121] (2) The hospital's review system must provide for the abstraction of data necessary to generate patient, practitioner, and institutional profiles. (3) For concurrent review purposes the hospital's review system must incorporate norms, criteria, and standards adopted by the PSRO.[122] This requirement has been an element of the PSRO review system engendering great opposition on the part of physicians and hospitals.[123] The old utilization review regulations gave "great weight" to the attending physician's opinion.[124] That provision supported the autonomy of the medical profession and may also have been advantageous to the patient. Presumably the attending physician is the one person most familiar with the patient's needs. Without primary reliance on him, review will be based primarily on review of records and the burden will be shifted to the physician to come forward and substantiate his findings. Even within the PSRO system retaining the weight of the attending physician's opinion could have been practically important to the patient. Consider the case where a physician orders services which, if approved, would entail an expansive application of norms, criteria, and standards; that is, the physician is utilizing services maximally within the limits of approval. Where a PSRO might disapprove coverage in a questionable case, a utilization review committee looking primarily to the attending physician's opinion might approve the services. The elimination of the weight of the attending physician's opinion, placing greater emphasis on norms, creates a more standardized system throughout the structure, but also strongly supports the cost control aims of the PSRO program.

(4) In order to be delegated review, each hospital must perform four medical care evaluation studies each year, and it must agree to participate in multiple hospital medical care evaluation studies conducted by the PSRO where they are appropriate.[125] This is the one criterion for delegation most obviously different from the utilization review requirements as conditions of participation. The utilization review regulations require only that one medical care evaluation study be performed each year.[126]

(5) Each hospital to be delegated review must be capable of providing the PSRO with information sufficient to monitor its performance.[127] (6) At least 25 percent of physicians with active hospital staff privileges must be members of the PSRO and participate in PSRO activities.[128] (7) Physicians must be excluded from review where financial or (8) professional conflicts of interest exist.[129] Finally, (9) the hospital shall include in its review plan provision for the inclusion of nonphysician practitioners in peer review activities.[130]

The *Program Manual* and the *Transmittal* suggest several sources of information for evaluating a hospital's past performance of its utilization review duties and estimating its capability to take on delegated review responsibilities.[131] These sources will obviously be very important initially, because, when the first determination of hospital review capability is made, hospitals will not have had the opportunity to use PSRO norms, criteria, and standards in utilization review—the principle demonstration of ability to perform review. Medicare state survey agencies, Medicare intermediaries, and Medicaid state agencies are three major sources suggested to the PSRO for evaluating a hospital's review performance.[132] Considering the role of fiscal intermediaries in usurping utilization review authority from hospitals and their own inability to perform their rightful responsibilities (see next chapter), combined with the failure of Medicaid utilization review as performed by state agencies (discussed above), these three sources of information may not be reliable; although, within the previously existing structure, they have had the greatest opportunity to develop relevant data. PSRO review of information received from the hospital concerning other types of review taking place in the hospital is also suggested.[133] Basic data generally maintained by all hospitals including number of beds; admissions per year; admissions of Medicare, Medicaid, and Title V patients per year; ownership; size of staff; teaching affiliations; and other information characterizing the institution are also recommended for consideration. Finally, other "specific information about the hospital's existing review systems including all narrative material concerning operating procedures, results and follow-up, and the changes needed to qualify for delegation"[134] should be taken into consideration by the PSRO.

The *Program Manual* suggests a five step process for implementing the delegation authority.[135] The more recent *Transmittal Letter* sets forth eight steps for review.[136] Presumably the more detailed, more recent *Transmittal Letter* supercedes the *Program Manual* during the interim period before further chapters in the *Manual* are issued and until final regulations are promulgated. Among other provisions, "Memoranda of Understanding," written documents outlining the hospital's responsibilities and the PSRO's duties, are required at various points in the process.[137] Cooperation is required between the PSRO and the hospital to develop a detailed plan for delegating review. "The PSRO has the responsibility to assure that the hospital's plan is put in place according to the agreed upon schedule."[138]

Incentives

Incentives operate on both PSROs and institutional committees, both for and against delegation of case by case review responsibility to institutional utilization review committees. The system creates two major incentives for PSROs to delegate review: (1) the need to ease their own workload because of overwhelming responsibilities not directly part of case by case review; and (2) the need to assure institutional compliance with PSRO procedures.

In addition to review of individual cases, PSROs have the responsibility to perform data processing, develop profiles, conduct hearings, and develop norms. Approval of institutional committees would lessen the PSRO's duties, thereby permitting it to operate more efficiently. The Senate Finance Committee, recognizing the enormity of PSRO responsibilities, suggested that hospital and local medical organization review committees be used to "maximize the productivity of physician review time without unduly imposing on his principal function, the provision of health care to his patient."[139] The report also recommended the use of automated screening of claims and initial review by registered nurses to facilitate physician participation in PSRO activities.[140] If the PSRO is to meet effectively the other requirements imposed on it, delegating review to hospital committees may significantly improve its ability to perform other activities.

Because the in-house committees themselves have incentives to seek approval for their review, the PSRO can use its approval authority as a technique to force cooperation and compliance by hospitals with the PSRO program. Approval of only those committees where the institution's staff participates in PSRO activities is a powerful incentive to providers to cooperate with the PSRO. Selective awarding of approval by PSROs could contribute to the intended revitalization of utilization review committees. A consumer-oriented PSRO could make approval of hospitals contingent on their meeting additional conditions relating to review of nontechnical aspects of care, patient grievance mechanisms, and generally greater responsiveness to total patient needs.

Finally, a negative incentive could push the PSRO toward indiscriminate approvals. If the physicians in the PSRO chose to sabotage the program, committee approvals could provide a swift technique for replicating the failures of the old utilization review system. The PSRO and its practitioner members are not formally separate entities: the structure of the PSRO system was designed to make them substantially the same. Physicians who are influential members of institutional utilization review committees will no doubt be involved in PSRO activities. If those same physicians, enjoying unique power and status within their own institutions and, consequently, within a PSRO itself, chose to minimize PSRO moves to reform institutional review, they could effectively destroy the system through indiscriminate approvals of nonfunctional, ineffective in-house committees. This potential could possibly be foreclosed through exercise of the fraud provisions of the Medicare and Medicaid statutes[141] or other regulatory action. Ultimately, though, machinations to defeat the PSRO system from within (through PSRO relations with in-house committees) would inevitably lead to a nonphysician-controlled program.[142]

Hospitals have two incentives to win the right to perform review for a PSRO: (1) political autonomy and (2) financial advantage. Once a hospital committee makes a review determination for a PSRO, it is not reversible or reviewable again by the PSRO. Although the hospitals' general review performance will be monitored by the PSRO, once review has been delegated to them, institutional committees are subject to less scrutiny than nonapproved committees. That hospitals desire such autonomy has been amply demonstrated in reported widespread hospitals' plans, very early in PSRO implementation, to develop qualifying in-house programs.[143]

Although earlier in this chapter the validity and effect of consumer participation in utilization review activities is set forth, it is important to note that the incentive to a hospital to be granted PSRO case by case review responsibilities can undermine any significant consumer role. The PSRO statute clearly permits no one other than physicians to review the activities of physicians for purposes of a final determination.[144] An in-house committee performing review in place of a PSRO is subject to the same restriction. "No [PSRO] shall utilize the services of any individual who is not a duly licensed doctor of medicine or osteopathy to make final determinations in accordance with its duties and functions"[145] as set out in the PSRO law. A hospital seeking PSRO approval has an incentive to disqualify consumers from participation in its PSRO activities. That restriction, however, does not mean a blanket prohibition on consumer membership in institutional utilization review committees. The restriction applies only to nonphysician participation in final determinations for PSRO purposes. Approved utilization review committees will engage in other activities open to consumer involvement. Expansive implementation of utilization review as the keystone to innovative hospital roles as community medical service centers does hold an important place for consumers. Their participation is critical to utilization committee work on reaching into the community, educating patients, confronting problems in finding public monies to finance care, and effectively evaluating nontechnical aspects of care.

The second incentive to hospitals to seek approval of their review activities for PSRO purposes is a financial one and it exists in two ways. Approved hospitals can be reimbursed for those activities which "are unique requirements made by the PSRO program and which will need to be initiated as a supplement to present hospital activities."[146] Costs of implementing the utilization review requirements as conditions of participation in Medicare and Medicaid are also available. Under Medicare, "Costs incurred in connection with the implementation of the utilization review plan are includable in reasonable costs and are reimbursable to the hospital to the extent that such costs relate to health insurance program beneficiaries. . ."[147] The *PSRO Manual* provision authorizing reimbursement for performance of unique PSRO requirements was written before the new utilization review regulations were issued. It now appears that anything a hospital does above and beyond basic utilization review requirements, in order to meet PSRO requirements, will be reimbursed; and, since most hospitals are approved for both Medicare and Medicaid (other than specialized children's institutions, for example), those basic costs would also be reimbursed.

In addition, under the "hold harmless" (waiver of liability) provision, a hospital with a functional, effective utilization review program, demonstrated in part by the PSRO's willingness to delegate review to it, would be indemnified by the government for the amount of otherwise noncovered services rendered to a patient.[148] Hospitals with delegated review would be reimbursed more often in questionable cases where hospitals without the delegation would not be.

Monitoring

Under the guidelines, committees, though approved for PSRO review, continue to be subject to on-going monitoring by the PSRO. In the

PSRO-hospital relationship, the need for monitoring hospital performance arises in two ways. (1) The statute gives the PSRO authority to accept the determinations of in-house committees "only for such time that such committees ... have demonstrated to the satisfaction" of the PSRO their capacity to review.[149] The provision, by implication, makes revocation of approval possible. Without the option to revoke approval, the PSRO would have little ability or power to enforce effective review. Monitoring will reveal when revocation of approval becomes necessary.

(2) Because those hospital activities which a PSRO accepts for review purposes are in place of its own review, the institution's determinations, in effect, become those of the PSRO for the limited terms of the acceptance. Were the various approved committees within a PSRO area to reach differing conclusions when faced with similar facts, the inconsistencies might lead the Secretary to terminate the PSRO's contract for failure to assure effective review. The guidelines emphasize, "After implementation of a hospital review plan, the PSRO is responsible for assuring that the hospital continues to perform review effectively."[150]

Once a hospital committee is approved by the PSRO, the statutory language appears to make PSRO acceptance of the committee's findings obligatory,[151] but the legislative history adds no further clarification. Although approval need only extend to those committee activities which satisfy the PSRO, the language suggests that *all* of the committee's approved activities must be accepted in place of PSRO determinations on the same issues. Because these individual decisions are then, in effect, the PSRO's, they could not, consistent with the intent to delegate, be subject again to PSRO scrutiny. Based on monitoring, if the PSRO is dissatisfied with a committee's determinations, by implication the approval mechanism requires the PSRO to withdraw its approval, rather than overrule individual hospital determinations.

Although the right of a PSRO to review an approved committee's individual determinations is not made clear in the statute, the legislative history, or the guidelines, it is important to consumers that the PSRO not be able to review approved committee decisions unless an appeal is filed. Without this interpretation, a PSRO could overrule a committee's decision to approve care, resulting in retroactive denials long after the fact. These denials would create severe financial hardship for patients. Nor would patients benefit medically if the PSRO reversed a committee's earlier denial of admission or continued stay. The monitoring process which might reveal a committee error would take so long that the value of the services might at that point be minimal. Finally, giving the PSRO the authority to overturn individual committee decisions would vitiate any reasons of convenience motivating the PSRO to substitute approved committee activities for its own.

The monitoring process initially will include on-site inspection of the hospital's committee to determine whether review is being performed and whether the process of review conforms to established guidelines. Later, monitoring will focus on the types of decisions made by the review committee, and the impact of these decisions on the quality of care and the utilization of services. The guidelines require the PSRO to develop written, objective criteria for effective performance, for use in the monitoring process.[152]

Although monitoring could utilize the provider profiles PSROs must develop anyway to examine the pattern of practices within an institution,[153] the *Program Manual* segregates these functions, and suggests instead other highly detailed data sources for use in monitoring.[154] The monitoring process itself will yield large quantities of information about individual hospitals. This information would be useful to consumers. For example, information needed by the PSRO in monitoring medical care evaluation studies will come from special reports by the hospital to the PSRO.[155] The guidelines do not proscribe the divulgence of material in these reports to consumers or the public, but the confidentiality provisions of the PSRO statute will probably be used to shield from outside scrutiny information which is critical of hospitals, but also demonstrates their efforts to improve.

PSROs AND HMOs

The discussion of the relationships between PSROs and providers has focused this far on hospitals. It is likely that nursing facilities may be able to achieve similar status for their utilization review committees where they are effective, once PSROs begin to monitor nursing home services. Other providers, though not specifically hospitals nor having institutional utilization review committees, may also be approved by the PSRO for delegated review duties.[156] The Senate Finance Committee noted two such organizations by name:

> Similarly a PSRO would be required to acknowledge and accept for its purposes, review activities of other medical facilities and organizations including those internal review activities of comprehensive prepaid group practice programs such as the Kaiser Health plans and the Health Insurance Plan (H.I.P.) in New York to the extent such review activities are effective.[157]

Prepaid health care delivery programs, with different financing mechanisms and utilization patterns, will require different treatment generally by PSROs, but also in the delegation of case by case review. The tensions created by the interaction of the fee for service–oriented PSROs with prepaid programs are problematic, if not totally unresolvable.

It is, admittedly, beyond the scope of this book to examine fully the relevant issues surrounding health maintenance organizations (HMOs), their advantages and disadvantages as health delivery mechanisms.[158] Indeed, a diversity of variations are included under the HMO rubric. Prepaid group practices and foundations for medical care are two predominant types, although different authorities dispute the definition of an HMO. There are, however, several characteristics common to the various types which, because they are pertinent, are discussed below. (The following description has been highly simplified in order to highlight those features which may create the greatest problems in PSRO–HMO relations.)

An individual enrolls in an HMO program by paying a single "capitation fee," usually paid annually to maintain enrollment before any services are delivered. For this fee, the HMO offers a variety of services, often at a single location, by its physician employees. The HMO subscriber pays the same fixed, basic fee to the HMO regardless of the services he will use, as contrasted with the fee for each individual service payment which traditional individual physicians ordinarily charge and receive. When the subscriber or enrollee is a Medicare or Medicaid patient, the government pays to the HMO a capitation fee on behalf of the Medicare or Medicaid patient. As a practical matter, the fees may be different from those charged to a private subscriber because the federal or state government can negotiate the fee with the HMO, and the fee may be paid for a group of subscribers rather than on behalf of an individual. But the capitation fee entitles the subscriber—private or public program beneficiary—to a benefits package similar in principle to the coverage which an insurance policy would provide. Unlike most indemnity–private health insurance policies, or even Blue Cross and Blue Shield, HMO plans usually cover many ambulatory services (those not requiring a stay in an institution) as well as hospitalization benefits.

Although some HMO physicians are salaried, others, especially those in foundations for medical care, are paid by the HMO on a fee for service basis. Under either payment scheme, the physician's HMO earnings are drawn only from the pool of capitation fees paid by the HMO subscribers. Simplistically stated, then, if an HMO wanted to increase its earnings, the financing system creates incentives both to increase the number of subscribers to the program and to decrease the amount of services provided, thereby lowering the costs of operation to the organization, while increasing the amount and availability of the pool of fees for payment to physicians. The incentives can operate to lead to underutilization—that is, delivering fewer services to individuals or as a pattern of care than optimal standards would call for.[159] There is substantial controversy over whether the potential for underutilization is consistently realized. For example, the Institute of Medicine of the National Academy of Sciences, in its policy statement on PSROs said:

> . . . When the financing mechanism is on the basis of a fixed amount per capita determined in advance, rather than fee-for-service, there may be an incentive to the providers for under-utilization as well as some patient-generated over-utilization. While this concern exists

about the incentives under an HMO arrangement, we note that in available analyses of prepaid group practice experiences, the prototype to the HMO concept, *there is little documentation of a problem with under-utilization or consumer overuse under this arrangement.* [160]

At the same time other studies show that HMO subscribers have lower hospital utilization rates than are characteristic of patients in the general population.[161] These lower rates have been attributed to a variety of factors. Relevant to PSRO-HMO relations are the following: greater availability of coverage for ambulatory care;[162] limitations of bed supply, intentional and unintentional[163] (some HMOs own their own hospitals, other contract with hospitals to provide care to HMO subscirbers when necessary); changed incentives to the physicians;[164] and the introduction of professional controls.[165] Whether underutilization exists or not, HMO proponents often emphasive, "One simply cannot say that under--utilization means poor quality of care. Organized prepaid health care systems (HIP, Kaiser, children and youth projects) have demonstrated that superior care is possible using less units (hospital bed days, for example) of health service."[166] Whether PSROs can have any impact on underutilization regardless of where it occurs has been discussed in Chapter Two.[167] Three separate problems arise from HMOs' differing payment mechanism and utilization patterns.

(1) Despite the fact that PSRO's are presently given jurisdiction to review care delivered by HMOs, PSRO norms based on fee for service patterns of care may not, in fact, be appropriate to review HMO care. Unless PSROs approve norms' modifications for HMOs, the effect of their being required to adhere to PSRO norms could financially cripple, if not bankrupt, an HMO. The HMO's capitation fee is set by projecting utilization patterns; unanticipated higher utilization rates would absorb the HMO's available resources in the delivery of care.[168] One HMO proponent has argued, "There is little chance that an HMO will over-utilize units of health care service, hence, no need for a PSRO to monitor an HMO,"[169] under any circumstances.

(2) HMO proponents charge that fee for service physicians are politically inclined to use their power through PSROs to kill HMOs altogether. One apologist for free market competition among HMOs and between them and other forms of health care delivery sees PSRO as "potentially the most effective anticompetitive device yet put in the hands of the medical profession."[170]

If, as is likely to be the case, PSROs are dominated by fee-for-service physicians, the temptation to make review of HMO care the first priority of the PSRO will be difficult to resist. Viewed from the standpoint of the fee-for-service doctor, the HMO's reduction in hospital utilization and other cost-saving measures may appear to sacrifice quality and to warrant regulation which will increase the

HMO's costs and diminish the HMO's ability to compete effectively with the fee-for-service system. [171]

In arguing against PSRO jurisdiction over HMOs Professor Havighurst claims, "HMOs have adequate incentives to limit their expenditures to effective treatments and to employ their resources efficiently. Indeed, this strength of the HMO highlights the very weakness of the fee-for-service system which necessitates introducing PSRO cost-control methods in the first place." [172]

To deal very briefly with these contentions, although theoretically HMOs do represent a financial threat to the fee for service physician, it is indeed questionable whether PSRO physicians, who must fulfill extensive requirements of the PSRO law, will have the time or the inclination to concentrate their attentions initially and fully on efforts to stifle HMO development. Even if self-interest is the primary force motivating fee for service physicians, presumably their efforts would be best focused on developing broadly liberal norms, permitting approval of whatever services they choose to deliver. Norms so drawn and liberally applied would much more directly benefit them than attempts to stifle fledgling HMOs. The well-established HMOs can presumably fend for themselves, since they have so far in the face of fee for service medicine which, Professor Havighurst asserts, "has never had great difficulty in slowing down the growth of prepaid group practice." [173]

Furthermore, Havighurst cites one of the strengths of HMOs, making PSRO's review of them superfluous, as incentives to limit costs through professional review mechanisms. In fact, the professional review experiences of HMOs served, in part, as models for PSROs. [174] But it is important to observe that the need for professional review to contain costs in an HMO arises because of the financial incentives to the participating doctors. If fewer services are utilized, more money in the pool of capitation fees is available to pay the doctors in the HMO. In one HMO model, that means that disapproval of services can result in higher salaries to physician employees. In another form, it means the physicians can raise the fees they charge to the HMO for their services. In either case, it is important to note that in an HMO the physicians who earn their incomes out of the pool of capitation fees also generally participate directly in the fee-setting mechanism. They have a direct interest in controlled costs, in order to maintain the financial viability of the HMO and their own incomes. This ability to set fees is significant to the question of whether HMOs served as valid models for PSROs, because PSROs, in contrast, have been specifically denied the authority to participate in fee-setting or other cost determinations for the Medicare and Medicaid programs. [175] Finally, recent reports raise questions about the validity of the proponents' assertions that HMO's are able to provide services more economically than fee for services delivery, where the patients are public program beneficiaries. [176]

Two techniques can mitigate the potentially stifling effect PSROs may have on HMOs: (1) participation by HMO physician members in all PSRO activities; and (2) approval of an HMO's in-house review program. The first approach presumably, would create at least a minimal dialogue between the representatives of the two major forms of health care delivery and financing, thereby preventing the immediate, complete emasculation of HMOs. The second technique would give to HMOs the autonomy they claim to need. At the same time, at least on an interim basis, delegation would give the PSROs the vital ability to monitor HMO patterns of care and review, and to develop aggregate data in order to create a reasonable, empirical base for evaluating the merits of the respective claims by both sectors of the health care delivery system. This function will be critical to an eventual resolution of the HMO vs. fee for service debate.

Professor Havighurst dismisses these approaches. On participation of HMO representatives in PSRO activities he says:

> Far from solving the problem, however, this proposed solution simply changes its nature without diminishing its seriousness. The PSRO would then become a forum for negotiating the differences between the fee-for-service sector and the HMOs represented in its councils. The PSRO would then function as a cartel, allocating markets, defining modes of competition, and denying competitive opportunities to new HMO entrants. . . . [177]

As to PSRO delegation of case by case review authority to an HMO, he says:

> While it seems likely that PSROs would delegate the task of utilization and quality review to some HMOs, subject to PSRO oversight, it is clear that the HMOs achieving this preferred status would be those which had negotiated treaties with the fee-for-service sector, and foresworn aggressive competition and price-cutting. New entrants and more vigorous competitors would be subjected to intensive supervision. [178]

Recognizing the merits of Professor Havighurst's and other's arguments, there is substantial question as to whether PSROs can appropriately review delivery of HMO services as they would hospitals and nursing homes. The reasons are quite different, and much more fundamental than those which Havighurst cites. Ultimately, the issue around HMOs and PSROs is whether PSROs can affect HMO practices in any way. PSRO review is predicated on a fee for service concept. By denying payment for those services not approved by the PSRO, the government intends to control costs in a direct and immediate way. Because the services which HMOs deliver have been prepaid, case by case review of HMO care with PSRO disapproval of unnecessary or inappropriate services will have no effect. PSROs have no power to impose on HMOs their determinations of no medical necessity because there is no payment to deny. If capitation rates on Medicare and Medicaid patients are paid after services are delivered and are based on actual costs incurred by the HMO in providing them, we are no longer talking about HMOs. [179] The prepayment mechanism is the essential characteristic of HMOs which will create significant obstacles to PSRO jurisdiction over them. Finally, if HMOs do emphasize ambulatory services in their benefits packages, unless and until PSROs choose to review ambulatory care (and a PSRO need never so choose) they will be powerless to affect a major component of the HMO delivery mechanism.

Without the clout of denied reimbursement, PSROs are powerless and ineffective to force compliance by any health care provider, solo practitioner, or HMO with their goals. But the educational value of peer review and participation in wide-scale efforts to develop statistics on health care delivery, including all financing and delivery mechanisms, are important, and, therefore, are factors pushing toward PSRO jurisdiction over HMOs. It seems, though, that some other mechanism will be necessary to review HMO health care delivery because PSROs are inherently ill-equipped to perform the task.

PSROs AND STATE MEDICAID AGENCIES

The relationships between PSROs and direct service providers—hospitals, nursing homes, HMOs—are governed and influenced by the provisions on delegating review authority to providers. The PSRO system is designed to create a direct link between the PSROs and those providers, so that the various review requirements under the differing programs are compatible with PSRO activities and goals. Given the necessity for a direct relationship between PSROs and providers, it is important to evaluate the role of state Medicaid agencies, effectively interposed between the PSRO and Medicaid providers in medical care review.

State Medicaid agencies (as discussed in this chapter) have primary responsibility for the administration of utilization review of Medicaid services delivered in their respective states. [180] If, because of faulty utilization review, the care provided to Medicaid patients exceeds that which is medically necessary and covered, the law provides for federal financial penalties to be invoked against the state. [181] The law inherently creates the potential for tension between the state's authority and that of PSROs, and the tension is further aggravated by the way in which Medicaid is financed. Unlike Medicare, which if financed solely by money collected by the federal government, [182] Medicaid is underwritten by federal and state contributions. [183] The participating states each contribute between 20 and 50 percent of the costs of the program with most of the states paying 50 percent. [184] The state Medicaid agency administering the program in each state is responsible to its state government for the expenditure of the state's share of the money. This financial accountability could prevent a state agency from relinquishing cost and quality review of Medicaid services to a PSRO.

The PSRO statute attempts to resolve the tension by requiring that state Medicaid plans be subject to PSRO authority. [185] The statute recognizes that in some states action by the state legislature will be required to relinquish authority from the state Medicaid agency to the PSRO; [186] but a PSRO itself has no authority to force compliance with the statute. Rather it is the federal government, through the HEW compliance process, that must enforce the provision. States which fail to submit their Medicaid plan to PSRO authority run the risk of losing all or part of their federal contributions for Medicaid. [187] As a practical matter, HEW may not enforce compliance against a state which eschews PSRO review, especially if that state's Medicaid agency is effectively controlling costs. The Medicaid utilization review regulations discussed earlier in this chapter fail to specify the respective authorities of PSROs and Medicaid agencies.

The interests of the Medicaid state agencies and PSROs coincide in their general goals. But in specific areas they can conflict, and in some areas the state agencies may seek to influence PSROs toward actions serving their own interests. The discussion below briefly touches on some of the areas of possible tension in the complex maze of administrative authority for cost and quality control through utilization review. [188]

Shortly after the PSRO law was enacted, the Medical Services Administration, responsible in part for the federal administration of Medicaid, sent a notice to state Medicaid agencies indicating how PSRO–state agency interaction might be mutually beneficial. [189] In addition to providing an opportunity to increase professional acceptance of the Medicaid program, [190] the memorandum presented PSROs as capable of helping state agencies in three ways.

> 8. Relieving the State of the cost of utilization review activites.
> 9. Relieving the State of responsibility of meeting HEW requirements for utilization review.
> 10. Relieving the State of administrative responsibility for conducting utilization review. [191]

The new utilization review regulations do not indicate a clear intent to use PSROs to relieve states of their mandated utilization control responsibilities, but the regulations *are* silent on the issue. The memorandum listed 13 activites under "How State Medicaid Agencies Can Help PSROs." Three of them were informational activities: (1) inform physicians of the intricacies of Medicaid; (2) respond to PSRO requests for advice; and (3) include PSRO representatives in planning for information system in the Medicaid agency. [192] All of the other activities actually represent attempts to ensure that state agencies' interests be adequately represented in the PSRO system. These include, for example, assuring that PSRO contracts emphasize cost containment, providing PSROs with Medicaid agency data, continuing to perform utilization review during a PSRO's conditional phase and in those areas not served by a PSRO, communicating with Medicare intermediaries and carriers on the PSRO's proficiency, monitoring PSROs; serving on Statewide PSR Councils, and urging PSROs to expand their review to all levels of care. [193]

The above-mentioned activities can influence the activities of PSROs to reflect the interests of state Medicaid agencies. But they must also be regarded in light of the fact that, after 1976, a state Medicaid agency can serve as a PSRO. [194] If it intends to seek such a designation, its activities relating to PSROs may reflect that motivation. Monitoring PSROs is in the interests of a state agency which does agree to accept PSRO authority. If it is to be held responsible for the state money it administers, it will need to watch the process by which some of it is allocated. But if in its monitoring the state Medicaid agency discovers lax PSRO review, that failure would no doubt be communicated to the Secretary for consideration as possible grounds for terminating the PSRO's contract; and showing the PSRO's inefficiency would pave the way for designation of the state agency itself to serve as a PSRO. [195]

Other suggested state agency activities vis-a-vis PSROs reflect the countervailing tensions between the two entities. Where a state agency tentatively accepts PSROs, service on Statewide PSR Councils assures direct input of state agency views. On the other hand, because state Medicaid agencies are charged with the responsibility to review all Medicaid services, in much the same way that PSROs have an incentive to delegate review to hospitals state agencies have an incentive to see that PSROs assume most of the responsibilities for review, especially review of long term care, which comprises a substantial portion of Medicaid expenditures. That many agencies have undertaken a vast reorganization of their data collection systems (with federal financial incentives to do so) [196] may predispose them to seek to control PSRO data activities, at least by supplying them with much of their data needs. [197]

Another unclear aspect of the PSRO-agency relationship is the effect of a PSRO's determinations during its conditional phase. The statute implies that PSRO determinations of issues for which the Secretary has given approval are to be binding even during the conditional period. [198] But any duties not performed by a PSRO will be performed as under the previous systems. [199] The state Medicaid agency is given at least residual power, which can be transmuted into preeminence through an agency's overruling those PSRO determinations it considers incorrect. One approach which has been considered would have the state agency enter into an agreement with the PSRO to conduct review as the state agency's agent. [200] This technique attempts to create a legal fiction giving the state agency a basis on which to accept PSRO authority. However, if state law, in fact, holds the state agency primarily responsible for expenditure of money (and federal law clearly requires the state to assure utilization review compliance), the proposed contract would not absolve the state of that responsibility.

The PSRO statute requires that a PSRO not be given full review responsibility unless it demonstrates a "capacity for improved review effort." [201] Any state agency seeking to prevent the Secretary's awarding the PSRO designation to another entity, or a state agency seeking a designation for itself, would need only maintain a better system than the PSRO could offer.

Other issues, including federal support for agency costs in administering utilization review or activities in connection with PSRO operations, will no doubt contribute to tensions in agency-PSRO relationships. The need for further study of these problems has been recognized in the consideration by the Social and Rehabilitation Service, which administers Medicaid on the federal level, of funding experiments to study potential solutions. Some of the areas of study would include assessment of state utilization control programs, definition of state Medicaid agency relations with PSROs, and possible development of minimum standards on the frequency and extent of utilization review by in-house committees. [202]

In the last analysis, the issues may be resolved through bureaucratic politics rather than academic study. If the Medicaid state agencies, represented in the federal bureauacracy through SRS, set out to thwart PSROs by encouraging state challenges to them, PSROs may not survive the pressure. The incentive to SRS to support such challenges stems from the federal agency's own vested interest in the maintenance of a functional bureaucracy with substantial responsibilities for it to administer. If federal agencies seeking the deominance of PSROs for similar reasons can, with the support of the Senate Finance Committee, resist such pressure, PSROs may ultimately supercede state Medicaid agencies.

Notes for Chapter Three

1. §1861(k)(1) of the Social Security Act; 42 USC §1395x(k)(1)
2. 20 CFR §405.1035(b)(2) (changed 1974). Because these regulations have in part been changed, in this chapter citations to the Federal Register will be given for the new regulations; old regulations which remain unchanged will be cited to the Code of Federal Regulations (CFR); and old regulations which have been changed will be cited to the CFR with the added notation "(changed 1974)."
3. Blue Cross of Philadelphia requires utilization review in its provider contracts for private patients. *Hospital Agreement with Delaware Valley Hospital Council*, July 1, 1971, at §11.2. Section 11.1.1 requires the presence of one nonphysician member of the hospital governing board on the utilization review committee. But see this chapter at xx *infra* for a discussion of incentives to utilization review committees to exclude consumers.
4. §1155(e)(1); 42 USC §1320c–4(e)(1).

5. "Because there are significant divergences in opinion among individual physicians in respect to evaluation of medical necessity for inpatient hospital services the judgment of the attending physician in an extended case is given great weight, and is not rejected except under unusual circumstances." 20 CFR §405.1035(g) (changed 1974).
6. See Chapter Five, n. 83 at 164 *infra*.
7. §§1879, 1158; 42 USC §§1395pp, 1320c-7. See this chapter at 87 *infra*. There are two separate provisions one for Medicare alone; the other as part of the PSRO law applies to Medicare and Medicaid patients. Regulations under Medicare have been issued. 40 FR 1022, January 6, 1975. Because the Medicare provision is more restrictive, it is unlikely the PSRO regulations will use identical procedures.
8. 20 CFR §405.195(a) (40 FR 1023, January 6, 1975). These regulations apply to the Medicare provision, but the effectiveness of institutional review will undoubtedly be part of the PSRO regulations.
9. Part A Intermediary Letter, No. 73–30, III A.1 at 4.
10. 45 CFR §250.20(a) (39 FR 41617, November 29, 1974).
11. *Sen. Fin. Comm. Rpt.* at 255.
12. §1151; 42 USC §1320c. *Sen. Fin. Comm. Rpt.* at 262.
13. §1155(g); 42 USC §1320c-4(g). *Sen. Fin. Comm. Rpt.* at 264.
14. §1156; 42 USC §1320c-5.
15. §1152; 42 USC §1320c-1.
16. See Chapter Seven.
17. Chapter Four fully examines the failures of these paying agents and their roles in the PSRO system.
18. *Sen. Fin. Comm. Rpt.* at 255.
19. Quoted in *Medicare and Medicaid Problems Issues and Alternatives* Report of the Staff to the Committee on Finance, U.S. Sen. (91st Cong., 1st sess. February 9, 1970), at 107. [hereinafter cited as *Medicare and Medicaid 1970*].
20. *Id.* at 108.
21. *Id.* at 106. The inadequate regulations referred to by the report involve conflict of interest and "cronyism" problems (refusal to discipline colleagues) primarily. The staff contended that regulations on the use of outside committees in smaller institutions and extended care facilities were not sufficiently specific to preclude conflicts of interest on financial grounds. *Id.*
22. *Sen. Fin. Comm. Rpt.* at 256.
23. Under the Hill-Burton hospital construction program (42 USC §291) nonprofit hospitals receiving direct grants for construction are required to render a certain amount of "uncompensated services" to poor people. Auditing and accounting phenomena like those described have been used to evade the law's free service requirement. See Rose, "The Hill-Burton Act—The Interim Regulation and Service to the Poor: A Study in Public Interest Litigation," 7 *Clearinghouse Rev.* 145 (July 1973); Schwartz, "Expanding the Quantity of Medical Services Available to the Poor," 7 *Clearinghouse Rev.* 587

(February 1974); Schwartz and Rose, "Opening the Doors of the Non-profit Hospital to the Poor," 7 *Clearinghouse Rev.* 655 (March 1974).

24. §1155 generally; 42 USC §1320c–4.
25. §1155(e)(1); 42 USC §1320c–4(e)(1).
26. *Id.*
27. §1155(e)(2); 42 USC.§1320c–4(e)(2).
28. §1155(e)(1); 42 USC §1320c–4(e)(1).
29. *Sen. Fin. Comm. Rpt.* at 263.
30. Technically, the statute designates the relationship between the PSRO and the committee as one of "approval" rather than "delegation." Although practically speaking the results may be the same under either label, the distinction may be relevant in arguments about whether the PSRO's activities constitute "state action." State action has been used as a prerequisite to establishment of special procedural hearing rights for consumers. See Chapter Five, n. 113 at 170 *infra*.
31. *Sen. Fin. Comm. Rpt.* at 262. This requirement is important to gaining utilization review committee cooperation with PSROs. See this chapter at 86 *infra*. The requirement is also critical to the enforcement process. See Chapter Seven at 245 *infra*.
32. *Sen. Fin. Comm. Rpt.* at 262.
33. The Senate Finance Committee has expressed concern that PSROs act "professionally."

> Objective and impartial review must be provided by a PSRO if it is to be effective and respected. Malice, vendettas, or other arbitrary and discriminatory practices or policies are by definition "non-professional," and in the unlikely event of such occurrences the Secretary is expected to promptly act to terminate the contract with the organization involved unless it immediately undertakes voluntary corrective measures.

> *Sen. Fin. Comm. Rpt.* at 267. The discussion related to application of sanctions by PSROs generally. See also Chapter Four at 120 *infra;* and Chapter Seven at 248 *infra*.

34. *Sen. Fin. Comm. Rpt.* at 262.
35. *Program Manual*, Chapter IV, §405.34(c) at 6, and Chapter V, §505.74(c) at 6.
36. In addition, both types of organizations, planning and conditional, are to assess in their area "the current quality assessment assurance and utilization review activities in each short stay hospital, and the willingness of each such hospital to perform review activities in conformance with PSRO guidelines and regulations." *Id.* Chapter V, §505.71(c) at 5.
37. (Emphasis added.) *PSRO Transmittal No. 11* HEW (Washington, D.C.: Bureau of Quality Assurance, November 26, 1974), at 4, c, 8, [hereinafter cited as *PSRO Transmittal* No. 11].

38. *Program Manual*, Chapter VII, §701 at 3.
39. *Id.* Chapter VII, §720.01 at 22.
40. *Sen. Fin. Comm. Rpt.* at 262.
41. *Program Manual,* Chapter VII, §710.2 at 21.
42. *Id.* Chapter VII, §705.11 at 5.
43. *Id.* Chapter VII, §705.21 at 10.
44. *Id.* Chapter VII, §705.31 at 13.
45. *Id.* Chapter VII, §710.22 at 21.
46. *Id.* Chapter VII, §710.23 at 21. Hospital review need not be performed exclusively by the body designated the "utilization review committee." Another committee or several committees may be approved as long as their review is effective. *Id.* Chapter VII, §720.03 at 22.
47. §1156(d)(1)(A); 42 USC §1320c–5(d)(1)(A).
48. §1156(d)(1)(B); 42 USC §1320c–5(d)(1)(B).
49. §1156(d)(2); 42 USC §1320c–5(d)(2). The 50th percentile represents that point in time at which 50 percent of similar patients with similar conditions will have been discharged. For example, if, out of a population of 100 patients having had appendectomies, 10 stay for three days, 35 stay for four days, 15 stay for five days, 30 stay for six days, and 10 stay for seven days, the 50th percentile is the fifth day because the 50th person was discharged by that date.
50. §§1861(e)(6),(j)(8), and (k); 42 USC §§1395x(e)(6), (j)(8), and (k) set forth the basic requirements for a utilization review plan as a condition of participation. 20 CFR §405.1035 established the finer details of the program.
51. §1902(a)(30); 42 USC §1396a(a)(30); 45 CFR §250.20.
52. 45 CFR §250.20(a)(1).
53. *Id.*
54. §§207, 237, P.L. 92–603.
55. §1903(i)(4); 42 USC §1396b(i)(4).
56. §§1903(i)(4), 1861(k); 42 USC §§1396b(i)(4), 1395x(k).
57. *Sen. Fin. Comm. Rpt.* at 246.
58. See 39 FR 41605 and 41610, November 29, 1974.
59. 39 FR 41610, November 29, 1974.
60. 20 CFR §405.1035(a) (39 FR 41605, November 29, 1974).
61. 20 CFR §405.1035(b) (39 FR 41605, November 29, 1974).
62. 20 CFR §405.1035(d) (39 FR 41605, November 29, 1974).
63. *Id.*
64. 20 CFR §405.1035(e) (39 FR 41605, November 29, 1974).
65. 20 CFR §405.1035(e)(3) (39 FR 41605, November 29, 1974).
66. Before the new regulations, only exclusions from review based on financial conflicts of interest were specified; and they could be overcome if there was no one else available to perform review. 20 CFR §405.1035(e)(2)(iii) (changed 1974).
67. 20 CFR §405.1035(c) (39 FR 41605, November 29, 1974).
68. The question of confidentiality of patient records may be raised when nonprofessionals participate in review. Deleting reference to patient identity can successfully answer the question.

69. See n. 5 *supra.*
70. 20 CFR §405.1035(e)(4) (39 FR 41605, November 29, 1974).
71. *Id.* at 39 FR 41606, November 29, 1974.
72. See Chapter Two at 35 *supra.*
73. 20 CFR §405.1035(e)(6)(ii) (39 FR 41606, November 29, 1974). This provision was the subject of intense pressure from hospitals. They asserted they could not meet the implementation deadline. On March 25, 1975, Secretary Weinberger extended the implementation deadline to July 1, 1975. With the extension, Secretary Weinberger announced that HEW would use the time until the deadline to "work out special problems that may be faced in small rural hospitals." *HEW News Release*, March 25, 1975. See also 40 FR 14591, 14597 (April 1, 1975).
74. 20 CFR §405.1035(f) (39 FR 41606, November 29, 1974).
75. 20 CFR §405.1035(f)(2) (39 FR 41606, November 29, 1974).
76. 20 CFR §405.1035(f)(1) (39 FR 41606, November 29, 1974).
77. 20 CFR §405.1035(f)(6) (39 FR 41606, November 29, 1974).
78. See Chapter Two at 38 *supra.* In psychiatric hospitals, the initial period may not extend beyond 30 days. 20 CFR §405.1035(f)(6) (39 FR 41606, November 29, 1974).
79. 20 CFR §405.1035(f)(7) (39 FR 41606, November 29, 1974).
80. 20 CFR §405.1035(g) (39 FR 41607, November 29, 1974).
81. See Chapter Two, at 38 *supra.*
82. 20 CFR §405.1035(g) (39 FR 41607, November 29, 1974).
83. 20 CFR §405.1035(j) (39 FR 41607, November 29, 1974).
84. *Id.*
85. *Id.*
86. *Id.*
87. 20 CFR §405.1035(f)(3) (39 FR 41606, November 29, 1974).
88. 20 CFR §405.1035(k) (39 FR 41607, November 29, 1974).
89. 45 CFR §250.18 (39 FR 41611, November 29, 1974).
90. §1903(g); 42 USC §1396b(g); 45 CFR §250.20(c) (39 FR 41617, November 29, 1974).
91. 45 CFR §250.18(a)(1)(i) (39 FR 41611, November 29, 1974).
92. 45 CFR §350.18(a)(1)(ii) (39 FR 41611. November 29, 1974).
93. (Emphasis added.) *Id.*
94. 45 CFR §250.19(a)(1) (39 FR 41612, November 29, 1974).
95. *Id.*
96. 45 CFR §§250.19(a)(1)(viii)(E), (x)(G) (39 FR 41613, November 29, 1974). Further requirements are provided specifically for inpatient mental hospitals although they also perform the three basic types of review. 45 CFR §250.19(a)(2) (39 FR 41614, November 29, 1974).
97. §1861(j)(8); 42 USC §1395x(j)(8). For a discussion of some of the general problems in reviewing nursing home care see *Developments in Aging 1973 and January–March 1974,* Report of the Special Committee on Aging, U.S. Sen., Pursuant to S. Res. 51. (Rpt. No. 93–846) (93d Cong., 2d sess.) at 37–79.
98. 20 CFR §405.1137 (39 FR 41607, November 29, 1974).

99. *Id.*
100. §1155(a)(1)(C); 42 USC §1320c–4(a)(1)(C).
101. §1155(a)(1)(B); 42 USC §1320c–4(a)(1)(B).
102. 20 CFR §405.1137(d) (39 FR 41607, November 29, 1974).
103. 20 CFR §405.1137(d)(2) (39 FR 41607, November 29, 1974).
104. *Id.*
105. 20 CFR §405.1137(d)(3) (39 FR 41608, November 29, 1974).
106. 20 CFR §405.1137(e) (39 FR 41608, November 29, 1974).
107. 20 CFR §405.1137(i) (39 FR 41608, November 29, 1974).
108. 45 CFR §250.19(a)(3) (39 FR 41615, November 29, 1974).
109. 45 CFR §250.18(a)(1)(iv) (39 FR 41611, November 29, 1974).
110. 45 CFR §250.18(a)(1)(iv)(A) (39 FR 41611, November 29, 1974).
111. 45 CFR §250.18(a)(1)(iv)(B) (39 FR 41611, November 29, 1974).
112. 45 CFR §250.18(a)(2) (39 FR 41612, November 29, 1974).
113. (Emphasis added.) 45 CFR §250.18(a)(4) (39 FR 41612, November 29, 1974).
114. 45 CFR §250.23.
115. 45 CFR §250.19(a)(4) (39 FR 41616, November 29, 1974).
116. 45 CFR §250.19(a)(4)(vi) (39 FR 41616, November 28, 1974).
117. 45 CFR §250.19(b) (39 FR 41617, November 29, 1974). When the Secretary extended the deadline for implementation of utilization review to July 1, 1978, (see n. 73, *supra*) the regulations said the new date would apply wherever February 1, 1975 had previously appeared. Waivers, then, will be evaluated after that date. See 40 FR 14597 (April 1, 1975).
118. *PSRO Letter* (no. 11), January 15, 1974, at 8.
119. *PSRO Letter* (no. 12), February 1, 1974, at 4.
120. *PSRO Transmittal No. 11* at 5.
121. *Id.* The *Transmittal* further emphasizes,

> Retrospective medical audit systems such as those of the Quality Assurance Program (QAP) of the American Hospital Association (AHA), the Trustee-Administrator-Physicians (TAP) Manual of the Joint Commission on Accreditation of Hospitals (JCAH), and the Medical Audit Study Method of the Commission on Professional and Hospital Activities (CPHA) meet the retrospective medical care evaluation study requirements.

> *Id.*

122. *Id.*; and *Program Manual,* Chapter VII, §710.3 at 21.
123. See "Interpreting PSRO 'norms of care'—cookbook medicine or textbook medicine?" *American Medical News,* May 20, 1974, at 19.
124. See 20 CFR §405.1035(g) (changed 1974).
125. *PSRO Transmittal No. 11* at 6.
126. 45 CFR §250.19(a)(xi)(A) (39 FR 41611, November 29, 1974); 20 CFR §405.1035(j) (39 FR 41607), November 29, 1974.
127. *PSRO Transmittal No. 11* at 6.

128. *Id.*
129. *Id.*; and *Program Manual,* Chapter V, §520.04(1) at 11.
130. *PSRO Transmittal No. 11* at 6.
131. Although the PSRO system is based on development of norms by PSROs, initially there was some support for the idea that norms emanate from hospitals. *PSRO Letter* (no. 15), March 15, 1974, at 3.
132. *Program Manual,* Chapter VII, §702.21 at 24; and *PSRO Transmittal No. 11* at 7.
133. *Id.* at 8. Included among these other review committees are (1) tissue committees which evaluate whether there was need for surgery based on comparison of a pathologist's findings about the specimen which was removed from the patient with the reason the surgeon operated. If the specimen proves to be normal the tissue committee might conclude there was no need for surgery; (2) medical audit committees which evaluate the treatment given against a list of recommended or required procedures appropriate to the patient's diagnosis or condition; (3) other review programs established under the auspices of other organizations. See n. 121 *supra.* For a summary of these types of programs and their roles in the PSRO system, see Farrell, "PSROs and Internal Hospital Review," *Hospital Progress,* October 1973, at 64; and "An Overview of Existing Quality Review Systems and Programs," 44 *Medical Record News* 40 (April 1973).
134. *Program Manual,* Chapter VII, §720.2 at 24; *PSRO Transmittal No. 11* at 8.
135. Step 1: Initial Assessment of Hospital; Step 2: Initial Expression of Interest by Hospital; Step 3: Joint Development of a Review Plan; Step 4: Approval by the PSRO; Step 5: Implementation of the Plan. *Program Manual,* Chapter VII, §720 at 24–26.
136. Step 1: PSRO Written Communication to Hospital; Step 2: The Hospital's Expression of Interest; Step 3: PSRO Initial Assessment of the Hospital's Capability for Review; Step 4: Hospital Development of a Review Plan with PSRO Technical Support; Step 5: PSRO Determinations of Review Functions, if any, to be Delegated; Step 6: Written Memorandum of Understanding Between the PSRO and Hospital; Step 7: Implementation of the Hospital's Review Plan; Step 8: PSRO Periodic Reassessment and On-site Inspection of the Hospital's Review Plan. *PSRO Transmittal No. 11* at 5–11.
137. In early considerations, those provisions were criticized by the Bureau of Quality Assurance. "The discussion of in-house review capacity provides for the development of new *written* UR plans by PSRO's in collaboration with *each* individual hospital—despite the fact that *written* UR plans have been in existence since the inception of Medicare. (As you know, the *written* plan never has and is not now the real problem,)" BQA Memorandum quoted in *PSRO Letter* (no. 16), April 1, 1974 at 6.
138. *Program Manual,* Chapter VII, §720.61 at 26.
139. *Sen. Fin. Comm. Rpt.* at 264.

140. *Id.*
141. See Chapter Seven at 248 *infra.*
142. Senator Bennett consistently emphasized the possibility of something less acceptable to physicians if this program fails. "Make no mistake, the direction of the House passed social security bill is toward more—not less—review for the need for and quality of health care." Speech of Senator Bennett, 116 *Cong. Rec.* S22475, July 1,1970.

> I sincerely believe that the amendment I now send to the desk represents the best and perhaps the last opportunity to safeguard the public's concern with respect to the cost and quality of medical care, while, at the same time, leaving the actual control of medical practice in the hands of those best qualified—American physicians.

> Speech of Senator Bennett, 118 *Cong. Rec.* S420, January 25, 1972. See also "Stop kidding yourself about PSRO," interview with Senator Bennett, *Medical Economics*, September 16, 1974 at 29.

143. One report indicates that by January 1974, 1100 hospitals were developing such programs. McMahon, "PSROs . . . implications for hospitals," 48 *Hospitals, JAHA* 55, January 1, 1974.
144. §1155(c); 42 USC §1320c–4(c).
145. *Id.*
146. *Program Manual,* Chapter VII, §720.09 at 23.
147. 20 CFR §405.1035(b)(3).
148. §1158(b); 42 USC §1320c–7(b).
149. §1155(e)(1); 42 USC §1320c–4(e)(1).
150. *PSRO Transmittal No. 11* at 11.
151. The PSRO "shall utilize the services of and accept the findings of" an approved committee. §1155(e)(1); 42 USC §1320c–4(e)(1).
152. *PSRO Transmittal No. 11* at 11.
153. §1155(a)(4); 42 USC §1320c–4(a)(4).
154. *Program Manual,* Chapter VII, §720.71 at 27–31.
155. *Id.* at §720.80A2 at 29, B2 at 30, C2 at 31.
156. Under the Social Security Amendments of 1972, Medicare and Medicaid can now reimburse for services provided by these organizations. §226, P.L. 92–603, §§1833, 1876, 1903(k) of the Social Security Act; 42 USC §§13951, 1395mm, 1396(k).
157. *Sen. Fin. Comm. Rpt.* at 262.
158. For an analytical summary of their characteristics and functions, see Klarman, "Analysis of the HMO Proposal—Its Assumptions, Implications and Prospects" in *Health Maintenance Organizations: A Reconfiguration of the Health Services System* (Proceedings of the Graduate Program in Hospital Administration and Center for Health administration Studies, Graduate School of Business, University of Chicago, 1971), at 24–38. Other wide-ranging studies of them are Donabedian, "An Evaluation of Prepaid Group Practice," VI *Inquiry* 3 (September 1969); and "Note—The Role of Prepaid Group

Practice in Relieving the Medical Care Crisis," 84 *Harv. L. Rev.* 887 (1971).

159. Obviously these tendencies are tempered by the populations enrolled. In other words, if poor people and old people utilize more services than the general population, gaining more poor and old subscribers would mean that more of the capitation fees would go toward costs of delivery, other than physician payment. Theoretically there would be no financial advantage to increased Medicare and Medicaid enrollments without a simultaneous decrease in the services provided.

160. (Emphasis added.) *Advancing the Quality of Health Care* (Washington, D.C.: Institute of Medicine, National Academy of Sciences, August 1974), at 45.

161. See n. 158 *supra*; Drucker, "Progress Report on the Utilization of Medical Care Services by Project Enrollees from February 1971 through February 1972" (Report to Seattle Community Health Board, March 20, 1973), in Arthur Young, *An Annotated Bibliography of HMO Utilization by Title XIX Recipients* (DHEW-HSA, August 1973), at 41–46; and Klarman, "Effect of Prepaid Group Practice on Hospital Use," 78 *Public Health Reports* 955 (November 1963).

162. *Id.* at 27. Klarman has found HMO hospitalization rates about 20 percent lower than the general population.

163. *Id.* at 29.

164. Donabedian, *supra* n. 158, at 16.

165. *Id.* The San Joaquin and Sacramento Medical Foundations cited in the Senate Finance Committee Report (at 264) have well-established review mechanisms. In fact, the experiences of foundations for medical care were among the primary models for PSROs. See *PSRO Oversight Hearings* at 119.

166. Fifer, "Point of View, Cost Containment and Quality Assurance: An Adversary Relationship," 1 *Health Services Information* 5 (December 2, 1974).

167. Chapter Two at 48 *supra.*

168. For a statement of the elements considered in setting capitation rates, see Van Steenwyck, "Actuarial Determination of Capitation Rates by Health Maintenance Organizations" (Health Services Division, Martin E. Segal Co., 730 Fifth Ave., New York 10019), September 1973.

169. Fifer, *supra*, n. 166.

170. Testimony of Clark C. Havighurst, Professor of Law, Duke University, *Hearings Before the Subcommittee on Antitrust and Monopoly of the Committee on the Judiciary*, U.S. Sen., "Competition in the Health Services Market" (93d Cong., 2d sess., May 17, 1974) at 1085.

171. *Id.*

172. *Id.*

173. *Id.* But see, "AMA Says it is Willing to Give HMOs a Trial" 8 *Internal Medicine News* 4 (January 15, 1975). In a recent study of

physicians' attitudes toward national health insurance, when asked "Would you prefer a plan that would support the development of prepaid group practice, where the patient gets complete care for a flat sum in advance . . .?" 33 percent said they supported prepaid group practice and 61 percent said they did not support it. In the same study it was found that 24 percent of AMA leaders supported a plan with prepaid group practice, 32 percent of their members supported prepaid group practice, but 58 percent of nonmembers would support a national health insurance plan which supported the development of prepaid group practice. See Colombotos, Kirchner and Millman, "Physicians View National Health Insurance, A National Study" (A preliminary report of findings presented to the Health Staff Seminar, Washington, D.C., September 23, 1974; available from Colombotos, Columbia University School of Public Health, Division of Sociomedical Sciences). The obvious implication is that organized medicine does not speak for all physicians. See Chapter Seven at 241 *infra.*

174. Existing medical organizations such as the San Joaquin and Sacramento Medical Foundations in California, and others have developed patient and practitioner profile forms and approval certification and other review methods which may provide the bases for development of uniform data gathering and review procedures capable of being employed in many areas of the Nation.

    Sen. Fin. Comm. Rpt. at 264.

175. "The PSRO would not be involved with questions concerning the reasonableness of charges or costs or methods of payment . . . ." *Sen. Fin. Comm. Rpt.* at 261.

176. See "Prepaid plans' costs exceed fee-for-service, GAO Reports," *American Medical News,* October 14, 1974, at 11; and "PHP savings unproved report says," *American Medical News,* November 4, 1974, at 3.

177. Havighurst, *supra* n. 170.

178. *Id.* at 1086.

179. Still, the possibility of reimbursement based on costs incurred seems to be contemplated by proposed regulations on Medicaid reimbursement to HMOs. 39 FR 20042, June 5, 1974. As proposed, 45 CFR §249.82(c)(2)(iii) would permit reimbursement on a prepaid basis to "at risk" HMOs and on a retrospective basis to "at cost" HMOs. These provisions are not expected to be changed in the final regulations.

180. §1902(a)(3); 42 USC §1396a(a)(30).

181. The state will lose part of the federal share of the program. §207, P.L. 92–603; §1903(g) of the Social Security Act; 42 USC §1396b(g).

182. Part A—hospital services are paid for by the Federal Hospital Insurance Trust Fund. §1817; 42 USC §1395i. Part B—physicians' services are paid for out of the Federal Supplementary Medical Insurance Trust Fund. §1841; 42 USC §1395t.

183. The formula for federal financial participation is complex. See §§1903 (a), 1905(b); 42 USC §1396b(a), 1396d(b).
184. Medical Services Administration (HEW) issues paper, "Medicaid—PSRO Issues and Problems," Winter 1973.
185. "In addition to the requirements imposed by law as a condition of approval of a state plan approved under any title [of the Social Security Act] under which services are paid for in whole or in part, with Federal funds, there is hereby imposed the requirement that provisions [of the PSRO law] shall apply to the operation of such plan or program." §1164(a); 42 USC §1320c–13(a).
187. §1904; 42 USC §1396c.
188. It is interesting to review which of the 1972 Amendments to the Social Security Act created many of the complexities of these interactions. Some of the sections relevant to utilization review include the following (citations are to P.L. 92–603, followed by the Social Security Act, and then the United States Code):

    —§207;§1903(g), (h); 42 USC §1396b(g), (h); part of the Secretary's authority to ensure that state utilization review procedures are effective includes sample on-site surveys of private and public institutions serving Medicaid patients.
    —§237(a); §1903(i)(4); 42 USC §1396b(i)(4); unifies the Medicare and Medicaid requirements by making the Medicaid institutional utilization review requirements conform to Medicare committees.
    —§239(b); §1902(a)(33); 42 USC §1396a(a)(33); requires the state agency to use "appropriate professional personnel" to review appropriateness and quality of care under a state plan; and that the state agency which is appointed to certify institutions for Medicare may perform the same functions under Medicaid. See §1864(a); 42 USC §1395aa(a).
    —§247(a), (b); §1814(a)(2)(C), 1905(f); 42 USC §1395f(a)(2)(C), 1396d(f); establishes uniform criteria for skilled nursing care.
    —§278, amends 38 separate sections of the Social Security Act, eliminating two separate designations of long term care institutions—"extended care facility" and "skilled nursing home"—for the single label "skilled nursing facility."

189. *Information Memorandum,* MSA–IM–73–14, June 1, 1973.
190. *Id.* at 3.
191. *Id.*
192. *Id.*
193. *Id.*
194. §1155(b)(1)(B), (C); 42 USC §1320c–4(b)(1)(B), (C).
195. The issues discussed in the text which follows are issues noted by the Medical Services Administration (MSA) in its issues paper "Medicaid—PSRO Issues and Problems," *supra* n. 184.
196. See Chapter Six, n. 53, at 214 *infra.*

197. The Surveillance and Utilization Review Subsystem of the Medicaid Management Information System (MMIS) will develop information specifically and directly relevant to utilization review activities. "Medicaid—PSRO Issues and Problems," *supra* n. 184 at 3b.
198. §1154(a); 42 USC §1320c–3(a).
199. §1154(b); 42 USC §1320c–3(b).
200. "Medicaid—PSRO Issues and Problems," *supra* n. 184, at 4b(1).
201. §1153; 42 USC §1320c–2.
202. *PSRO Letter* (no. 34), January 1, 1975, at 6.

Chapter Four

PSROs and Paying Agents

Under the old review requirements, while utilization review committees made determinations of medical necessity of services, paying agents for Medicare and Medicaid administered fiscal review. They determined the amount, reasonableness, and appropriateness of payments for medical services. Not only had these organizations (described more fully below) usurped the role of utilization review committees by second-guessing medical determinations, but, as this chapter will demonstrate, they also did not perform their statutory duties or their usurped responsibilities properly. Dissatisfaction with the failure of payment claims review was one of the principal motivations for the creation of PSROs.[1] As a result of congressional dissatisfaction with their performances, the roles of these institutions in review of Medicare and Medicaid services have been drastically reduced, although paying agents will still operate within the PSRO structure.

Under the PSRO statute, no payment may be made for medical care rendered to Medicare and Medicaid beneficiaries where a PSRO has disapproved the provision of services.[2] But the determinations of the actual amount of payment to be made will continue to be the jurisdiction of state agencies and other designated organizations referred to here collectively as paying agents. The significance of the role of paying agents in the PSRO system is twofold: (1) to be effective PSROs must overcome the demonstrated failures of paying agents; and (2) in determinations of medical necessity and therefore allowable costs, the PSRO system as a whole must be responsive to the Medicare or Medicaid patient's interests. The Senate Finance Committee recognized the basic tensions in the PSRO system when it stated that the government's responsibility for review is "to the millions of persons dependent upon medicare and medicaid, to the taxpayers who bear the burden of billions of dollars in annual program costs, and to the health care system."[3]

The consumers of the PSRO program—the patients to whom the Finance Committee referred—are primarily concerned with receiving high quality medical care and having the costs of services paid without inconvenience. In evaluating the roles of paying agents in the PSRO system, it is important to note that the consumer's interests cannot be adequately served unless his medical care is reviewed by an organization which: (1) is professionally competent to make accurate and consistent medical review judgements; (2) employs a method of review which is timely and least inconveniences patients; (3) places a priority in its review on the quality of care received; (4) harbors no interests conflicting with the patient's which could unfairly influence its decisions; and (5) operates within a system which selects capable participants to perform those tasks and ensures their proper performance. The previous review system, and paying agents' performances within it, have been deficient in each of these areas. This chapter examines the vulnerability of PSROs to these deficiencies, and elucidates how the PSRO system was designed to overcome them. Second, the discussion sets forth the functions and roles of paying agents under the new structure, to the degree that PSROs do not replace them in the review of medical care.[4] Basically, PSROs will not replace the fiscal administration functions which paying agents have performed,[5] including the processing of claims for payment. On the contrary, the data handling capabilities which paying agents have already developed will in many instances be utilized by PSROs in applying norms, developing profiles, and judging the ability of providers to perform case by case review.[6]

In order to better understand the changes to paying agents presented by the PSRO structure, a brief description of the duties of paying agents is necessary. The paying agents for each of the Medicare and Medicaid programs have different titles: "fiscal intermediaries," for Part A of Medicare (the hospital insurance program); "carriers," for part B of Medicare (supplementary medical insurance); and "fiscal agents," for Medicaid.

Under Part A of Medicare, reimbursements for in-patient hospital services, post–hospital extended care services, and post–hospital home health services[7] are made by fiscal intermediaries that are designated by providers.[8] Pursuant to a contract with the Social Security Administration (SSA), fiscal intermediaries are to "assist the providers [i.e., institutional utilization review committies] . . . in the application of safeguards against unnecessary utilization of services."[9] In actual practice, it is the fiscal intermediaries themselves which determine whether the care rendered to a Medicare patient was medically necessary or constituted a noncovered level of care.

Under Part B of Medicare, payments for physicians' services, drugs, out-patient hospital services, and home health services,[10] are made by carriers designated by the Secretary.[11] Carriers, like fiscal intermediaries, enter into a contract with HEW.[12] But, unlike fiscal intermediaries, carriers are charged, under the terms of their contracts, with the responsibility for reviewing medical care. Regulations stipulate further that they institute utilization safeguards to assure the medical necessity of services for which payments are made[13] and, in other ways, assist providers in their utilization review activities.[14]

Payments for services offered under a Medicaid plan may be made by the state agency administering the plan or by a fiscal agent under contract to the state.[15] State agencies administering Medicaid plans must seek to ensure that utilization control is implemented for all services offered under the plan.[16] Under the old system, to reduce the cost of administering the plan, state agency utilization review functions could be delegated to Medicare "fiscal intermediaries" or "carriers."[17] Since Medicare carriers and intermediaries are also the "fiscal agents" in many states, the same organization often performs both claims processing and utilization review functions. Initially, it was intended that fiscal intermediaries not review the coverage or medical necessity of services provided under Part A of Medicare. The statutory language calls only for their assisting providers in the application of utilization safeguards. It was intended that the determinations of utilization review committees would be final and unreviewable.[18] The system did not perform as intended.[19] Studies by the Social Security Administration (SSA) in 1968 and by the staff of the Senate Finance Committee in 1970[20] found that utilization review was not being performed in many instances. In lieu of salvaging the system as designed, through enforcement, HEW authorized fiscal intermediaries to review retroactively the care received by Medicare patients and, when appropriate, to deny payment for unnecessary medical care.[21] With this administrative change, the utilization review committee's decisions were not even required to be given primary weight in retrospective review.[22] The grounds for denying claims were either that the service was not medically necessary or constituted custodial care.[23] Although in the establishment of PSROs the failures of paying agents primarily in reviewing claims for payment to control costs were cited, these fiscal agencies were responsible for a panoply of professionally related activities.

> While the major responsibility of intermediaries and carriers involves the prompt determination and payment of benefit amounts, the other functions performed by these organizations are of considerable importance. Both carriers and intermediaries are responsible for the full range of professional relations activities: i.e., continuing an effective liaison with medical societies, provider medical staffs, utilization review committees, and individual physicians. Carriers are heavily involved in the review and investigation of potentially fraudulent claims, in the operation of an appeals process for beneficiaries dissatisfied with decisions on claims, and in the coordination of certain program activities with State agencies .... In addition, the carriers' beneficiary services section furnishes information to beneficiaries about the program and serves, on the local level, as the focal point for coordination with Social Security Administration (SSA) district and regional offices.[24]

Considering the emphasis on professional and public relations in the duties with which they were charged, it is significant that the organizations serving as paying agents have been drawn primarily from the health insurance industry. Blue Cross and Blue Shield have been the primary participants.[25] Approximately 95 percent of the hospitals providing short term care nominated the Blue Cross Association as their intermediary and are served under subcontracts by local Blue Cross plans,[26] and they serve similarly more than one-half of participating skilled nursing homes.[27] Of the 47 Part B carriers, 32 are Blue Shield plans, 13 are commercial (for-profit organizations), and there are two other organizations serving as carriers.[28] As of spring 1974, Blue Cross and Blue Shield plans were also the fiscal agents for 22 state Medicaid plans.[29]

The failures of paying agents, like those of the utilization review system generally before PSROs, were both inherent in the design of the system and compounded by poor performance. The next section examines each of the oversights and derelictions, and explicates the role of PSROs with regard to the same responsibilities.

PRIOR PROBLEMS, PRESENT RESOLUTIONS

Professional Competence to Review

After HEW's change in the administration of Medicare so that paying agents could examine medical records and decide whether payments should be made, the final decisions were often not made by medically skilled personnel.[30] The burden of incompetence fell most often on patients, when reviewers decided to disallow coverage for services which would have been approved by appropriate personnel with medical expertise. Likewise, where a claim was erroneously approved, the patient might have benefited financially, but the provision of medically unnecessary services could not be considered proper medical care. Also, from a systemic perspective, erroneous approvals were counterproductive because they increased program costs. Professional incompetance, therefore, benefitted no one, and all participants in the PSRO system have an interest in assuring that determinations are made by appropriately qualified people and methods.

The PSRO approach confronts this problem through the proscription against utilizing "the services of any individual who is not a duly licensed doctor of medicine or osteopathy to make final determinations . . . with respect to the professional conduct of [any act performed by] any other duly qualified doctor of medicine or osteopathy . . . ."[31] That requirement was intended to improve the quality and accuracy of evaluation.[32] As a practical matter it is unlikely that the proscription can be uniformly applied. In using norms as the "principal points of evaluation and review,"[33] computer processing or other screening techniques will be used to select for professional review only those cases in which the care provided does not satisfy the evaluative criteria. If cases which pass this initial screening are approved for payment, it will be clerical personnel, conducting the screening, who will, in fact, make final determinations of approval. It is legitimate to ask to what extent physician involvement and medical competence in decisionmaking will be compromised by the need for expeditious handling of claims. The legislative history is both instructive and troubling in this regard. The Senate Finance Committee endorsed the "automated screening of claims by computers ... carried out under review specifications and parameters set forth by the PSRO," noting the need to economize on physicians' time spent in review in order to liberate them to spend time in direct patient care.[34] The Committee conditioned the use of non-physician screeners, saying, "in no case could any final *adverse* determination by a PSRO with respect to the conduct or provision of care by a physician be made by anyone except another qualified physician."[35] Allowing PSROs to rely on a favorable screening report for approving payments may save the reviewing physician's time, but by implication it will entail mechancial, standardized application of norms.[36] Whether PSRO medical review is to assure flexible application of standards, and, therefore, high quality care, while containing costs will depend on the active participation of physicians in review. The Senate Finance Committee has recognized the burden this places on physicians, but finds the balance better struck in the concept that "only physicians are, in general, qualified to judge whether services ordered by other physicians are necessary,"[37]

Finally, in assuming the desirability of having professionals perform review, the question arises as to which professionals they should be.[38] In making their evaluations, the doctors serving on PSROs are authorized to make "arrangements to utilize the services of persons who are practitioners of, or specialists in, the various areas of medicine ... or other types of health care."[39] The balance between interspeciality review and intraspecialty review is a difficult one. Using surgeons to review the services provided by other surgeons, for example, may offer some advantage in the common professional knowledge brought to bear in evaluating a case, but may impede objective determinations. Similar specialists may be less likely than others to question the judgement of a colleague in the same specialty. If review which is critical and exacting will improve the quality of care rendered, then it is in the patient's interest to ensure strict review. But at the point where strict review cuts back on approval of services, solely to save money, strict review is contrary to consumer's interests. These factors are legitimate in constructing a reasonable system of review which will not be vulnerable to the abuse suffered under the previous structure.

Consistency of Judgement
Delegation of review authority to paying agents without thorough and uniform guidance on the parameters to be used necessarily resulted in the application of varying criteria with correspondingly varying results. In some instances, paying agents applied no criteria at all,[40] or were left to develop their own standards.[41] The effect of discontinuities in review outcomes was to make

some patients liable for bills which should have been paid by the government, while others with similar medical conditions had the cost of their services paid. In addition, unless verified standards are applied, the educational function of the reviewing process, bringing questionable practices to the physician's attention for corrective action, is lost.

PSRO use of norms will contribute to greater uniformity in the reviewing system, at least within a PSRO area. The resulting standardization of reviewing criteria can promote consistent results and, therefore, fairness to patients. It may also, however, lead to the exclusion of innovative approaches. But the risk of unsubstantiated, indiscriminate application of review criteria has been significantly minimized under the PSRO system.

Retroactive Denials of Payment

The timing of review is of great importance to the patient. The burdensome effect of a retroactive denial of payment on the patient has been a questionable element of the utilization review program[42] and the old hearings and appeals process.[43] When payment for services already rendered is suddenly denied, the patient has no time to plan to meet the expense of medical care. Considering the high cost of health care today, the financial impact of an unexpected medical bill is often disastrous. Patients have been powerless to prevent a retroactive denial because they usually have had no basis on which to challenge a physician's recommendation of medical care. At the same time, providers fearing a retroactive denial of payment, deny them access to services which would, in fact, have been covered. Recent changes in the Social Security Amendments have attempted to alleviate this problem through "hold harmless" or "waiver of liability" provisions (discussed elsewhere in this book.)[44]

Retroactive denials of payment had other adverse effects on patients aside from the uncertainty of liability for payment. Skilled nursing homes, fearful of admitting a patient for whom payment might at some later date be denied, were under a considerable incentive to deny access to treatment in cases where reimbursement was not certain. The old law provided a mechanism, administered by paying agents, which offered an opportunity to be assured of payment. But its use was conditioned to qualified homes,[45] and its improper implementation often thwarted the procedure's ability to reduce retroactive denials.[46] Uncertainty of payment as a result of experience with retroactive denials also led many skilled nursing homes to withdraw from the Medicare program.[47]

PSROs may have the capability to bring nursing homes back into the publicly financed programs through the norms requirement on the basis of which homes may have greater certainty about admission decisions. Futhermore, the explicit emphasis in the PSRO law is on approving appropriate care, and considering whether it can be "more economically [provided] in an inpatient health care facility of a different type."[48] The clear implication is that nursing homes are expected to provide that care which they are qualified to render, and the administration of the statutory language will entail efforts to woo those providers who have dropped out of the program because of the previous mismanagement.

Prospective Review

Review and approval of medical services before they are rendered has been a component of the Medicaid review system, rather than Medicare. The decision of whether to approve or disapprove care was made by the state Medicaid agency or its designated fiscal agent. The federal *Medical Assistance Manual* authorizes the establishment of a mechanism whereby qualified professionals review the medical necessity, economy, and propriety (in view of accepted community standards of practice) of certain types of nonemergency services—those which are elective, costly, or of long duration. This prospective review led to advance determinations of whether payment for those services should be made. They were not to be used to meet fiscal emergencies through denial or postponement of needed services, but rather, determinations were to be made quickly (with provision for automatic approval in the event that no determination was made within a specified time). The guidelines required systematic evaluation of a state's implementation of the prior review system for cost effectiveness, rates of rejection of claims, rates of modification of requests, and the effect of the plan on promoting attention to treatment by diagnosis, rather than only alleviation of symptoms.[49]

Although prospective review administered by paying agents offered the certainty that payment would or would not be available, it could be a harsh system, without accurate, professional determinations. Patients were denied access to care, or the approval of care took so long that vital hospitalization or treatment had to be deferred until the patient suffered physically as a result.[50] The implementation of prior authorization employed unlicensed clerks to make medical decisions.[51]

PSROs are given the authority to review in advance any elective admission or service involving extended or costly treatment, to determine (1) its medical necessity and (2) whether the service could be provided more economically in another type of institution or on an out-patient basis.[52] Implementation of the system is purely discretionary with the PSRO. Hospitals, too, may employ preadmission certification which has the same effect. If a hospital does choose to engage in prior review, regulations prescribe it shall be utilized "at least for those categories of elective admissions which produce unusually high costs, or which have frequently been found to be of questionable necessity, or which have been proposed by physicians whose patterns of care have been found questionable."[53] By using PSROs, or hospitals to whom they have delegated case by case review, to make prior authorizations, several of the criticisms of the old system are met: norms provide a medical basis for making determinations, and determinations will usually be made by qualified medical personnel. But in order to assure that advance determinations do not penalize patients whose care is reviewed by them, the PSRO system must provide for speedy determinations and automatic approval of services in the event of administrative delay. Implementation should also employ evaluation of the effects of advance determinations through follow-up studies where authorization was denied.

The use of prospective review to limit admissions when demand on available facilities was high was a problem under the old system. Because PSROs, unlike paying agents, are barred from reviewing fiscal considerations, and are not directly concerned with demand on the facilities of particular institutions, the pressure for reducing admissions will not be generated from within the PSRO. But where demand for medical facilities is high throughout the PSRO's area, the physicians serving may be tempted to be more exacting in exercising their advance determination authority. In addition, external pressure from HEW for cost control may result in use of prospective determinations to the detriment of patients.[54]

Conflicts of Interest

Structural weaknesses in a review system can undermine its effectiveness, like those failures of the system discussed above. The performance of the system depends equally on the reviewing authority's willingness to perform its responsibilities thoroughly and impartially. The health insurance industry, from whose ranks paying agents have primarily been drawn, had a substantial business interest in maintaining amicable relationships with practitioners and providers. The paying agent's interest in preserving this relationship proved contrary, however, to an effective review program.[55] There was also a financial conflict of interest between the paying agent as private entrepreneur and as public program fiscal administrator. Reimbursement arrangements with hospitals where a fiscal intermediary first pays the costs of Medicare and then, as private insurer, pays the hospital on behalf of its regular subscribers creates a financial incentive to maximize the costs chargeable to Medicare.[56]

HEW pressures for cost control have sometimes counteracted a paying agent's laxity in review,[57] especially when those pressures carried with them the implied threat of revocation of the paying agent's contract.[58] The threat has worked because paying agents have had an interest in continued participation in the government programs because of the government's subsidy of their administrative costs.

In contrast, patients' interests barely influenced the reviewing process, if at all. Patients may have had bills gratuitously paid by a paying agent reluctant to subject a provider or practitioner to close scrutiny; but that was not the result of any concern for the patinet. To the extent that proper medical determinations can improve the quality of care, the paying agents' interest in perfunctory, lax review was at odds with patients' interests, and more significantly, was given greater weight in the operation of the system.[59]

Physician PSRO members will, in some ways, have interests similar to those that paying agents have had. Whether they will be eager to closely examine their peers' medical judgements is questionable, and the past failures of institutional utilization review committees discourages confidence that they will.[60] Specific physician bias in individual cases is supposed to be eliminated by the requirement that no physician review any case where he was involved in the provision of services or has a financial interest in the institution where care was being provided.[61] His institutional identification, however, is given sanction through the delegation of case by case review to institutional utilization review committees. Also, like paying agents, physicians' closer ties to hospitals may again tend to bring the care furnished in skilled nursing homes under comparatively closer scrutiny.[62] The "fox guarding the chicken coop" analysis which has often been used to criticize the PSRO structure will be a valid one unless enforcement of the program's goal is achieved through education, voluntary cooperation, and, if necessary, imposition of sanctions.[63]

The design of the PSRO structure establishes an implicit checks and balances system. Were physicians in PSROs to adopt completely the program values and goals of efficient fiscal administrators, quality of medical care would undoubtedly suffer. The system is predicated on the understanding that physicians will bring to their review countervailing biases and incentives in favor of more care and more services. In a review structure involving practicing physicians, it would be impossible to eradicate those biases, and consumers have a vital interest in assuring their maintenance.

Administrative Accountability

Accountability to consumers is discussed in a later chapter.[64] HEW control of PSROs through their selection, monitoring, and sanctions on them is a critical element of an accountable system where proper implementation is a priority. The preceeding discussion has touched on those apsects of the PSRO system which have the potential to serve the patient's interest while overcoming the failures of the preexisting program—e.g., use of professionals in making final determinations, elimination of retroactive denials of care, and the use of norms to achieve objectivity in review. The realization of potential service depends not only upon the tendencies of individual participants, but also upon how closely HEW supervises the program. It is, of course, critical that HEW be committed to making the program work. The Senate Finance Committee said, ". . . only a full implementation effort will provide the impetus needed to establish effective and equitable comprehensive professional review throughout the Nation."[65] The blame for the failure of the old system, they recognized, "must be shared between failings in the statutory requirements and the willingness and capacity of those responsible for implementing what [was] required [by the old] law."[66]

In order to translate a willingness to implement into action, there must also be established effective administration procedures for evaluating PSROs and supervising their performance. The following discussion compares the previous system with the PSRO approach.

Selection. General criteria for the selection of fiscal intermediaries and carriers have been specified by statute, but the requirements are not further elaborated in regulations. Nor have regulations specified any procedure for prospective evaluation of the competence of those agencies.[67] Nomination of fiscal intermediaries is by providers, not by the Secretary; consequently, selection can be made on the basis of favoritism or expected leniency in performing review.[68] There are no standards for the selection of fiscal agents by state Medicaid agencies.[69]

Selection of PSROs offers a substantial improvement over the methods by which paying agents are selected.[70] PSROs will be chosen on the basis of a "formal written plan" subject to evaluation by the Secretary to determine that the organization is "willing and capable of performing, in an effective, timely and objective manner and at reasonable cost."[71] Selection by the Secretary eliminates some of the problems raised by provider nomination under Part A of Medicare. The Secretary is, however, required to give notice to all physicians in a PSRO area of the intent to enter into a PSRO agreement, and, if 10 percent of the physicians object to the prospective PSRO as unrepresentative, all physicians in the area must be polled.[72] That a PSRO is not representative of practicing physicians in the PSRO area is the only grounds for challenging designation. But, as a practical matter, the system cannot prevent objections actually based on the expected stringency of the prospective PSRO's review or other extraneous grounds. While HEW will have to be flexible during the implementation phase of the program in order to encourage innovation,[73] past experience with paying agents demonstrates the need for detailed criteria for evaluation of PSRO plans. The *Program Manual* has published such criteria. Those requirements relate to both organizational structure and review responsibilities.[74]

The most significant difference in PSRO selection, as compared to selection of paying agents, is the trial period during which conditionally designated PSROs assume their duties as their proficiency allows.[75] Each PSRO will increase its review responsibilities according to a plan approved by the Secretary, and will assume each new duty only with HEW approval.[76]

Monitoring. The frequency and scope of HEW monitoring have not ensured the performance of paying agents. The Senate Finance Committee noted that Medicare and Medicaid have "suffered from the lack of a dynamic and ongoing mechanism with specific responsibility for continuing review ... of the effectiveness of program operations ... ."[77] The Committee proposed to deal with this problem by creating an office of Inspector General for Health Administration. The provision was dropped during later stages of the legislative process.[78] Without such a central agency with responsibility for assuring program operations, HEW monitoring of the operations of Part A fiscal intermediaries has been minimal and sporadic: of the Blue Cross plans serving as fiscal intermediaries for the District of Columbia, Texas, Southern California, Puerto Rico, and New York City, during 1970–71 only the New York plan received a contract performance review.[79] As of December 1972, HEW had issued 251 audit reports on the activities of the Blue Cross Association and 74 of its member plans as fiscal intermediaries.[80] HEW offered the presence of on-site representatives as justification for not performing more contract performance reviews. Such informal monitoring, however, is more akin to liaison than inspection and cannot be expected to provide the detailed scrutiny and corrective action that should result from formal evaluation and written reports with subsequent sanctions. The effectiveness of contract performance review reports in achieving remedial action was further reduced by HEW's policy of keeping them confidential. Congress, recognizing that public access to such reports would itself generate pressure for improvement, amended the statute to require disclosure of these and similar reports.[81]

Studies of the review of Part B carriers reveal similar problems. In a recent study by the Advisory Committee on Medicare Administraton, Contracting and Subcontracting, inadequate monitoring techniques were specifically cited for criticism and recommendations. Criteria for measuring carrier performance must be refined, the Advisory Committee suggested.[82] Incentives to better performance were recommended,[83] and, significantly, dissemination of information about carriers was included as a noteworthy possibility.[84]

Infrequent monitoring has also been undermined by its own narrow scope. Carriers and fiscal agents have been required by HEW to establish utilization controls for payments to physicians under Part B of Medicare and under Medicaid; but, for the most part, HEW has made no effort to evaluate the effectiveness of the various plans in operation nor to guide contractors in implementing effective systems.[85] The focus of HEW's monitoring efforts with regard to the utilization control requirements has been only on whether required controls were established, not on whether established systems were working.[86]

PSROs' performance must be monitored, under the law. The National Professional Standards Review Council will review the operations of PSROs to determine their effectiveness and compare their performances.[87] The findings of their studies, together with their recommendations for program improvement are to be reported annually both to the Secretary and to Congress.[88] In addition Statewide Professional Standards Review Councils will assist the Secretary in evaluating the performance of each PSRO.[89]

PSROs will be subjected to more intense scrutiny than audit reports alone. The system will generate data which can be used for statistical comparisons and other analyses to evaluate performance on a regular and continuing basis.[90] Provider and patient profiles, which each PSRO is required to develop and maintain, offer a ready basis for comparing PSROs.[91] The minimum frequency for formal comparative appraisals of PSROs is contained in the requirement that the National Council issue annual reports "contain[ing] comparative data indicating the results of review activities . . . in each state and in each of the various areas."[92]

The effectiveness of monitoring procedures may depend on how the assessor is chosen. Past problems in the process of reviewing fiscal intermediaries are illuminating. The Social Security Administration (SSA) has a prime contract with the Blue Cross Association (BCA) as fiscal intermediary for Part A. BCA then lets subcontracts to the local Blue Cross plans which, in fact, perform the fiscal intermediary responsibilities. BCA's intermediate position has been used to insulate local plans from direct SSA supervision. At one point, SSA personnel had to channel all but the most routine inquiries through BCA headquarters in Chicago in lieu of direct communication with the local plan.[93] There were instances where a local plan refused to comply with a federal directive until it received BCA's approval to do so.[94] A provision was added to the 1970 contract, however, which permitted direct communication between SSA and local plans regarding matters in the subcontract, with BCA receiving prior notice of such communications.[95] The prime contract–subcontract approach forced SSA into an "all or nothing" posture regarding the local plans: SSA could not terminate a subcontract, because there was no provision in the prime contract allowing it to do so; nor had BCA itself ever rejected a local plan for inefficiency.[96] To use BCA, SSA had to accept the local plans regardless of the quality of their performance.

There is nothing in the PSRO statute which could conceivably lead to a similar dilemma. Early proposals that statewide PSROs subcontract the actual performance of medical review to local PSROs would have replicated the problem;[97] but those moves were resisted during early implementation phases. The regulations' creation of Statewide Support Centers,[98] for which there was no specific statutory authority, could create problems reminiscent of the SSA-BCA struggles, depending on how much substantive review responsibilities they assume.

Sanctions. Under the Medicare laws, the only available sanction against an inefficient paying agent has been termination of the contract.[99] HEW, however, has demonstrated considerable reluctance to exercise this authority despite wide variations in the performance of individual contractors.[100] Recent studies of carrier performances have recommended that termination of contracts be made more workable as a sanction, and that mechanisms to spur competition among agencies vying for contracts be developed.[101] Termination of the contract is also the only sanction which the Secretary has against errant PSROs, and it may be similarly infrequently exercised.

The Secretary may terminate a PSRO contract by nonrenewal at the end of a term or midterm, with notice and opportunity for a hearing, if the PSRO "is not substantially complying with or effectively carrying out the provisions of [its] agreement." [102] The legislative history makes clear the intent that the Secretary alert himself to poor performance and terminate agreements with derelict PSROs if timely efforts to effect improvements fail. [103] Impeding the effective assumption of that responsibility, however, is the cumbersome process entailed in qualifying a new PSRO. Neither the statute nor the legislative history specify who would perform interim review functions until a new PSRO became conditionally qualified to assume review duties. The Senate Finance Committee has recommended that the Secretary approach other review organizations in the state and the state medical society for suggestions regarding a willing and capable replacement, if a conditional PSRO does not qualify for full duties. [104] State or local health departments could be approached if medical groups failed to respond. [105] But the only consideration given to the possible failure of a PSRO was that "[a] PSRO agreement would include provisions for orderly transfer of medicare and medicaid records, data and other materials developed during the trial period to the Secretary or such successor organization as he might designate in the event of termination of the initial agreement." [106] None of these considerations confronts the problem of who is responsible in the interim.

One possibility would be to allow the original PSRO to continue until a replacement is fully qualified, but this would subsidize incompetence. Another interim replacement could be a neighboring PSRO; although for a quick transfer of responsibility to be feasible the reviewing mechanisms would have to be highly standardized [107] and some technique would have to be found to permit the personnel at the replacement PSRO to absorb the increased burden of review for two areas. The administrative implications of imposing termination of its contract on a PSRO are so troublesome that PSROs and HEW would best expend their efforts on assuring proper compliance by educating individual practitioners and gaining their cooperation, combined with efforts to use dissemination of information about PSROs to the public in order to create a meaningful incentive to comply. [108]

PAYING AGENTS IN THE PSRO PROGRAM

Although ineligible in most cases to serve as PSROs, paying agents will continue to review medical care to the extent that their functions are not superceded by PSROs. The PSRO law provides that "any review with respect to [Medicare, Medicaid, and Title V] services which has not been designated by the Secretary as the full responsibility of [a PSRO], shall be reviewed in the manner otherwise provided for under law."[109] The scope of PSRO review is itself limited to "health care services provided by or in institutions," unless the Secretary approves a PSRO's request for expanded responsibility.[110] Initially, this authority has been used to let PSROs review acute care only in short stay hospitals. Whether ambulatory care delivered by institutional out-patient departments was contemplated in the initial drafting of the law is unclear. It is clear there was a decision not to include services delivered in physicians' offices or in the patient's home, unless the PSRO affirmatively seeks such authority. Because of the restriction on PSRO review (to institutional care) some services covered by Medicare and Medicaid will continue to be reviewed by paying agents, as under the system before PSROs. Review of physicians' services in the office or the home will still belong to paying agents; review of drugs and other ancillary services will be divided according to where they were provided. Paying agents will also continue to perform review in those areas where a PSRO has not yet been given full review responsibility. For example, an initial conditional designation could extend only to the review of admissions and performance of medical care evaluation studies. Concurrent extended stay review and retrospective review might be left to the jurisdiction of paying agents until the PSRO demonstrates its ability to take on more responsibility for review.

In addition to retaining responsibility for review functions not assigned to PSROs, the law implies that paying agents may, under certain circumstances, perform review of the same services PSROs are reviewing, but only in an advisory capacity. In order to avoid "duplication of functions and unnecessary review and control activities" the Secretary is authorized to waive "any or all of the review certification or similar activities" otherwise required under the Social Security Act, if he finds on the basis of "substantial evidence" that other review activities "are not needed for the provision of adequate review and control."[111] The Senate Finance Committee stated that the Secretary would be expected to waive these review requirements when a PSRO had satisfactorily demonstrated its effectiveness.[112] The statute and the legislative history imply a bias in favor of the previous system because a PSRO must show that its review is *superior* to existing systems before it will be given exclusive responsibility. The statute provides that existing review systems will remain in effect "pending the assumption of capacity [by PSROs] for improved review effort."[113] The Senate Finance Committee specifically preserved the role of paying agents.

> In a number of areas of the country, carriers and intermediaries—even though their activity is limited to retrospective review—are doing a reasonable effective job of controlling unnecessary utilization of health care services. Such effort should not be terminated in any area until such time as a PSRO has satisfactorily demonstrated the willingness, operational capacity, and performance to

effectively supplant and improve upon existing review work. Even where the PSRO becomes the paramount review organization, the existing review, if it is efficient and effective, should not be dismantled, if the PSRO can benefit by utilizing its experience and services.[114]

Where a functional PSRO exists, the experience and services to be offered by efficient paying agents would at least be advice. But beyond advice, from the language, it appears that some carriers and fiscal intermediaries may continue to operate as reviewing entities, notwithstanding the existence of a fully qualified PSRO in the same area. By implication, then, a PSRO's demonstrated ability to perform its duties will not be the sole, sufficient criterion for a decision to dismantle the paying agents' review authority in that area. Whether or not the PSRO's execution of review responsibilities is functionally superior to the old system as implemented in that area, if the existing review is "efficient and effective" it can be maintained.

The potential for confusion in this dual system is obvious. Which organization's determination is binding is not clearly stated. The Finance Committee suggests that even where a PSRO is "the *paramount* review organization," paying agents can perform parallel activities. The Committee suggests that the PSRO's needs be given priority in making the decision to retain a role for paying agents in review of care. Unless that consideration is predominant, the PSRO structure could be undermined by paying agents' overruling PSRO determinations. To eliminate the potential for paying agents to second-guess PSROs, their advisory role should be limited to the overall performance of the program and not to case by case advice.

Until PSROs are capable of assuming 'paramount' responsibilities, they will operate side by side with paying agents for considerable time. Without coordination of review, a PSRO could find in a particular case that proposed services are medically necessary but could be most economically furnished to the patient at home, while the paying agent, in carrying out its responsbility to review noninstitutional services, determines retroactively that services were not medically necessary and, therefore, disallows payment. The statute requires the Secretary to provide by regulations "for such correlation of activities, such interchange of data and information, and such other cooperation" among PSROs and other review organizations as is "consistent with economical, efficient, coordinated and comprehensive implementation" of the PSRO program.[115] Standardized record formats, and standardized review criteria within each parallel system will be essential to avoid discontinuities in review like those posed above.

Claims Processing and Coverage

Aside from problems of allocating case by case review responsibility between paying agents and PSROs, paying agents will continue to act as the fiscal administrators of the Medicare and Medicaid programs. In exercising their responsibilities, those organizations must determine whether the appropriate program offers coverage for the services for which a claim is made. Some of the statutory bases for disallowance (exclusion from coverage) are nonmedical and therefore should be within the exclusive purview of paying agents. An example is services which are paid for under a workmen's compensation plan.[116] However, other statutory exclusions from coverage, notably exclusions for lack of medical necessity, and because care was custodial,[117] involve medical judgements which are now within the PSRO's jurisdiction.

Although the use of paying agents to administer payments for Medicare and Medicaid services is essential, division of review responsibility between and fiscal judgements will be difficult because the statutory exclusions do not fall clearly within one or the other category. Basic determinations that care is or is not medically necessary will now be based on PSRO norms, critera, and standards, which paying agents should be expected to honor. Custodial care, however, is an administrative category. Never defined in the statute, it has been defined through administrative processes as "care designed essentially to assist an individual to meet his activities of daily living . . . and which does not entail or require the continuing attention of trained medical or paramedical personnel."[118] If a PSRO determines that care not requiring continuing attention of trained personnel is, nonetheless, medically necessary, the law would deny payment for those services regardless of their medical necessity. Conflict will arise where a PSRO approves care as medically necessary without employing the magic words of the definition of "custodial care." A paying agent then determining that the PSRO's approval was for care, in effect, custodial would be crossing that fine line between medical and fiscal judgements.

Also implicated in this dilemma is the PSRO's responsibility to determine whether proposed in-patient care could be provided on an out-patient basis, or in another type of in-patient care facility.[119] These are so-called "level of care" decisions—which facility provides the appropriate level of care for that patient. PSROs will necessarily discover cases where, consistent with their norms, criteria, and standards, the patient requires neither in-patient nor out-patient care—care, then, which according to the administrative definition is custodial. If the only way to determine whether care is custodial is through the use of PSRO norms, criteria, and standards, then level of care determinations, and application of the custodial care exclusion, are medical determinations. Because the premise of the PSRO law is that physicians, not insurance companies, should make medical judgements, this whole category of decisions should be designated exclusively the PSRO's responsibility.

Data Processing

The PSRO system in many ways is predicated on sophisticated data handling techniques to develop norms, and to compile and analyze profiles of care; and much of the program's effectiveness will be a function of its technology. Because the way in which a PSRO reviews individual cases and compares profiles will be heavily influenced by the data it receives, a critical issue is who will determine the structure and content of that data. Paying agents have concentrated much of their attention on seeking control of the PSRO data systems.

The paying agents for Medicare and Medicaid have accumulated years of experience handling data for Medicare and Medicaid. The Blue Cross Association has developed nationwide statistics, and Blue Shield has emphasized its previous experience as well.[120] In part, their eagerness to offer their data services to PSROs is motivated by a desire to minimize the expected loss of federal subsidies which will result from their replacement by PSROs. Beyond the issue of PSROs, control of those operations in a national health insurance program will undoubtedly be based, at least in part, on experience gained from the PSRO program. Because PSROs in so many ways represent a direct threat to paying agents, the Senate Finance Committee gave extensive and detailed consideration to the scope of activities paying agents should be permitted to control:

It is expected that where economical and efficient computer and other resources already exist in carriers and intermediaries they would be utilized to the extent feasible and that operations would be consolidated and coordinated wherever possible . . . .

The committee would stress that the approach recommended does not envisage Blue Cross or Blue Shield or other insurance organizations or hospital or medical association review committees, assuming the review responsibilities for the professional standards review organizations. Where Blue Cross or Blue Shield or other insurers, or agencies have existing computer capacity capable of producing the necessary patient, practitioner, and provider profiles in accordance with the parameters and other requirements of the PSRO, on an ongoing expeditious and economical basis, it would certainly be appropriate to employ that capacity as a basic tool for the professional standards review organizations; but that mechanism would be employed essentially to feed computer printouts to the review organizations which would be responsible for their evaluation. Where it would facilitate administration, the Secretary could designate a specific carrier or intermediary as "lead" carrier or intermediary for purposes of coordination with PSROs in an area. The responsibility for handling requests for such prior approval of hospital admissions, elective procedures and services as might be required, as well as the administrative mechanism for processing such requests, would lie with the PSROs. A "lead" carrier or intermediary would not interfere with nor interrupt direct contact between the Secretary and the PSROs.[121]

Unless PSROs delegate only the physical tasks of electronic data collection and processing to paying agents, more extensive control of data could subvert the program. Medical evaluation of data should be left to the discretion of PSROs if this aspect of the PSRO system is to be consistent with the intent of the legislation. In addition, because of the demonstrated failures of paying agents, especially with regard to their data processing capabilities which have been specifically singled out for criticism,[122] each PSRO should develop a system for monitoring the data processing performance of paying agents. Based on information gained through monitoring, PSROs should be able to specify their data needs, suggest and anticipate change and improvements, and report paying agents' failure to produce to HEW. Since PSROs will not be given their own data processing systems, they must at least be able to assure the integrity of the data they must use in order to safeguard the operation of the program. Because HEW's monitoring of paying agents' performance has at best relied on information generated by the subjects themselves, an added PSRO monitoring capability will better assure the system's effectiveness by supplying a source of information outside of the paying agents themselves.

Paying Agents as PSROs

Although organizations which have served as paying agents, will be eligible to serve as PSROs only as a last resort, (like state Medicaid agencies already discussed) the potential may be sufficient to motivate them to bring it to realization.

No organization which is not a nonprofit physicians' association, representative of medical practice in the area, voluntary, and open to all area physicians may serve as a PSRO prior to January 1, 1976.[123] After that date, other professionally competent organizations found by the Secretary to be capable of performing the duties of a PSRO may be eligible, but only if there is no qualified voluntary physicians' association in the area.[124] In no case may physicians' services be reviewed by anyone other than physicians, nor may the Secretary renew a PSRO contract with any alternate organization if a voluntary physicians' association is willing and able to assume the duties of a PSRO.[125]

If all the above contingencies are met and an alternate organization must be designated, the legislative history emphatically states that paying agents should be considered last.

> Physician organizations or groupings would be completely free to undertake or decline assumption of the responsibilities of organizing a PSRO. If they decline, the Secretary would be empowered to seek alternative applicants from among other medical organizations, State and local health departments, medical schools, and failing all else, carriers and intermediaries or other health insurers.[126]

Paying agents, then, are presented with the possibility of becoming PSROs themselves, and therefore have an incentive to subvert initially designated organizations. A different strategy would depend on the requirement that PSROs must demonstrate superior review ability: a massive campaign of reform within the administration of the paying agents themselves would better assure their futures as PSROs, because such action would make it harder for PSROs to be effectively superior to them. Faced with the threat of PSROs, combined with the threat of some of the national health insurance proposals which would eliminate many of those agencies from substantive roles in health care insurance, paying agents have considerable interest in remaining as entrenched as they are. These incentives, and actions based on them, must be carefully watched if PSROs are to survive the political challenge of paying agents.

Notes for Chapter Four

1. *Sen. Fin. Comm. Rpt.* at 255.
2. §1158(a); 42 USC §1320c–7.
3. *Sen. Fin. Comm. Rpt.* at 256.
4. §1153; 42 USC §1320c–2.
5. The Senate Finance Committee stated that PSROs would "assume responsibility for the review of service (but not payments) provided through the medicare and medicaid programs." *Sen. Fin. Comm. Rpt.* at 257.
6. See Chapter Three at 84 *supra.*
7. §1812(a); 42 USC §1395d(a).
8. §1816; 42 USC §1395h.
9. §1816(b)(1)(B); 42 USC §1395h(b)(1)(B).
10. §§1832, 1861(m), 1861(s); 42 USC §§1395k, 1395x(m), 1395x(s).
11. §1842(a); 42 USC §1395u(a) sets out the duties of carriers which include assisting providers and practitioners in the development and application of utilization safeguards, making studies on the effectiveness of such procedures, and determining provider compliance with the utilization review conditions of participation. §1861(k); 42 USC §1395x(k).
12. *Id.*
13. 20 CFR §405.678(c).
14. §1842(a)(2); 42 USC §1395u(a)(2).
15. 45 CFR §249.82. This regulation allows the contractor to process and audit claims on behalf of the state (fiscal agent arrangement), or to receive monthly premiums from the state and make payments for services from these premiums (health insuring arrangement). For simplicity, the contractor in both cases will be referred to in the text as a fiscal agent to differentiate it from a fiscal intermediary or carrier.
16. §1902(a)(30); 42 USC §1396a(a)(30).
17. 45 CFR §250.20. This applied only to monitoring of utilization review of in-patient hospital and skilled nursing home services. The state is

nevertheless responsible for all utilization review plans and activities. This regulation has recently been changed to make the state responsbile for monitoring utilization review. It makes no mention of delegation or of paying agents. 45 CFR §250.20 (39 FR 41617, November 29, 1974).

18. Wilbur Cohen, then Undersecretary of HEW, explained to the House Ways and Means Committee that a utilization review committee determination was comparable to a "supreme court decision." "If the [utilization] review board makes a mistake, there is nothing we can do about it, because that is the decision of the doctors." *Hearings on H.R. 1 Before the House Ways and Means Committee* (89th Cong., 1st sess., 1965), pt. 1, at 68. Shortly after the passage of Medicare, Arthur Hess, then Director of the Bureau of Health Insurance (BHI), spoke of the role of the fiscal intermediary,

> When the fiscal intermediary comes on center stage in the near future, we will rely heavily on the intermediary to participate with the medical profession in the long-run measures that will result in assurance that utilization review does in fact function in the ways that it was indicated it would function at the time of certification of the institution .... We will look to the fiscal intermediary, the hospital administrative staff, and the medical community for primary assurance of effective functioning. This assurance, we believe, may be fully supported by statistical analyses and consultations based on questions arising out of day-to-day claims administration, rather than requiring audits of the individual case judgment of review committees.

> Address of Arthur Hess, Seventh Annual Medical Services Conference, American Medical Association, Philadelphia, November 27, 1965, as quoted in Associated Hospital Service of New York, *Medicare Advance Information Letter No. 12*, March 24, 1966.

19. The Social Security Administration found that extended stay cases were not being reviewed by 10 percent of the hospitals studied, and that 47 percent of the hospitals did not maintain any summary of medical records as a basis for evaluation of utilization by diagnosis or other common factors. Quoted in *Medicare and Medicaid Problems Issues and Alternatives*, Report of the Staff to the Committee on Finance, U.S. Sen. (91st Cong., 1st sess, 1970) at 107 [hereinafter cited as *Medicare and Medicaid 1970*].

20. *Id.* at 105. The staff concluded that "utilization review requirements, generally speaking, have been of a token nature and ineffectual as a curb to unnecessary use of institutional care and services. Utilization review in Medicare can be characterized as more form than substance."

21. BHI Intermediary Letter No. 237, August 14, 1967, quoted in *Hearings*

on H.R. 12080 Before the Senate Finance Committee (90th Cong., 1st sess., 1967), pt. 2, at 1042.

22. "Although consideration should be given to the view of a utilization review committee, the final decision regarding reimbursement rests with the intermediary." *Part A Intermediary Manual*, HIM–13, §3421.1.

23. §§1862(a)(1), 1862(a)(9); 42 USC §§1395y(a)(1), 1395y(a)(9). Custodial care is a conclusory term which is most often applied to exclude payment for services which are not skilled nursing services. For the definition of skilled nursing services see 20 CFR §405.127.

24. Report to the Secretary of Health Education and Welfare and the Commissioner of Social Security by the Advisory Committee on Medicare Administration, Contracting and Subcontracting, June 21, 1974, at 16 [hereinafter cited as *Perkins Report*].

25. The role of Blue Cross in Medicare and Medicaid is given a thorough analysis in Sylvia Law, *Blue Cross: What Went Wrong?* (New Haven: Yale University Press, 1974), a Health Law Project book. This chapter has made extensive use of this analysis, particularly in the discussion to follow on retrospective review and on selection and monitoring of paying agents. The author's cooperation is gratefully acknowledged.

26. *Perkins Report* at 16, n. 1.

27. *Medicare and Medicaid 1970* at 113.

28. *Perkins Report* at 26.

29. *CCH Medicare and Medicaid Guide* ¶¶15,550–660. Blue Cross–Blue Shield plans do not process claims for all services in these states, and they have been removed as the agents in Michigan.

30. A Social Security Administration contract performance review team's study of Associated Hospital Services, Inc., (a Blue Cross plan serving as the fiscal intermediary for New York City) found that basically clerical personnel review claims submitted for payment. The review team felt that these claims processors, who received only twenty hours of instruction in medical terminology, and who had no screening standards to follow, were not qualified to pass judgment on the medical necessity of services provided. Social Security Administration, Bureau of Health Insurance, "Status of Implementation of Contract Performance Review Recommendations Made in March 1970," May 20, 1971, at 5 [hereinafter cited as *New York Contract Performance Review*].

A study made in 1972 by the General Accounting Office (GAO) of six carriers and fiscal agents found that one of them did not use the services of medical consultants to determine the medical necessity of physician services. Comptroller General's Report to the Congress, No. B–164031, "More Needs to Be Done to Assure That Physician's Services—Paid for by Medicare and Medicaid—Are Necessary," August 2, 1972, at 30–33 [hereinafter cited as *1972 GAO Report*].

31. §1155(c); 42 USC §1320c–4(c).
32. However, there is no necessary conclusion that physicians as the final arbiters will generally be more vigorous in undertaking an impartial, critical review of the medical profession. See Chapter Seven, at 234 *infra.*
33. §1156(a); 42 USC §1320c–5(a).
34. *Sen. Fin. Comm. Rpt.* at 264.
35. (Emphasis added.) *Id.* at 260.
36. See Chapter Two at 50 *supra.*
37. *Sen. Fin. Comm. Rpt.* at 257. This burden does not seem unjust since "ever since medicare began, physicians have expressed resentment that their medical determinations are challenged by insurance company personnel." *Id.*
38. See Chapter Two at 32 *supra* for a discussion of the appropriate roles of nonprofessionals in reviewing care.
39. §1155(b)(1); 42 USC §1320c–4(b)(1).
40. In New York, the fiscal intermediary was found not to have applied screening criteria to hospital bills (e.g., length of stay in relation to diagnosis, high ancillary charges in relation to diagnosis and/or length of stay, or questionable diagnosis indicating unnecessary admissions). Home health agency bills received no review for necessity of service, nonskilled service, or therapy rendered on a long term basis. *New York Contract Performance Review* at 6.
41. It was left to carriers and fiscal agents in reviewing physician services to define for themselves what constitutes an unusual pattern of services (i.e., what circumstances indicate a need for further review of the necessity of services which a physician has ordered). Accordingly, these paying agents varied considerably in their identification of questionable utilization patterns, assigning different weight to the patient's medical history and to the number of physician visits as elements of this calculus. *1972 GAO Report* at 16, 20.

    A further problem has been the lack of coordination in review efforts between Medicare and Medicaid, resulting in instances where a physician's bills are paid without question by one program, while the same physician is under investigation for fraud by the other program. *Id.* at 36–39.

    The paying agents were not exclusively to blame for this patchwork quilt of criteria. Lack of supervision and guidance from HEW was also a major factor.
42. See Chapter Three at 71 *supra.*
43. See Chapter Five at 147 *infra.*
44. See Chapter Three at 87 *supra* and Chapter Five at 145 *infra.*
45. Under the "Assurance of Payments procedure," a patient could be presumed to qualify for post–hospital extended care services during a reasonable time required for the intermediary to process a request for determination of coverage, or from the time of admission if the request is filed within forty-eight hours. However, this procedure

was available only for those nursing homes which the intermediary had found to be qualified, considering the adequacy of utilization review; effectiveness in determining whether a patient received covered care and accordingly limiting requests for payment; effectiveness in use of the assurance of payments procedure; and the adequacy of medical information furnished by the nursing home. 20 CFR §405.129 (changed 1974). See Chapter Five at 144 *infra*.

46. The Contract Performance Review Team evaluating the intermediary in New York City found that all extended care facilities operated under this procedure, but most were unable to comply with its requirements. Many submitted their requests for coverage determinations together with the first bill, a practice that destroyed the ability of the assurance of payments mechanism to reduce retroactive denials through determination of coverage early in the patient's stay. *New York Contract Performance Review* at 11.

47. "The retroactive denial of claims is a basic underlying reason for the decline in ECF use. Moreover, the decline in use has resulted in the decline in the number of participating ECFs by about 700 or 64,000 beds between December 1969, and December 1971." Comptroller General, "Study of Health Facilities Construction Costs," report to the Congress of the United States, December 1971, at 799–800.

48. §1155(a)(1)(C); 42 USC §1320c–4(a)(1)(C).

49. *Medical Assistance Manual,* §§5–30–10, 5–30–20. See Chapter Five at 139 *infra* for a discussion of the legal implications for consumers of prior authorization.

50. See Brian, "Government Control of Hospital Utilization: A California Experience," 286 *NEJM* 1340, 1342 (June 22, 1972).

51. "Doctors' Views of Medi-Cal," 287 *NEJM* 618 September 21, 1972). The success of prior authorization in reducing hospital utilization has also been disputed, as have the costs of its operation in relation to the savings achieved. See "Screening Program Effects Disputed," *American Medical News,* October 16, 1972, at 8; Somers, "Hospital Utilization Controls: What is the Way?" 286 *NEJM* 1362 (June 22, 1972).

52. §1155(a)(2); 42 USC §1320c–4(a)(2).

53. 20 CFR §405.1035(f)(3) (39 FR 41606, November 29, 1974).

54. For example, when the intermediary for New York City was reviewed by an SSA Contract Performance Review Team, it was recommended that the intermediary consider the informational and educational aspects of its utilization review program as secondary, and proceed to use the program to deny or reduce bills. *New York Contract Performance Review* at 5.

55. For example, in response to an SSA instruction to identify doctors to whom over $25,000 had been paid under Part B of Medicare, many Blue Shield plans serving as carriers refused initially to furnish this information on the grounds that such disclosures had not been authorized by the physicians concerned. *Medicare and Medicaid*

1970 at 120. The interest of these carriers in keeping the good will of physicians conflicted with SSA's purpose of identifying cases where overpayment may have been made.

56. *Medicare and Medicaid 1970* at 116. Since the cost of patient services reflects the cost of operating the entire hospital, overutilization of services by Medicare patients can reduce the amount which would otherwise be payable by Blue Cross as private insurer.

57. See n. 54 *supra.*

58. See this chapter at 120 *infra* on sanctions against paying agents.

59. In some instances, a fiscal intermediary has subjected skilled nursing home bills to closer scrutiny than hospital bills. The Blue Cross intermediary for New York was giving medical review to 100 percent of bills from skilled nursing homes, at a time when review of hospital bills was virtually nil. *New York Contract Performance Review* at 6. This could be the result of Blue Cross' traditionally close association with hospitals. It is obvious that determining the strictness of review on the basis of where the patient received medical care is against the patient's interest.

60. See also Chapter Seven.

61. §1155(a)(6); 42 USC §1320c–4(a)(6).

62. See n. 59 *supra.*

63. See Chapter Seven at 231 *infra.*

64. See Chapter Six at 173 *infra.*

65. *Sen. Fin. Comm. Rpt.* at 259.

66. *Id.* at 256.

67. The statute requires that the Secretary shall not enter into an agreement with a fiscal intermediary unless "to do so is consistent with the effective and efficient administration of the program." §1816(b); 42 USC §1395h(b). A fiscal intermediary must also be "willing and able to assist the providers . . . in the application of safeguards against unnecessary utilization of services," and must furnish the Secretary with any information which the latter may require. *Id.* The regulations state that a nominated organization must have "the overall resources and experience to administer effectively and efficiently [its] responsibilities" as intermediary. This competence is presumed if the intermediary has had five years' experience in "paying for or reimbursing the cost of health services." 20 CFR §405.660.

Criteria for selection of Part B carriers are generally similar. §1842(b)(2); 42 USC §1395u(b)(2).

Broad criteria such as these are subject to widely varying, possibly inconsistent interpretations in individual cases. The presumption of competence on the basis of five years' experience may in some cases be unwarranted, as longevity need not be synonymous with ability.

68. The statute requires that providers nominate fiscal intermediaries. §1816(d); 42 USC §1395h(d). This provision was originally intended to ensure that Medicare would be administered by

organizations familiar with and acceptable to providers. However, providers could nominate the organization least likely to be vigorous in curbing overutilization, and prospective intermediaries could be deliberately lax in their duties in order to obtain a nomination, or ensure against its withdrawal by a dissatisfied provider. *Medicare and Medicaid 1970* at 114.

69. The only provision in the regulations relating to a fiscal agent contract requires merely that the contract specify the duties to be performed and the payment the fiscal agent will receive; that payments will be made pursuant to the state's regulations; that records will be kept and reports made as required by the state; that the amount paid the fiscal agent will be periodically renegotiated; and that the term of the contract and provisions for termination will be specified 45 CFR §249.82(b)(2). For health insuring arrangements, it is further required that the contract will state the premiums and the scope of benefits and fee schedules by which payments will be made. 45 CFR §249.82(b)(1).

70. See Chapter Six at 196 *infra* for a discussion of consumer accountability in the selection process.

71. §1152(b)(2); 42 USC §1320c–4(b)(2).

72. §1152(f); 42 USC §1320c–1(f). Regulations on physician polling have been published. 42 CFR §101.101 *et seq.* (39 FR 16201, May 7, 1974).

73. [I]t is recognized that the successful development of professional review organizations can encompass a variety of prototypes and that changes in technology can be expected to result in continued modifications in procedures, and that much remains to be done in the area of the development and refinement of professional norms. It is believed, though, that the proposal can be implemented within an overall framework of innovation and flexibility. *Sen. Fin. Comm. Rpt.* at 259.

74. *Program Manual* Chapter Five generally for conditional designations; Chapter Four for planning grants; Chapter Six describes the actual selection and agreement process.

75. §1154; 42 USC §1320c–3. See Chapter Six at 196 *infra* for a discussion of the implications for consumers of conditional designations.

76. §1154; 42 USC §1320c–3.

77. *Sen. Fin. Comm. Rpt.* at 278.

78. Social Security Amendments of 1972, Conference Report, H.R. Rep. No. 92–1605, (92d Cong., 2d sess.), at 49.

79. See Law, *supra* n. 25 at 44; and letter from Robert M. Ball, Commissioner, of social security, June 15, 1971 (on file at the Health Law Library, 133 So. 36th Street, Philadelphia, Pa. 19174). Also Program Review and Evaluation Project (PREP) teams have conducted reviews of Medicaid operations, but a 1969 HEW Audit Agency Report on Medicaid administration in 16 states found PREP reviews had not

been done with sufficient frequency to identify, on a timely basis, areas in need of improvement. Furthermore, the study found delays of up to nine months in follow-up on PREP reports by HEW regional offices. Supervision by HEW regional offices, apart from participation in PREP reviews, was found to be limited, in some cases due to an inadequate number of staff. *Medicare and Medicaid 1970* at 237, 238, 242.

80. See Law, n. 25 *supra*, at 186, n. 256.
81. §1106(d); 42 USC §1306(d). *Sen. Fin. Comm. Rpt.* at 306.
82. *Perkins Report* at 2.
83. *Id.* at 3.
84. *Id.* at 56.
85. Comptroller General's Report to the Congress, No. B–160431(4), August 2, 1972, "More Needs To Be Done to Assure That Physicians' Services—Paid For By Medicare and Medicaid—Are Necessary," at 17.
86. *Id.* at 25.
87. §1163(e)(3); 42 USC §1320c–12(e)(3).
88. §§1163(e)(4),(f); 42 USC §§1320c–12(e)(4),(f).
89. §1162(c)(2); 42 USC §1320c–11(c)(2). To meet the deficiencies of past monitoring, regulations should establish clearly the respective responsibilities of Statewide Councils, the National Council, and HEW for monitoring PSROs' performances.
90. *Sen. Fin. Comm. Rpt.* at 260.
91. §1155(a)(4); 42 USC §1320c–4(a)(4).
92. §1163(f); 42 USC §1320c–12(f).
93. *Medicare and Medicaid 1970* at 115.
94. HEW Audit Agency Report (No. 10036–07), Blue Cross Hospital Service, Inc., of St. Louis, November 30, 1970.
95. Hospital Insurance Benefits for the Aged, *Agreement with Intermediary Pursuant to 42 USC §1816*, 1970, Art. XVIII. HEW may also inspect and evaluate the local plans, again with prior notice to BCA. *Id.* Art. XX. Nevertheless, BCA still has considerable power over SSA's ability to supervise the operations of local plans. No regulation or instruction may be prescribed by the Secretary without prior consultation with BCA. *Id.* Art. VII, §B.
96. *Medicare and Medicaid 1970* at 115. The report cited criticism of BCA's position as "an additional, artifical, costly, duplicative and sometimes unnecessary layer of administration."
97. See Chapter Six at 180 *infra*.
98. 39 FR 10204, March 18, 1974; *Program Manual*, Chapter II generally. See Chapter Six at 181 *infra*.
99. Under Part A of Medicare, a fiscal intermediary contract may be terminated only if the Secretary finds, after notice to the intermediary and opportunity for a hearing, that the intermediary has substantially failed to carry out the agreement or that continuation of some or all of its functions would be disadvantageous or inconsistent with

efficient administration. §1816(e)(2); 42 USC §1395h(e)(2). Grounds for termination of Part B carrier contracts for cause are the same. §1842(b)(4); 42 USC §1395u(b)(4). Carrier contracts may also be allowed to lapse, by giving the carrier notice of the Secretary's intent not to renew, 90 days prior to the expiration of the contract term. 20 CFR §405.675.

Grounds for termination of a fiscal agent contract by a Medicaid state agency must be specified in the contract, but what the grounds are to be is not stated in federal regulations. 45 CFR §§249.82(b)(1)(vi), 249.82(v)(2)(v). Also, a state which fails to implement a satisfactory plan of utilization review is subject to a one-third reduction in federal financial participation for care provided beyond 60 days in a hospital, skilled nursing home, or intermediate care facility, or beyond 90 days in a mental hospital. §1903(g)(1); 42 USC §1396b(g)(1).

100. See *Medicare and Medicaid 1970* at 115, regarding variations in fiscal intermediary performance. Contracts with carriers have, as a rule, been renewed automatically, despite wide variations in carrier performance, although some renewals have been made contingent upon the correction of certain deficiencies. *Id.* at 117–119.

101. *Perkins Report* at 3.

102. §1152(d); 42 USC §1320c–1(d).

103. *Sen. Fin. Comm. Rpt.* at 261.

104. *Id.*

105. §§1153, 1154; 42 USC §§1320c–2,3.

106. *Sen. Fin. Comm. Rpt.* at 266.

107. Development of statewide standardization of operating procedures and data collection is a duty of the Statewide Council. §1162(e)(1); 42 USC §1320c–11(e)(1).

108. See n. 84 *supra*; and Chapter Six at 189 *infra*.

109. §1153; 42 USC §1320c–2.

110. §1155(g); 42 USC §1320c–4(g).

111. §1152(e); 42 USC §1320c–1(e).

112. *Sen. Fin. Comm. Rpt.* at 260.

113. §1153; 42 USC §1320c–2.

114. *Sen. Fin. Comm. Rpt.* at 258.

115. §1165; 42 USC §1320c–14.

116. §1862(b); 42 USC §1395y(b) excludes such services from Medicare coverage.

117. §§1862(a)(1),(a)(9); 42 USC §§1395y(a)(1),(a)(9) prohibit reimbursement for services which are not medically necessary or which constitute custodial care.

118. Part A Intermediary Manual, HIM–13, §3159.1. See Chapter Five n. 83 at 164 *infra* for the legal applications of the custodial care exclusion.

119. §1155(a)(1)(C); 42 USC §1320c–4(a)(1)(C).

120. Blue Shield of California claims to be saving its subscribers $100 million a year. That savings combined with its claims processing abilities are

asserted as supporting a Blue Shield role in PSROs. See "Blue Shield plan says control saving $100 million a year," *American Medical News,* March 11, 1974, at 8. See also Chapter Six at 184 *infra.*

121.   *Sen. Fin. Comm. Rpt.* at 265.
122.   See *Perkins Report* generally.
123.   §1152(b)(1)(A); 42 USC §1320c–1(b)(1)(A).
124.   §§1152(b),(c); 42 USC §§1320c–1(b),(c).
125.   §1152(c)(2); 42 USC §§1320c–1(c).
126.   *Sen. Fin. Comm. Rpt.* at 259–260.

Chapter Five

Hearings and Review

Of the separate PSRO provisions, the hearings and review section of the PSRO statute (and the provisions on norms[1]) will have the most direct effects on patients. The importance of implementing the hearings and review provisions with special consideration for consumers' needs cannot be overemphasized, because it is hearings and review mechanisms which provide the means for guaranteeing and safeguarding the rights of patients throughout the PSRO system.

Although the Medicare and Medicaid programs have both held up the doctor-patient relationship to some degree of scrutiny, PSROs will intrude more directly in the delivery of medical care to the poor and aged populations. These two primary programs[2] subject to PSRO jurisdiction have already in some ways estranged the patient from his physician through inevitable bureaucracies and hierarchical review of individual physician determinations—through utilization review and paying agents' activities. In some cases these trends have denied to patients the freedom of choice in their medical care they might otherwise enjoy if they could pay for their care or afford good private health insurance. With the additional developments brought by PSROs, it is crucial to ensure that hearings and review mechanisms are properly established so that patients have at least this minimal ability to assert themselves as individuals in PSRO processes.[3]

The language of the statute establishes a formal procedure by reference to other existing systems of review: primarily to Old Age and Survivors Disability Insurance hearings (Social Security)[4] and, by implication, to the Medicare appeals system. The PSRO program's hearings and review provisions do not confront at all the problems in creating a unified appeals mechanism in a single system of review over medical services rendered under two different programs— Medicare and Medicaid.[5] The beneficiaries of those programs have, until now, been subject to two very different procedural systems for review of determinations of medical necessity and coverage. There is no elucidating legislative history on the PSRO provision (and therefore no explanation for the apparent choice of the Medicare review system model for PSROs).

The different appeals systems of Medicare and Medicaid will continue to function on issues over which PSROs have no authority.[6] But, because PSROs were created in part to coordinate review and management of *all* medical determinations affecting coverage of Medicare and Medicaid patients, proper interpretation of §1159[7] through regulations must consider an orderly analysis of each of the preexisting systems, an analysis the apparent statutory choice seems not to have taken into account. To look to one program alone as the model for the PSRO appeals structure not only fails to incorporate the advantages of both programs (and so avoid replication of previous failures and disadvantages), but also may severely diminish rights of one class of recipients which are already firmly established. For example, from the earliest history of Medicaid, recipients have established rights to hearings and judicial review of most determinations affecting them, based on their judicially recognized statutory entitlement to benefits.[8] But Medicare traditionally has been regarded by its administrators as an insurance program, and courts have not found in the Medicare program the same kind of legal entitlements to benefits. Accordingly, Medicare patients have never been able to win for themselves the kind of wide-ranging procedural rights Medicaid recipients have enjoyed, but may lose under the PSRO scheme.[9] This is not to imply that Medicaid patients have been given favored treatment, nor that in practice they receive "fairer" hearings; only that the letter of the law provides more opportunities for Medicaid patients to pursue determinations adverse to them.

The formalities and technical procedures granted by law (and labeled "fair hearings" by lawyers and bureaucrats) do not *necessarily* guarantee fairness or a favorable outcome to the party seeking the hearing. A hearing examiner's prejudices, the patient's inability to obtain or understand relevant medical records, a physician's refusal to testify for the patient, and the patient's inability to obtain a lawyer are all factors which can influence the process and outcome of a "fair" hearing. While those are critical factors in ensuring the patient's ability to present his case effectively, the premise of this discussion is that without at least the legal obligation to provide patients with procedural opportunities to present their cases, there will be no chance to challenge governmental decisions; and those decisions and their makers will then be entirely unaccountable. Without procedural rights there will be, then, no context in which to attempt to solve the problems of factors which unfairly influence the course of a hearing, such as those cited above.

To further the interests of consumer-patients faced with adverse PSRO determinations, this section (1) outlines the process and deficiencies of the Medicaid and Medicare hearings and review systems, (2) suggests possible interpretations of the PSRO statute, and (3) on the basis of those analyses proposes actions which the Secretary should implement to begin to resolve past inequities and to serve better the interests of patients in the PSRO process.

MEDICAID

The Medicaid program has generally guaranteed more procedural rights to recipients than the Medicare program has. Disputes over Medicaid claims arise retrospectively and prospectively. Prospective claims are claims for services brought under the "prior authorization" mechanism. Under federal regulations a state may provide for authorization for payment of medical services before they are delivered, where the services are those which could not be required on an emergency basis (often these include eyeglasses, dentures, or prosthetic devices). In order for a Medicaid patient to obtain those specified services (varying from state to state), the prior authorization from the state must be granted. When it is granted, a denial of coverage after services are rendered is precluded. If the authorization is denied, the recipient can appeal that determination to the same extent that appeals are generally provided for in the Medicaid program. Although the state has discretion in determining whether and under what circumstances to use prior authorizations, once the state program provides for their use they are mandatory. Patients can be penalized by the state's refusing to pay for services at all, if the services for which a claim is presented should have been authorized before they were rendered.[10] Although a prior authorization can give the patient a definite answer on coverage before he or she might incur liability for uncovered services, in practice prior authorizations can be a harsh review system, effectively denying patients access to institutions when authorizations are denied, and requiring long waits and bureaucratic red tape, in some cases until the patient's condition is so serious a prior authorization can no longer be used.[11] Retrospective review—after services have been rendered and a claim for payment for them is presented—is more commonly used.

Medicaid "fair hearings" have been available "to any applicant who requests a hearing because his claim for financial or medical assistance is denied, or is not acted upon with reasonable promptness, and to any recipient who is aggrieved by agency action resulting in suspension, reduction, discontinuance, or termination of assistance."[12] The statutory authority for that regulation requires a state to provide ". . . for granting an opportunity for a fair hearing before the State agency to any individual whose claim for medical assistance under the plan is denied or is not acted upon with promptness."[13]

Who seeks a hearing depends on the situation. Review of determinations denying a prior authorization (claims for services) are generally sought by the patient-recipient. Appeals from retrospective determinations (claims for payment) are ordinarily brought by "vendor-providers"—physicians or institutions rendering medical services—because under federal Medicaid laws (except for highly unusual circumstances) payments are made directly to providers, not to patients.[14]

Although there is no recognized federal law on the subject, because Medicaid patients are indigent by definition, some state courts have imposed strict requirements of "self-help" on health service providers seeking payment from patients when administrative appeals have been adverse to the provider's interests. Federal law, through regulation, requires Medicaid providers to accept the state's payment for covered services and forbids providers to look to the patient for additional payment if the state pays less than the amount requested.[15] Although the provider may seek payment from a recipient for non-covered services, there are cases which have considered suits against recipients for payment improper, regardless of the effect of coverage determinations. In *Knickerbocker Hospital* v. *Downing*,[16] the hospital sought to recover payment from indigent parents for services provided to their infant son. The infant was the Medicaid recipient and the hospital was aware of that fact, but sought to recover the payment on a theory of parental responsibility for necessary services supplied to an infant. The court held for the parents and said, "The commencement of the lawsuit itself against these defendants is improper since it requires an indigent, unable to pay for his medical care and assistance, to defend himself in a lawsuit brought to recover the charges for the very thing he is too indigent to pay."[17] In a similar case, *Society of New York Hospital* v. *Mogensen*,[18] the hospital sought to recover payment from a Medicaid recipient who had obtained a prior authorization for services. The court held that the hospital must look to the state agency for payment. Recognizing that there was no federal law on the point, the court said,

> The Social Services Law does not specifically address itself to the question of whether a Medicaid vendor who treats a recipient can bill the recipient for services rendered. However, it is clear that such a proposition is totally incompatible with the stated purposes [of the program] which were to provide . . . a comprehensive program of medical assistance for needy persons . . . which will assure a uniform high standard of medical assistance throughout the state.[19]

A more recent case also held a hospital responsible for helping a patient complete processes which would establish his right to coverage; because the hospital failed to meet that responsibility it could not later seek payment.[20] Because of the duties imposed on them, provider institutions and physicians most often seek review of Medicaid determinations denying payment, although the relevant federal authorities give that right to patients as well. As a practical matter, many Medicaid patients are judgment-proof: they have no assets against which a court could execute an order to pay the provider, even if the provider won in a suit against them. The provider, therefore, has good reason to seek his rights vigorously against the state. Many other Medicaid patients, however, are not judgment-proof and their right to appeal adverse determinations is an important one; of these nondestitute patients many are the so-called "medically needy," who do *not* receive welfare or other state assistance, but whose medical expenses are so great compared with their income that they qualify for Medicaid.[21] The "medically needy," in particular, have an interest in seeking to assure coverage by the state to protect their minimal assets.

Through the fair hearing mechanism, the Medicaid recipient, or the provider derivatively, seeks to establish his or her rights to participate in the program (eligibility) and to receive its benefits (entitlements), and the amount of benefits to be covered. The federal regulations[22] specifically require states to provide for these hearings in accordance with standards set forth in the case of *Goldberg* v. *Kelly*.[23] Notice of determinations and of the right to a hearing must be given in writing to the patient; representation must be permitted at the hearing; a record must be kept; cross-examination of adverse witnesses must be permitted; and an impartial hearing examiner must conduct the hearings. These elements which characterize a "fair hearing" were found by the court in *Goldberg* to be constitutionally required and to provide the best context for assuring fairness.

Recent changes in the federal Medicaid regulations may have conditioned the *Goldberg*-required elements in an unconstitutional way. In *Goldberg,* the court held that welfare recipients must be given an opportunity to challenge agency action to be taken against them *before* the agency executes its decision. The new regulations change this broad principle in two ways: (1) They permit a state to provide either a hearing before the state agency itself[24] or an evidentiary hearing at the local level with a right of appeal to a state agency hearing.[25] The hearing immediately before the state agency can put an additional hardship on recipients by requiring them to travel to an office less convenient to them; but, more important, it eliminates the additional chance for review which the local hearing with appeal to the state agency can provide. (2) In addition, the new regulations permit a change in the notice requirements established in *Goldberg.* Under that case "timely" notice of agency action— *before* the agency acts on its decision—must be given to the patient in written form. Under the new regulations, under certain circumstances timely notice may be dispensed with in favor of "adequate notice," given at the time the agency executes its decision.[26] Among those permissible situations especially relevant to Medicaid patients whose care is reviewed by PSROs are (a) when "the recipient has been placed in skilled nursing care, intermediate care or long-term hospitalization";[27] or (b) when "a change in level of medical care is prescribed by the recipient patient's physician."[28]

Under the Medicaid program, rights to judicial review of state agency decisions are liberal. Claims may be presented in state court, where no jurisdictional amount applies, or in federal court, where a claim worth $10,000 must be presented with other appropriate claims for jurisdiction.[29]

MEDICARE

Detailed consideration of issues in Medicare hearings and review must focus on the two separate Medicare programs: Part A—Hospital Insurance,[30] and Part B— Supplementary Medical Insurance.[31] Within both contexts, Medicare generally affords fewer rights to beneficiaries in comparison with Medicaid. The statutory language establishing the hearings and appeals mechanisms is, however, very similar to that of the PSRO statute, as is discussed in further detail below.

The first obstacle to better Medicare hearing rights has been the federal government's insistence on a claim for payment before granting the right to a hearing, based on its. characterization of Medicare as an insurance program. The government has claimed that the requirement established in *Goldberg* v. *Kelly* that the claimant has a right to a hearing *before* final agency action (prior review) does not apply in Medicare because appeals of determinations of claims for services do not "involve termination of monies since" patients are not at the point "in payment status."[32] Essentially, then, the argument is that since no payments have yet been made, no termination is effected by the agency's action, so no need for a hearing arises. The government considers the decision on the claim for payment to be the "initial determination" under the law in a Medicare case. The government asserts it is not until then that a hearing need be provided. In one case where a Medicare beneficiary claimed the right to a hearing before the state denied him nursing home benefits following his hospital stay, the government made the following distinction:

> In contrast to Title XVIII (Part A) payments which are not predicated on need, in the welfare context need is the essential criterion to establish the substantive right to payment of benefits; in the Part A, Title XVIII context ... the criterion to establish the substantive right to payment of benefits is that the insured wage earner receive ... services of a medical nature to be covered under the Act.[33]

Therefore, in Medicare, the government has required the delivery of services and a claim for payment for them before it will hold a Medicare hearing. This insistence may be unconstitutional under *Goldberg* v. *Kelly*. In *Goldberg* v. *Kelly* the state had provided for a hearing *after* it had terminated the welfare recipient's benefits. Part of the Court's reasoning in establishing the right to a prior hearing rested on the fact that the applicability of due process was not at issue. Welfare benefits are a matter of statutory entitlement for persons qualified to receive them. The Court specifically noted that "... [i]t may be realistic today to regard welfare entitlements as more like 'property' than a 'gratuity.' "[34] Prior hearings have also been required in Medicaid, based on the same analysis. The government's asserted distinction in Medicare (that no "entitlement" exists), although more semantic than substantive, has been successful so far. The effect of the claim for payment requirement is that all appeals of Medicare determinations involve retroactive denials of coverage for services already rendered. The burden on the patient is enormous when he expected Medicare would cover those services and is unprepared to pay for them himself.[35]

Separate doctrines govern the retroactive appeals under Part A and Part B situations. Under Part A, the appeals process is initiated by submitting to the Social Security Administration (SSA) a "Request for Reconsideration," of the fiscal intermediary's initial determination.[36] SSA reconsiders its determination without giving the beneficiary opportunity to present evidence or cross-examine adverse witnesses.[37] If the amount of benefits in controversy under Part A (the cost of the services being disputed) is $100 or more, the beneficiary is advised of his right to a hearing by the Secretary, if he wants one because he is dissatisfied.[38] The hearing is conducted by a hearing examiner from the Bureau of Hearings and Appeals of the Social Security Administration.[39] Any party to the determination (anyone affected by the decision), including the government, can then request a review of an adverse hearing decision before the Appeals Council of SSA.[40] The Appeals Council also may initiate review of a hearing decision on its own motion. When the amount in controversy is $1,000 or more, the beneficiary has the right to judicial review of an Appeals Council decision (or review of its failure to review a hearing decision when requested).[41] Federal courts have original jurisdiction of Medicare claims cases, as in Title II (Social Security),[42] so, unlike Medicaid patients, Medicare beneficiaries cannot choose state court review; but they can get access to federal court without meeting the requirement of presenting a claim equal to $10,000.

Part B Supplementary Insurance Benefits appeals begin with the carrier's review of its own initial determination by the same carrier.[43] If the beneficiary is still dissatisfied, and if the amount in controversy is $100 or more, he may request a fair hearing conducted by the Social Security Administration.[44] The beneficiary may present evidence in person and may examine witnesses.[45] The hearing is final, subject only to reopening to correct procedural or substantive defects in the proceedings.[46] It is generally accepted that there is, now, no judicial review of a Part B determinations, per se.

The 1972 amendments clarify the exclusion of Part B determinations from judicial scrutiny. Judicial review is now available in three specific classes of cases: (1) entitlement disputes—whether the beneficiary qualifies as a wage earner for any benefits; (2) enrollment controversies—whether the patient is eligible to enroll in the program or has enrolled; and (3) disputes concerning "the amount of benefits under Part A (including a determination where such amount is determined to be zero)."[47] Prior to the change, the issue in the few court cases considering whether Part B disputes could be reviewed was distinguishing between controversies over "entitlement" and those on "amount of benefits."[48] The change in the law clearly restricts even further the beneficiary's ability to challenge an adverse Part B determination.

Because the Medicare beneficiary, unlike the Medicaid recipient, is responsible for portions of bills not paid by the government, beneficiaries are usually the parties seeking review of adverse determinations.[49] Under Part B, however, provision is made for optional assignment of claims to the physician.

As a practical matter the option is the physician's and nothing can force him to accept assignment. When the physician accepts assignment, payment is made directly to him according to carrier standards, eliminating liability of the beneficiary.[50] When the assignment is made, the physician cannot collect from the beneficiary any unpaid amounts of that bill.[51] As a result of the assignment, the physician gains, however, the same appeal rights the beneficiary would have enjoyed. Without assignment, any disputes over determinations are disputes between the patient and carrier, as in any insurance system. With assignment, the physician steps into the beneficiary's shoes and disputes are then between the physician and the carrier.

The Part A and Part B procedures just described apply to all retrospective Medicare hearings and review of entitlement, eligibility, coverage, and amount of benefits. The only Medicare procedure similar to prior Medicaid authorization was "Assurance of Payment." Under the "Assurance of Payment" procedure[52] whenever an extended care facility (ECF) (now called "skilled nursing facility") has reason to doubt the Medicare coverage of a newly admitted patient or the coverage of a patient's reduced level of care, the facility submits to its intermediary detailed information on the type and medical necessity of services provided. This procedure must begin within 48 hours of admission or whenever a dispute arises on a change in level of care. The intermediary then processes "promptly" such information and informs the facility of its decision on coverage. If in the intermediary's opinion the facility has, in the past, conscientiously followed the procedure, then even though the information presented might not clearly support coverage, the provider will be covered for a "reasonable number of days." The procedure, however, is limited in application to eligible, restricted institutions and doubtful coverage circumstances only. (It cannot be invoked where there is an outright refusal by the facility to accept the patient or its automatic provision of a lesser amount of services.) The procedure is conducted between provider and intermediary. The patient cannot appeal the determination even though as a practical matter he may be denied access to a skilled nursing facility on the basis of the intermediary's decision of no coverage.

The procedure has been deleted from federal regulations.[53] Since PSROs will be making level of care determinations for purposes of Medicare coverage, the "assurance of payment" mechanism will not be necessary if PSROs work effectively.

PSRO PROVISIONS

In addition to general principles of fairness, due process, and accountability, the nature of the PSRO system inherently creates the need for hearings and review. The need for administrative and judicial review of PSRO determinations exists because of the authority of PSROs to disapprove services and supplies as medically unnecessary, or inappropriate, thereby establishing that no federal moneys will be available for payment for those disapproved services or items.

When a PSRO makes a determination adverse to the interests of the patient, physician, or provider, that dissatisfied party will seek to establish either (1) that the determination was incorrect according to appropriate standards, or (2) that he was without fault in accepting or ordering such services. The first type of showing has been typical in Medicare and Medicaid hearings in the past, although now PSRO norms, criteria, and standards will provide part of the basis for evaluating the propriety of determinations. The second showing would be made because of 1972 changes in the law.

> The Senate Finance Committee established a second ground for overthrowing a decision of no medical necessity. Generally, where the PSRO disapproved items or services furnished under Medicare and Medicaid, payment for such items and services could not be made by these programs. However, provision is made for the Secretary to make payment for disapproved items and services where he determined that a claimant was without fault with respect to the provision of items or services. This provision is needed to prevent making individuals liable for payment for the disapproved services when they accepted services under the impression they would be paid by Medicare and Medicaid.[54]

The PSRO provision is in addition to a separate, similar Medicare "hold harmless" provision written into the 1972 Social Security Amendments.[55] Although the provisions are independent, the legislative history on the Medicare provision is indicative of how liability under the PSRO provision will be determined. Who failed to exercise due care is the basic test. If the beneficiary acted in good faith and had no notice that services would not be covered, he will be "held harmless," and will be absolved of liability; but the burden will then shift to the provider or the government. If the provider knew services would not be covered, the provider will be liable. If the provider acted in good faith, the government will bear the burden of the costs of the noncovered services. But when the provision is invoked, notice of noncoverage must be provided to beneficiary and provider, indicating that services of that type are not covered. Once such notice is given, in any future similar situations all participants will be deemed to have notice and thereby will not qualify for the "hold harmless" provision in the future in that type of case. The intent is to limit progressively the government's liability for such uncovered services.[56] The PSRO provision (subject to implementation through regulations issued by the Secretary) would apply to Medicaid patients, too.[57]

The Statutory Language

All PSRO hearings are provided for under the same provision. The process begins similarly to the Medicare procedures:

> Any beneficiary or recipient who is entitled to benefits under this Act (other than Title V) or a provider or practitioner who is dissatisfied with a determination with respect to a claim made by a Professional Standards Review Organization in carrying out its responsibilities for . . . review . . . shall, after being notified of such determination be entitled to a reconsideration thereof by the Professional Standards Review Organization . . . .[58]

Where the local PSRO affirms the original determination, and where the matter in controversy (disputed services) is $100 or more, the professional members of the Statewide Council will review the reconsidered determination; and if they so decide the determination will be revised.[59] Where the Statewide Council's determination is adverse to the beneficiary or recipient "such beneficiary or recipient shall be entitled to a hearing thereon by the Secretary to the same extent as is provided in section 205(b) . . . ."[60] In states where there is no Statewide Council,[61] the beneficiary has the right to an immediate hearing by the Secretary, if the amount in controversy is at least $100. The Secretary's decision may be rendered "only after appropriate professional consultation on the matter."[62] If the amount in controversy is $1,000 or more, after the Secretary's decision, the beneficiary is entitled to judicial review as provided in section 205(g), Social Security (Old Age, Survivor's Disability Insurance), and previously available under the Medicare provisions.[63] Hearings and review under the PSRO statute preempt any other review on the same issue;[64] so that a decision made by a PSRO cannot be appealed through the Medicare or Medicaid processes; nor may an appeal which has gone through the PSRO structure be brought again through either of the other two systems.

To the same extent, then, that the PSRO program supercedes both the Medicare and Medicaid systems for making determinations of medical necessity, quality, appropriateness, and availability of medical services, review of those determinations is preempted. The Medicare and Medicaid hearings and review structures will continue to function on questions of eligibility, entitlement (§1159 is not triggered until an entitlement under the new definitions is established),[65] and coverage (for example, whether the recipient exhausted coverage for that year, or whether allowable Medicare days in the hospital have been exhausted).[66]

The PSRO hearings and review scheme can deal with two major types of claims—claims for services *and* claims for payment—because the language in the statute refers to review of any "determination with respect to a claim."[67] As this chapter has discussed, under the Medicare system the government has always considered a claim to be a claim for payment for services already rendered.[68] On the other hand Medicaid, with its prior authorization mechanism and its generally broader procedural rights, has permitted review of claims for services as well. The PSRO statute links availability of review to whether the determination is part of the PSRO's authority to make determinations of past medical necessity, quality of care (both of which must be retrospective determinations), and, "where services are proposed" on an in-patient basis, that the facility is appropriate to supply the proposed services (clearly a prospective determination).[69] More explicitly, PSROs have the authority "to determine, in advance"[70] in cases of elective admissions or extended or costly courses of treatment, whether the proposed care meets the criteria on medical necessity and appropriateness of facility. It is clear, then, that review can be sought on PSRO determinations of claims for services as well as claims for payment—prospective and retrospective denials—giving to Medicare beneficiaries greater review rights than they enjoyed in the past.[71]

The general review scheme as laid out in the statute bears more resemblance to the Medicare system than to that of Medicaid. The only difference is that instead of the Social Security Administration (in Part A claims), or the carrier (under Part B), it is the PSRO itself which reviews its own decisions,[72] and responsibility for establishing the regulations on PSRO review are given to the same agencies which administered the old Medicare system—the Bureau of Health Insurance (BHI) and the Bureau of Hearings and Appeals (BHA).

Constitutional Challenges

The basic deficiencies in the PSRO hearings and review process are (1) the jurisdictional amount requirements in order to gain access to administrative review and judicial review, and (2) the preclusion to Medicaid recipients of state court review. The terms of the provision refer to and rely on the hearings and review system as established for Old Age Survivors and Disability Insurance (Social Security). But under that program there is no financial restriction on administrative review[73] and judicial review is provided for "any final decision of the Secretary, made after a hearing, *irrespective of the amount in controversy.*"[74] Although there is no legislative history discussing the obvious congressional decision to limit review, the usual explanation is that "Congress did not want to overburden HEW and the courts with small claims."[75]

The hearings and review provision can be challenged on several grounds as ignoring significant consumer interests and needs in an attempt to alleviate HEW's and the court system's administrative burdens. Medicaid recipients are necessarily unable to afford medical services. They have never been subject to jurisdictional amount conditions for administrative review or judicial review in state court. (They are, of course, subject to federal court restrictions.) A so-called "small claim," up to $100, can mean to them the difference between being able to buy their basic necessities and struggling to provide for themselves out of the meager sums left to them after an unfavorable judgment. (For many Medicaid recipients this can mean they will have to use their welfare moneys to pay a medical debt levied on them as a result of an adverse PSRO determination. Others will pay the debt from incomes which were so low that they qualified as "medically needy." [76]) Many Medicare recipients live on fixed incomes (Social Security payments, small pensions) and the effect to them would be similar. Although providing a hearing does not *necessarily* guarantee a decision favorable to the beneficiary or recipient, it does grant the patient the best opportunity to present his case effectively and to challenge the PSRO's. Where the claim involved is less than $100, the only reconsideration available to the patient is by the very entity (the PSRO) which acted against him in the first instance. The provision also has the effect of penalizing healthier patients who do not need more than $100 worth of services.

Some may argue that with today's high costs of health care few patients will be unable to meet the $100 amount even after only one episode of care. But PSROs are also expected eventually to review ambulatory services, which generally do not entail such high costs. Is there to be no fair hearing on any dispute involving ambulatory care? If we assume that most patients reviewed by PSROs will use medical services more than once, the effect of the jurisdictional amount requirements is to "nickel and dime" the patient "to the wall."[77]

The effect of the PSRO preemption of hearings and review is to foreclose to Medicaid patients the ability to bring claims in state court. Medicaid is financed with state and federal funds (unlike Medicare which is purely federal)[78] and the program is administered through a state plan scheme; jurisdiction in state courts over issues of coverage based on medical necessity has always been available. The PSRO provision eliminates Medicaid patients' rights to state court review which is exercised more easily than the right to sue in federal court. Not the least significant distinction between state and federal courts is the state court's more local nature and greater proximity to recipients.[79]

Whether or not, as a practical matter, the $100 restriction is a bar to administrative review, two legal issues arise for the consumer advocate: (1) a challenge to the restriction on administrative review, and (2) a challenge to the $1,000 amount restriction on judicial review.

The Need for Administrative Review. The argument against the amount in controversy limitation on administrative review begins with a list of the circumstances when appeal from a PRSO determination would be necessary. One of the goals of the PSRO review process is to eliminate most retroactive denials of coverage, which are unfair to the patient as well as the provider. In order to effect that reduction, the emphasis in review is on prospective review (determinations of coverage before services are rendered) and concurrent review (determining while the patient is in the institution whether he should stay longer or go elsewhere). These types of review encompass those decisions which have been labeled "level-of-care determinations."[80] (e.g., Does the patient need acute care in a hospital, extended care in a skilled nursing facility, or a lower level of care in an intermediate care facility?) Applying the labels for the levels of care now may be even more difficult, because PSRO review will be based on norms and medical necessity. But the effect of the PSRO's decisions will be similar to simple label application. The following chart below demonstrates the range of situations where disputes will arise.

Chart I

When the request is made:	*What is requested*	*PSRO Decision*
Prior to any access	Hospital admission	Denied
	Hospital admission	Other facility
	Nursing home admission	Denied
While in the hospital	Extended stay	Denied
	Extended stay	Other facility
	Nursing home admission	Denied
While in nursing home	Hospital admission	Denied
	Extended stay in nursing home	Denied

If the PSRO approves the request, no need for an administrative hearing will arise. But, in each of the situations above, the beneficiary, at least, (and in some cases the physician) will seek to press the claim for services. The alliance of the physician in the patient's appeal will be necessary because the law implies that a physician's order is required before the PSRO can entertain the claim in the first place.[81] It appears from the nature of the scheme that if the physician and patient disagree among themselves, the PSRO is not in a position to resolve the dispute. The PSRO can only evaluate professional, medical judgments which adjudicate the beneficiary's rights derivatively by their effect. This reliance on, and the weight given to, physician determinations in the delivery of health care is a trend which has been given judicial sanction. Under the old system, the physician's opinion was given great weight by law[82] and the support of the physician's opinion alone often changed the court's decision to favor the patient.[83] Also, in judicial review of other types of health care issues the role of the physician has been critical, as in the recent abortion cases, for example, where courts have held that the only allowable condition on the patient's right to abortion in the first three months of pregnancy is the concurrence of the physician.[84]

The $100 restriction on administrative review means that patients must challenge the restriction itself or find a way to combine the value of proposed services (or past services and those which would continue past treatment in the future) to reach the $100 amount. The ability to use such an aggregation of claims will depend on the Secretary's regulations. There is nothing in the law or legislative history precluding such action. But why is it so important for a patient to have an adverse decision reviewed in the context of a "fair hearing" *before* the PSRO's determination becomes effective and final? Again, reference to *Goldberg* v. *Kelly* provides the answer. In that case, where the court held that only a hearing prior to termination of benefits could assure due process, the Supreme Court reiterated the lower court's reasoning:

> While post-termination review is relevant, there is one over-powering fact which controls here. By hypothesis, a welfare recipient is destitute, without funds or assets. . . . Suffice it to say that to cut off a welfare recipient in the face of . . . "brutal need" without a prior hearing of some sort is unconscionable, unless overwhelming considerations justify it.[85]

In the PSRO context, the patient's "brutal need" is a need for medical services to prolong or sustain life itself. In any situation where proposed services are involved, whether of a value of $100 or not, that "brutal need" is present. Where retrospective review alone is involved, the patient will have already received the medical services, and his need becomes somewhat different. His need is to obtain a decision which will not force him to use his minimal assets to meet a judgment which might be reversed anyway. (Whether the patient faced with a retrospective denial presents sufficiently brutal need, will be a decision for the courts.) But because PSROs, if effective, will eliminate most retroactive denials, most patients will face a situation of brutal need when a PSRO denies them services which they and their physicians have proposed. In *Goldberg* the court held that a judicial or quasi-judicial hearing was not necessary at the pretermination stage; in the PSRO's review that stage occurs at the points indicated in Chart I after the PSRO's initial decision. The required elements previously referred to—timely and adequate notice, detailed statement of the reasons for the agency's decision, an effective opportunity to defend by confronting adverse witnesses, and a right to present an oral defense—should be provided to the recipient at those points. Under the law as it is written, that hearing will take place only if the matter in controversy is $100 or more.

Two recent cases directly relevent to PSROs held that prior hearings according to *Goldberg* standards were required where levels of care were changed.[86] In *Bell* v. *Heim*,[87] a Medicaid case in New Mexico, a PSRO-type review system had been established.[88] The court entered a stipulated order that a *Goldberg* hearing must be held for each patient subject to a change in his level of care as a result of redefinitions of nursing home levels of care. In *Martinez* v. *Richardson*,[89] a pre-PSRO Medicare case, (although the class claim was denied) the court held similarly to *Bell* when it said that the beneficiary must be afforded a *Goldberg* hearing where reduction or termination of home health care benefits was involved.

It is precisely because of the needs and interests recognized in these three cases—*Goldberg, Bell,* and *Martinez*—that changes in the federal Medicaid regulations may be vulnerable to attack on constitutional grounds. The elements guaranteed in *Goldberg* were minimal elements. At least those must be provided, according to the due process clause of the Constitution. Although *Goldberg* required timely and adequate notice, one of the new Medicaid regulations permits the agency to dispense with timely notice as long as adequate notice is provided when the recipient has been placed in skilled nursing care, intermediate care, or long term hospitalization, or when a change in level of care is prescribed by the recipient patient's physician.[90] Under the new regulations, timely notice means 10 days before the intended change would be effective;[91] adequate notice means a written notice stating the intended action and reason for it, the right to request a hearing, and a statement on whether assistance is to be continued.[92] When the agency does dispense with timely notice, adequate notice is to be sent "not later than the date of action."[93] The regulations give no indication of their application to PSRO determinations, although clearly the types of situations involved are those situations where PSROs will have authority to act. The regulations are vague. Does notice "not later than the action" mean that as the patient is being transferred to a different facility he or she will be told that a hearing about that very transfer is available? To which action does the regulation refer? Action can mean the determination that the agency will, at a later point, execute its determination or it can mean the execution itself. The regulation refers to the authority to dispense with timely notice when the recipient "has been placed" in a long term care facility.[94] Of what value is notice when the recipient has already been transferred?

In order to ensure that the dictates of *Goldberg* v. *Kelly* are followed, the Secretary must provide that the PSRO hearings regulations guarantee the presence of three additional elements in the hearing: (1) timeliness of review; (2) an impartial examiner; and (3) adequate and effective patient participation.

Timeliness will be a critical factor in all the situations indicated in the chart.[95] In each of those circumstances, if the PSRO's determination is incorrect, failure to act quickly can result in serious and irreparable injury to the patient. The value of a swift and equitable determination to the patient is beyond measurement, and should, therefore, be stringently required of PSROs. In the Medicaid prior authorization system the need for immediate consideration has been noted by the federal guidelines on such programs. Because prior authorizations may not be required by any state for those services ". . . which generally need to be performed on an emergency or immediate basis, patients should not suffer from the short delay involved in securing the necessary professional approval."[96] The guidelines further provide that requests not acted on in sufficient time should be automatically approved.[97] Similar timing standards should be applied appropriately to PSROs; furthermore, when the initial determination is made by the utilization review committee and an inappropriate delay results, the committee should be held to the same standard as the PSRO. Automatic approval precluding a retroactive denial should result from inordinate delays.[98] At that point, however, the patient may have already suffered the injury.[99] The primary emphasis in the Secretary's regulations must be placed on establishing a swift and efficient review process. It may well be that patients' needs for quick review are so great that an adversary process which may serve to delay a decision should be dispensed with in favor of a different, but equitable, expedited procedure.

An impartial hearing examiner is essential. An examiner with a direct interest in the decision (e.g., the attending physician, a member of the staff of the institution involved) will not be likely to make an objective determination. Similarly, the likelihood that the reviewer who made the initial decision would overrule himself is minimal. The PSRO statute does exclude from review responsibilities those physicians with conflicts of interest in cases being considered at the *initial* stages of review.[100] Similar restrictions must be imposed in regulations on later review. Of particular importance is the fact that in those cases where the statute denies the patient the right to a hearing by the Secretary, the only review available under the statute is a reconsideration by the same PSRO which initially reviewed the case. At the very least, the Secretary should assure that a group of PSRO members different from those rendering the initial determination exercise the reconsideration responsibility. Although there still may exist incentives to reaffirm their colleagues' original judgment for nonprofessional reasons (out of cronyism or a desire to avoid polarization and dissent within the PSRO), the chances will be greater that, if good reasons are presented, a reversal of the initial decision will result.

The third element which the Secretary should guarantee is the patient's effective participation in the hearing. The *Goldberg* court offered to the recipient the right to bring counsel to the hearing.

> Counsel can help delineate the issues, present the factual contentions in an orderly manner, conduct cross-examination and generally safeguard the interests of the recipient. We do not anticipate that this assistance will unduly prolong or otherwise encumber the hearing.[101]

In review of a PSRO's determination, effective representation is even more important because most of the information at issue will be highly technical. (It should go without saying that for the hearing the patient (or at least his representative) must be given access to his medical record, and in every situation where he is given notice that a hearing is available, he must also be told that his medical record can be made available to him.

The patient's attending physician, who, by the nature of the scheme, [102] will support the patient in all prior review cases (and may often have concurrent interests in retrospective review), is in the best position to be a true advocate for his patient. Clearly, he can be expected to have mastery over the essential facts in the case. Unfortunately, physician participation in such hearings usually has been only at the request of the patient. In some cases where the service-oriented physician seeks to establish good will or feels particularly strongly about the medical aspects of the case, he or she will voluntarily set forth information on the patient's behalf. The PSRO statute does provide for direct, immediate notice of PSRO denials to be sent to the physician or provider and requires that notice be given of the basis for the determination and an opportunity be given for discussion and review of the matter. [103] This provision should greatly facilitate informal resolution of disputes. If the adverse determination can be resolved easily, without a formal appeal, by correcting misinformation or supplementing incomplete information, the physician can provide the necessary data without undue burden on the patient to initiate such activity. Of course, notice of all such transactions should be sent to the patient contemporaneously.

But voluntary participation by the physician to the benefit of the patient will depend on a highly motivated service-oriented physician who has the time and inclination to engage in activities which may not directly redound to his benefit. Such a system would cast many patients into a situation of distinct disadvantage. Should their physician be unable or unwilling to advocate for them they will have no adequate way to ensure that their interests are properly represented. As the court noted in *Goldberg*, [104] self-representation in a procedure which depends heavily on the written word is unfeasible, unrealistic, and unfair for poor, elderly people who lack the medical expertise they need in this process.

Several types of programs could ameliorate this situation. A small claims court for health issues, informally run, with special assistants and assistance available to help the patient with his claim might further the patient's interest while facilitating communication between physician and patient. When a patient must look outside his doctor-patient relationship for help which could be easily provided by the physician, it is a reasonable assumption that good communication is lacking.

A different type of patient advocate program could be implemented. Patient advocates whose responsibility it would be to initiate immediate appeals of PSRO denials, acting as liaison between patient, provider, and physician, would need some medical training to deal with the complexities of the information required in the hearings and review process. Where the PSRO review mechanism itself is not equipped to handle physician-patient or patient-provider dispute, patient advocates could function as independent grievance arbitrators in a system where patients may feel they have been estranged from their physician. If they were based in the hospital (or nursing facility) itself, the advocates would

be accessible to patients and able to obtain cooperation from the staff of that
institution with regard to the claims in which they are involved. With a medically
trained person reviewing the information in the case with an eye toward the
patient's interest (a nurse, paramedic, or specially trained paralegal could serve),
physicians and providers might lose some of the fears—that records would be
misunderstood—often cited to preclude their release to patients. Provision of
office space and cooperation by the hospital (or other facility) could be imposed
as conditions for participation in the Medicare and Medicaid programs as well as
preconditions to delegation of duties by the PSRO to the institutional utilization
review committee. By imposing those conditions, compliance would be assured
and the advocates would achieve the requisite credibility and respectability
necessary for cooperation by physicians. Location in the institution would
facilitate quick processing of appeals involving extended stays or transfers to a
different type of facility, minimizing harm and anguish to the patient as a result
of delay.[105]

 A variety of approaches might be taken, the details of which should
depend on demonstrated evidence of patient needs. After some initial experience
with PSROs, identification of specifically needed reforms will be possible. It is
safe to predict, however, that some technique will be necessary to facilitate
liaison between patients and physicians, and patients and institutions, if the
PSRO system is to act in the patient's interests quickly, efficiently, and
simply. [106] In addition, it will undoubtedly be necessary to teach physicians and
consumers how to use the hearing and review system. No participant can
properly decide to press for review unless he understands the jurisdiction, scope
of review, and purpose of the appeals mechanism.[107]

 Due Process. Policy considerations alone may be sufficient to
persuade the Secretary to issue regulations as indicated above. The interests
advocated in the discussion of the need for administrative review are legitimate
and important and should be persuasive in themselves. The strongest arguments,
sufficient to *compel* such action, would rest on legal doctrines. The following
discussion examines those arguments and considers potential obstacles to their
success.

 The Fifth Amendment of the United States Constitution guarantees
that "No person shall be . . . deprived of life, liberty, or property, without due
process of law . . . ." This amendment applies to the federal government. The
PSRO law is a federal law passed by the United States Congress. The
bureaucracy it establishes is a *federal* bureaucracy. As a practical matter, this was
made clear by the Senate Finance Committee: "Where the Federal Government
has paid for or supplied necessary equipment to the review organizations, title to
such property would remain with the government." [108] No aspect of the PSRO
program is administered by any of the 50 states as the scheme is presently
created. [109] The Secretary of HEW administers and governs the program. He

issues regulations controlling the activities of each of the three levels of PSRO administration: national, state, and local. Every entity in the PSRO scheme—from the National Council to the local PSROs—has only that authority to review Medicare and Medicaid services expressly given to it by the federal statute and the Secretary's interpretation of the statute. The contracts between the Secretary and the local PSROs legally bind the PSROs to perform those activities which the Secretary chooses to contract for, and their fulfillment of those contracts is governed by the Secretary's regulations.[110]

The activities of the PSRO system are governed exclusively by federal law and, therefore, the Fifth Amendment will apply to the program's operations. The requirements of due process—that is, the substance of what is *due* to a beneficiary or recipient—is governed by a flexible standard. "[W]hether the Constitution requires that a particular right obtain in a specific proceeding depends upon a complexity of factors . . . the nature of the alleged right involved, the nature of the proceeding, and the possible burden on that proceeding."[111] Courts will apply that principle in any litigation seeking to interject into the PSRO hearings and review process any of those elements which would make the system more consumer-responsive (e.g., elimination of jurisdictional amount requirements, requirements for patient advocates). In order to apply the principle, courts must determine whether any challenge to the PSRO system alleging denial of due process presents a showing of deprivation of life, liberty, or property. In the situation where a patient is denied a prior approval of services and is precluded from a hearing because of failure to meet the $100 amount requirement, he or she can allege deprivation of life. (No court, however, has yet held the right to medical services per se to be a constitutionally protected fundamental right.) In addition, the patient's interest in government health benefits is in the nature of a property right, and denying benefits without due process would violate the Fifth Amendment.[112]

The challenge to the $100 exclusion on administrative review based on the Fifth Amendment due process clause can rely on several legal grounds: (1) Those patients who cannot meet the amount are entitled to no *legal* process governed by legal standards and precedents at all. They have only the reconsideration of the PSRO itself, a process not subject to any specific strictures to guarantee fairness; or, if their state has a Statewide Council, they can have an additional review by the Council. At no time, under the present scheme, do patients needing less than $100 worth of services have access to a hearing subject to specific standards established in *Goldberg* v. *Kelly*. (2) There is no compelling state interest sufficient to override the patient's right to a fair hearing. The only interest so far asserted is that in not overloading the hearings mechanism with petty claims. The additional burden of providing full hearings to that class of patients unable to meet the $100 exclusion is not so great for the government that it should be permitted to resist successfully giving to that class the hearing rights the law requires it to offer to others. (3) The preemption of a substantial portion of Medicaid hearings, never before so conditioned, is not based on a compelling state interest. The government, therefore, should be required to meet the standards it was previously held to before PSROs. Because the PSRO hearing system is unified, once granted to Medicaid recipients, those rights under the PSRO scheme must also be given to Medicare beneficiaries.[113]

The Condition on Judicial Review. The arguments relevant to the $100 precondition to administrative review are applicable to the PSRO statute's restriction on judicial review. The law places a condition of $1,000 amount in controversy on the patient's right to obtain judicial review of the Secretary's decision adverse to him (or her). Similarly, patients seeking judicial review may find it necessary to aggregate claims to reach the $1,000 amount,[114] subject to the Secretary's regulations.

Review by a court of law, in the American judicial system, provides the satisfaction of finality which can never be fully achieved in an administrative hearing. Also, any defects which occur in the hearings process can only be dealt with through litigation; because even the Secretary himself cannot unilaterally alter the hearing or change the procedures governing its process in order to correct a defect alleged to have existed during the process. Only a court or a legislature can remedy that situation. But the single greatest problem with the $1,000 exclusion lies in the preemption in the PSRO statute of state court review of Medicaid claims. Dual jurisdiction (by statutory amendment) or elimination of the exclusion are the two courses which would correct the existing statutory choice to better serve patients.

The Fifth Amendment's due process clause provides the basis for a challenge to the statute. The success of a challenge, however, is by no means sure. As the Supreme Court has stated, few cases alleging denial of due process raise the issue of actual access to the courts.[115] *Boddie* v. *Connecticut,*[116] the most favorable Supreme Court decision to date on the right of indigents to access to judicial review, accepted the plaintiff's equal protection argument. The indigent plaintiff asserted that Connecticut's $50 filing fee requirement for divorce actions denied equal protection of the laws and due process to indigents unable to pay the fee. Although that case is different from the PSRO law because it involved action by the state of Connecticut, and therefore the Fourteenth Amendment,[117] the Supreme Court has held that "[t]he 'equal protection of the laws' is a more explicit safeguard of prohibited unfairness than 'due process of law.' "[118] So if the Fourteenth Amendment requires specific procedures, the Fifth Amendment should require at least those.

Boddie v. *Connecticut,* seemed to establish the broad principle that government cannot exclude poor people from access to a government service through the imposition of financial eligibility conditions (1) if the right being conditioned is a constitutionally protected fundamental right and (2) if the government has a monopoly over the service. In *Boddie,* because there was no way to dissolve a marriage in Connecticut but through a divorce suit, the state could not limit poor people's ability to obtain a divorce by requiring a $50 payment to file a divorce suit. While there is a distinction between a requirement to pay a fee out-of-pocket before gaining access to review (as in *Boddie*), and a precondition of incurred liability without necessarily having paid anything (as under the PSRO system), the basic factor of a financial condition on entitlement to due process is common to both situations. An additional distinction between *Boddie* and the PSRO context is that under the PSRO law, while the class discriminated against is poor, they are treated separately as a class because they are healthier than those patients needing more than $1,000 worth of services.

Despite the apparent appeal of *Boddie* for use in a challenge to the PSRO judicial review provision, the Supreme Court issued a contrary decision in a case similar to *Boddie*. In *U.S.* v. *Kras,* [119] the Court dealt with the issue of a $50 filing fee required prior to discharge of bankruptcy. Distinguishing *Kras* from *Boddie,* the Court held that the filing fee did not violate the equal protection rights of indigents because "[g]aining or not gaining a discharge will effect no change with respect to basic necessities" [120] for an indigent. Bankruptcy, the Court said, was not the only method to resolve debts, and was not a fundamental right. Despite the distinctions between filing fee and amount in controversy preconditions on the right to judicial review, after *Kras* it seemed that a successful challenge to the PSRO statute (relying on *Boddie*) might be mounted by distinguishing the PSRO system from bankruptcy actions. Those arguments might include the following:

Like the divorce court situation, PSROs are entirely government-created, and by virtue of their preemption of Medicare and Medicaid review are the only effective means of resolving disputes around adverse PSRO determinations. Because the PSRO law does not provide a full administrative hearing to all beneficiaries and recipients suffering adverse decisions, the judicial system is the *only* forum available to them to pursue their rights. In light of the fact that Medicaid recipients are, by their status, unable to pay their medical bills (and that many Medicare patients are poor and live on meager fixed incomes), their incurring the risk of liability for $1,000 is so great for them that it can jeopardize their ability to obtain the "basic necessities"[121] in life.[122] The PSRO statute's condition on the right to judicial review raises a question of the fundamental fairness of the PSRO system. Even though all patients are not denied judicial review (only if their claims involve less than $1,000), neither was the $50 fee in *Boddie* a complete bar to judicial review. (In *Boddie* the fee denied access only to those who could not have afforded $100.) Finally, the fact that access is restricted only at the higher levels of review in no way defeats the argument, because, as the *Boddie* court recognized, the right to appeal is an essential part of the right to be heard in the first instance.[123] Limiting judicial review to those situations where the matter in controversy is $1,000 or more similarly violates the rights to due process and equal protection of the laws, with particularly pernicious effects for Medicaid recipients.

A court still may find those arguments persuasive. Unfortunately, though, the Supreme Court, most recently, has followed the *Kras* course. In *Ortwein* v. *Schwab*, [124] the Court held that Oregon's judicial filing fees were not unconstitutional when applied to a poor person, unable to afford the fee, who sought review of a welfare agency's decision. The Court said the recipient's interest in welfare benefits was of less constitutional significance than an interest in obtaining a divorce; and that the administrative hearing that Oregon had provided was an acceptable alternative to judicial review. The decision in *Ortwein* emphatically demonstrates the critical, bottom line need for an administrative hearing on every determination adverse to the patient.[125]

Further Considerations

Opening access to judicial review will not, in itself, solve the problem of granting meaningful due process rights to a patient seeking review of adverse administrative decisions. Chart I [126] presents those circumstances when an administrative hearing will be necessary. In each of those circumstances, if after a full hearing (or another type of expeditied procedure) the determination is still adverse to the beneficiary or recipient, he will often seek to pursue his rights further. But the American judicial system is maladapted to expedited processes. With crowded dockets and protracted procedures, judicial review may be of no value to the patient seeking PSRO approval of his proposed admission to a nursing home. As more patients, physicians, and providers avail themselves of their due process rights it will undoubtedly become necessary to devise new and better avenues and techniques to provide them with due process rights worth pursuing. Just as in the future attention should be devoted to the need for informal PSRO administrative hearings, further study and development of the system will be necessary to give meaning to the concept of due process in PSRO judicial review.

Notes for Chapter Five

1. §1156; 42 USC §1320c–5. See Chapter Two at 29 *supra.*
2. Title V recipients are also subject to PSRO authority. See Chapter One at 1 *supra.*
3. As Chapter Six discusses, consumers have been excluded from direct participation in the program. Because of the exclusion, there is little opportunity for systemic accountability generally. See Chapter Six at 177 *infra.* The hearings and review system will provide the sole method for ensuring accountability of the program to individual consumers, even if accountability to consumers generally has been foreclosed.
4. "...[S]uch beneficiary shall be entitled to a hearing thereon by the Secretary to the same extent as is provided in section 205(b), and, where the amount in controversy is $1,000 or more, the judicial review of the Secretary's final decision after such hearing as is provided in section 205(g)." §1159; 42 USC §1320c–8(b).

5. PSROs will review both Medicare and Medicaid cases, using the same standards for quality and necessity despite the differences in coverage which the two programs provide. See Chapter Two at 46 *supra.*

6. See this chapter at 146 *infra* for further elaboration on the extent of PSRO authority.

7. 42 USC §1320c–8.

8. §1902(a)(3); 42 USC §1396a(a)(3); see this chapter at *xx infra.*

9. See generally "Defendant's Brief in Support of Motion to Dismiss and/or Motion for Summary Judgment," *Allen v. Weinberger,* Civ. No. 39125, E. D. Mich., May 30, 1973, on file with the author. Opinion issued *sub nom. Allen v. Richardson,* E. D. Mich., Civ. No. 39125, October 25, 1973, reported in *CCH Medicare and Medicaid Guide* ¶26,793 (Chicago: Commerce Clearinghouse,) [hereinafter cited as *CCH M&M*].

   The author's analysis pertaining to Medicare processes is based on Health Law Project work which can be found in Health Law Project, "Medicare Level-of-Care Determinations," VI *Clearinghouse Rev.* 235 (August-September 1972). This study updates that previous work. The general principles enunciated here on the need and requirements for better procedural hearing rights for consumers have been central to the work of groups like the Health Law Project, the Center on Social Welfare Policy and Law, and the National Senior Citizens Law Center. However the research in the discussion which follows and the analysis of its relevance to PSROs are the author's.

10. See *Pazdera v. Department of Health and Social Services,* Wisc. Cir. Ct., Civ. No. 139–372, February 4, 1974, *CCH M&M* ¶26,967, where a patient was refused coverage for orthodontic treatment which should have been reviewed before care was rendered.

11. See n. 99 *infra.*

12. 45 CFR §205.10(a)(5).

13. §1902(a)(3); 42 USC §1396(a)(3).

14. §1902(a)(32); 42 USC §1396(a)(32).

15. 45 CFR §250.30(a)(6).

16. 317 NYS 2d 688 (1971).

17. *Id.* at 691.

18. 165 *NYLJ* 20 (#4, 1971), N.Y. Cir. Ct., March 13, 1971, *CCH M&M* ¶26,237.

19. *Id.* at 9605.

20. *Mt. Sinai Hospital v. Kornegay,* 342 NYS 2d 807 (1973), reported in *CCH Poverty Law Reporter* [hereinafter cited as *Pov. L. Rpt.*], at ¶18,423.

21. §1902(a)(10)(B); 42 USC §1396(a)(10)(B); 45 CFR §248.1(a)(2). The decision to offer coverage to these "medically needy" people is discretionary with the state and not all states include the medically needy populations in their medical assistance programs.

22. 45 CFR §205.10(a).

23. 397 US 254 (1970).

24. 45 CFR §205.10(a)(1)(i).
25. 45 CFR §205.10(a)(1)(ii).
26. 45 CFR §§205.10(a)(4)(ii)(A),(B).
27. 45 CFR §205.10(a)(4)(ii)(D).
28. 45 CFR §205.10(a)(4)(ii)(H). See this chapter at 151 *infra* for a more detailed discussion of the implications of these changes in the context of PSROs.

> The author knows of only one case to date which has considered the constitutionality of these changes. *Harrell* v. *Harder,* Civ. No. 13,800, D. Conn., January 11, 1974, *CCH Pov. L. Rpt.* ¶18,487 held that both changes were constitutional.

29. In federal court, in order to have the suit heard, the case usually must involve at least $10,000 worth of damages. This restriction does not apply in state courts. The restriction is intended to assure that federal courts hear major cases and not inconsequential ones. Most suits by Medicaid patients in federal court have been brought as class actions challenging the constitutionality of various state and federal agency actions and laws. The extent to which such suits may be brought in the future may have been seriously undermined by two recent cases.

> *Zahn v. International Paper Co.,* 414 US 291 (1973) held that each member of the plaintiff class must satisfy the requirement of a claim having a value of $10,000. In that case, where the named plaintiffs met the requirement but it could not be shown that the unnamed members of the class did, the class action could not be maintained in a diversity suit. At this writing, how or whether this decision would affect class actions brought by welfare or Medicaid recipients was unclear because their suits are usually brought, not under the diversity of citizenship jurisdiction, but under the federal question jurisdiction of federal courts. If the Supreme Court were to extend the requirement to federal question jurisdiction, fewer class actions could be brought in federal court.

> Even if a class action can be maintained, *Eisen* v. *Carlisle & Jacquelin,* 42 USLW 4804 (May 28, 1974), requiring individual notice to all members of the class who can be identified, with costs borne by the plaintiffs, could present a prohibitive financial obstacle to poor plaintiffs. The effect of this decision is also not yet clear.

30. Part A, §§1811–1817 of the Social Security Act; 42 USC §§1395c–i.
31. Part B, §§1831–1844; 42 USC §§1395j–m.
32. "Defendant's Brief," *supra* n. 9, at 14.
33. *Id.* at 17.
34. *Goldberg v. Kelly,* 397 US 254 (1970) at n. 34. See also *Hill v. State Department of Public Welfare,* Mo. S. Ct., No. 57,683, December 10, 1973, *CCH Pov. L. Rpt.* ¶18,266, where the court held that welfare benefits *were* a property right and therefore, subject to constitutional protection as a fundamental right.

35. See "Constitutional Issues in Social Security," 8 *Clearinghouse Rev.* 79 (June 1974).
36. §1869(a); 42 USC §1395ff(a); 20 CFR §§405.710–714; *Part A Intermediary Manual,* §§3783–3783.2 and 3792.
37. 20 CFR §405.715.
38. §1869(b)(2); 42 USC §1395ff(b)(2); 20 CFR §405.716; *Part A Intermediary Manual* §3784.
39. *Part A Intermediary Manual* §§3786(A),(B), 3794; 20 CFR §§422.201, 203.
40. 20 CFR §§405.724, 422.205; *Part A Intermediary Manual* §3786D.
41. §1869(b); 42 USC §1395ff(b); 20 CFR §§405.703, 422.210; *Part A Intermediary Manual* §3786D.
42. §205(g); 42 USC §405(g).
43. 20 CFR §405.801(a), §405.807.
44. 20 CFR §405.820; *Part B Intermediary Manual* §3794.
45. 20 CFR §405.830.
46. 20 CFR §405.841.
47. §1869(b)(1)(C); 42 USC §1395ff(b)(1)(C).
48. Prior to the Social Security Amendments of 1972 it was commonly accepted that there was no judicial review of Part B determinations, despite the absence of specific language excluding Part B judicial decisions. See, for example, *Kunstler* v. *Occidental Life Insurance Co.,* 292 F. Supp. (C.D. Calif. 1968). In that case, under the old provisions, the applicable law permitted judicial review of determinations "as to entitlement under Part A or Part B, or as to amount of benefits under Part A . . . ." Old §1869(b); 42 USC §1395ff(b). In *Bohlen* v. *Richardson,* (E.D. Pa., Civ. No. 70–2559, June 19, 1972) *CCH M&M* ¶26,493, the court found that judicial review of Part B entitlement controversies was available by using this definition: "It is our view that a question of entitlement is one which raises the issue of whether, regardless of the question of benefits in question, the claimant has the right to receive any payment for services rendered, or conversely, whether the claim is to be excluded entirely." (In contrast, "entitlement" in the Medicaid context has encompassed both entitlement and amount of benefits disputes.) A recent case on the new Medicare sections is *Hamilton* v. *Blue Cross of North Dakota and HEW,* (D. N. Dak., Civ. No. 4885, May 23, 1974), *CCH M&M* ¶27,013, where the distinction between the issues of "entitlement" and those on "amount of benefits" is analogized to the distinction between "liability" and "damages."

    The difference in the law under the new amendments, may not be as restrictive as they appear if courts apply rulings similar to that in *Wilson Coe, Admr.* v. *Sec. of HEW,* (4th Cir., No. 74–1215, September 24, 1974), *CCH M&M* ¶27,098. In that case the court held that an appellate court must apply the law in effect at the time it renders its decision, rather than the law in effect at the time the claim arose, *unless to do so would result in manifest injustice* or there is statutory direction or legislative history to the contrary. In that case the law had been liberalized under the 1972 amendments, providing more coverage than had been available to the claimant in 1970 when her claim arose; but the court applied the 1972 statutory approach. One can argue that the provision on Part B judicial review is more restrictive, and so in those cases where the claim arose before the 1972 amendments, the old provisions would apply. There is some question as to whether the effect of the *Coe* decision is unconstitutional because it creates ex post facto law, despite its apparently liberal, humane approach.

49. §1866; 42 USC §1395cc provides for conditions imposed on provider-institutions as a result of their participation in the program. Circumstances under which they can collect unpaid amounts for covered services are included and would be appealed under Part A procedures. There is no provision precluding to practitioners under Part B the right to collect from the beneficiary any unpaid portions of a bill for services.

50. §1842(b)(3)(B)(ii); 42 USC §1395u(b)(3)(B)(ii).

51. However, see *CCH M&M* ¶11,145; *Part B Intermediary Manual* HIM–14 §6318 on breaches of assignment contracts.

52. 20 CFR §405.129(c),(d); originally issued as Insurance Letter No. 328, reported at *CCH M&M* ¶4115.

53. New regulations eliminate the assurance of payments mechanism. 20 CFR §405.129 is revoked in its entirety. See 40 FR 1022, January 6, 1975.

54. *Sen. Fin. Comm. Rpt.* at 268.

55. §213, P.L. 92–603; §1879(a); 42 USC §1395pp.

56. Under the new regulations, there will be a presumption of coverage if the provider complies with utilization review requirements and demonstrates that it "effectively distinguishes between cases where items or services furnished . . . are covered . . . and cases where they are excluded from coverage." 20 CFR §405.195(b)(4). Interim procedures had held the provider to a standard of no more than 5 percent denial of bills submitted for payment under Medicare, but the regulations do not repeat this specific standard. *Part A Intermediary Letter* No. 73–30; *CCH M&M* ¶24,353.34.

   It is also important to note that the regulations under the Medicare hold harmless provision restrict its use for patients to instances where there has been an assignment. 20 CFR §405.330(a)(1). Despite the fact that comments on this issue were received, the Social Security Administration claimed the assignment requirement was in the statute and had to be embodied in the regulations. See 40 FR 1022, January 6, 1975. The relevant portion of the statute reads:

Where—

(1) a determination is made that, by reason of section 1862(a)(1) or (9), payment may not be made under part A or part B of this title for any expenses incurred for items or services furnished an individual by a provider of services or by another person pursuant to an assignment under section 1842(b)(3)(B)(ii) . . . .

§1879(a)(1); 42 USC §1395pp(a)(1).

There is no basis at all in the legislative history to interpret the statutory language restrictively, and, in fact, the legislative history specifically and explicitly states its liberal intent. See *Sen. Fin. Comm. Rpt.* at 294–295. The provision as written should be interpreted to hold the patient harmless where services have been furnished either by a provider directly or by another person pursuant to an assignment. There are no statutory restrictions on the PSRO hold harmless provision. §1158(a); 42 USC §1320c–7(a).

57. *Id.*
58. §1159(a); 42 USC §1320c–8(a). Note that Title V recipients have no hearing rights under the PSRO provision.
59. *Id.*
60. §1159(b); 42 USC §1320c–8(b).
61. Statewide Councils exist where there are three or more PSROs. §1162(a); 42 USC §1320c–11.
62. §1159(a); 42 USC §1320c–8(a).
63. *Id.*
64. §1159(c); 42 USC §1320c–8(c).
65. See n. 49 *supra.*
66. Although on its face the statute appears to provide more hearing rights to beneficiary-recipients (giving them review beyond the Statewide Council to the Secretary), but by omission apparently precluding that review to physicians and providers, the legislative history demonstrates an intent to afford higher review rights to all participants in the tripartite system.

The statute says,

Where the determination of the Statewide Professional Standards Review Council is *adverse to the beneficiary or recipient,* (or in the absence of such Council in a State and where the matter in controversy is $100 or more), such *beneficiary or recipient* shall be entitled to a hearing thereon by the Secretary . . . and where the amount in controversy is $1,000 or more, to judicial review of the Secretary's final decision after such hearing . . . .
(Emphasis added.) §1159(b); 42 USC §1320c–8(b).

The legislative history provides no distinction among participants:

A Medicare beneficiary, Medicaid recipient, *provider of services or health care practitioner* who was dissatisfied with a determination by a PSRO under this provision would be entitled to a reconsideration of the determination by the PSRO; where the matter in controversy is $100 or more, the reconsideration would be subject to review, on appeal, by a State Professional Standards Review Council or by the Secretary. Where the amount in question exceeded $1,000, the Secretary's final decision would be subject to judicial review. (Emphasis added.) *Sen. Fin. Comm. Rpt.* at 267–8.

67. §1159(a); 42 USC §1320c–8(a).
68. See this chapter at 142 *supra*.
69. §1155(a)(1); 42 USC §1320c–4(a)(1).
70. §1155(a)(2); 42 USC §1320c–4(a)(2).
71. Although the statutory language does not deal with challenges to the norms guidelines themselves, PSRO review may be available in a third type of situation. Issues of the inherent medical validity of a norm are probably beyond the jurisdiction of this particular review mechanism. "A determination with respect to a claim" can, however, be said to include a determination that a specific norm, criterion, or standard is applicable to a claim. It may be possible, through that type of analysis, to raise the question of the validity of the norm within the specific context of a particular case. The major obstacle to such a challenge would be the ability to discover what the norms are. See Chapter Six at 189 *infra*.
72. From the statutory language, it appears that once reconsideration is requested of the PSRO, affirmation automatically results in State-wide Council Review. The statute says that if the PSRO affirms its own decision, and the matter in controversy is $100 or more, the determination "shall be" reviewed by the professional members of the Statewide Council. This apparently self-generating review is not present in the Medicare scheme, but does mitigate the burden of requesting review which presently lies with the dissatisfied party. See §1159(a); 42 USC §1320c–8(a).
73. §205(b); 42 USC §405(b).
74. (Emphasis added.) §205(g); 42 USC §405(g).
75. *Bohlen v. Richardson*, n. 48 *supra* at 10,274.
76. See n. 21 *supra*.
77. *Sniadach v. Family Finance Corp. of Bay View*, 395 US 337 (1969).
78. See Chapter Three at 94 *supra*.
79. See Chapter Six at 181 *infra* for relevant analogous arguments on the issue of local or statewide PSROs.
80. See Health Law Project, *supra* n. 9. See n. 83 *infra*.
81. The PSRO is charged with the review of "professional" activities. §1155(a)(1); 42 USC §1320c–4(a)(1). The obligations which the law imposes are obligations on physicians and providers. §1160; 42 USC §1320c–9.
82. See Chapter Three at 68 *supra*.
83. Most determinations on appeal in which the physician's opinion has made the difference (between a decision favorable to the patient and one

where the patient would bear the financial responsibility) are "custodial care" cases. These Medicare determinations arise under the provision which provides that no payment may be made under Part A for "any expenses incurred for items or services . . . where such expenses are for custodial care." §1862(a)(9); 42 USC §1395y(a)(9). See also 20 CFR § §405.126–129. Custodial care has never been explicitly defined. (For a history of the exclusion, see Health Law Project, n. 9 *supra* at 240–242.)

Courts have been increasingly liberal in construing the Medicare law in favor of the patient, against the Secretary, where the physician's opinion supports the patient. Even now that the regulatory mandate of giving great weight to the physician's opinion has been removed in favor of norms, criteria, and standards, some courts still believe the physician's opinion carries great weight, particularly in a case of extended stay in a hospital. See *Dye v. Weinberger* (E.D. Okla., Civ. No. 74–92–C, August 16, 1974), *CCH M&M* ¶27,094.

There are four basic tests which have been used recently. Some of the cases rely on several of the four theories. (For earlier cases see Health Law Project, n. 9 *supra*.)

1. *Direct Primary Reliance on Physician's Opinion:* Typical of these cases is *Caudelle* v. *Weinberger* N.D. Ga. (Civ. No. 17547), August 28, 1973) *CCH M&M* ¶26,764, where the court held the Secretary "must accept uncontradicted, unimpeached and unanimous opinion of the treating physicians." See also, *Stephens* v. *Weinberger,* N.D. Ohio (Civ. No. C72–1330y, August 23, 1973), ¶26,763; *Blacker* v. *Richardson,* D. Mont. (Civ. No. 2055, November 21, 1972), *CCH M&M* ¶26,696; *Wilson* v. *Winberger,* E.D. Tenn. (Civ. No. 8105, June 29, 1973), *CCH M&M* ¶26,985.

2. *Physician's Opinion Supported by Institutional Utilization Review Committee: Collins v. Weinberger,* N.D. Iowa (Civ. No. 72–C–3075, (August 24, 1973), *CCH M&M* ¶26,744; *McKinley* v. *Richardson,* W.D.N.Y. (Civ. No. 1972–32, February 8, 1973), *CCH M&M* ¶26,623; *Sheck* v. *Richardson,* W.D.N.Y. (Civ. No. 1971–554, February 22, 1973), *CCH M&M* ¶26,641; *Tylka* v. *Weinberger,* N.D. Ohio (Civ. No. C72–1016–y, June 21, 1973), *CCH M&M* ¶26,745.

One important case has held that where a utilization review committee has not functioned effectively, the physician's opinion will still carry great weight. *Hultzman* v. *Weinberger,* No. 73–1917 (3rd Cir., April 18, 1974). See also National Health Law Program column, 8 *Clearinghouse Rev.* 275 (August 1974).

See also *Ingram* v. *Weinberger,* S.D.W.Va. (Civ. No. 72–157–CH, September 26, 1973), *CCH M&M* ¶26,769, where the utilization review committee failed to consult with the physician although it had expressly said it would. The court held that reliance on nurses' notes to prove the care was "custodial" was not sufficient evidence to overcome the doctor's opinion. *Harris* v. *Richardson,* E.D.Va.

(Civ. Act. No. 232-72-R, April 12, 1973), *CCH M&M* ¶26,656 also held that absence of nurses' notes was not conclusive evidence and could not overcome the physician's opinion.

3. *Physician's Opinion and Totality of Condition:* Two trends developed in judicial evaluation of custodial care determinations, based on an analysis of the type of services rendered. *Ridgely* v. *Secretary of HEW,* 345 F. Supp. 483 (D. Md. 1973) *aff'd.* 472 F. 2d. 1222 (4th Cir., 1972), *CCH M&M* ¶26,636 looked to the "course of treatment": which discrete services were rendered and how often they were rendered. This test yields a higher percentage of unfavorable results for recipients. An earlier case, *Sowell* v. *Richardson,* 319 F. Supp. 689 (D.S.C. 1970), said the test was the "total patient condition." The "total condition" or "total needs" test is more liberal, more favorable to the patient, and more often used. See *Edgington v. Richardson,* E.D. Mich. (Civ. No. 39069, November 30, 1973), *CCH M&M* ¶26,817; *Daniell v. Richardson,* D.N.H. (Civ. No. 72-172, February 6, 1973), *CCH M&M* ¶26,628; *Beever v. Weinberger,* S.D.W.Va. (Civ. Act. No. 3029, May 14, 1973), *CCH M&M* ¶26,662; *Fuller v. Secretary of HEW,* D. Md. (Civ. No. 72-972-M, June 4, 1972), *CCH M&M* ¶26,675; *Pantano v. Richardson,* E.D. Mich. (Civ. Act No. 38873, June 11, 1973), *CCH M&M* ¶26,713; *Allen v. Richardson,* E.D. Mich. (Civ. No. 39125, October 25, 1973), *CCH M&M* ¶26,793; *White v. Richardson,* W.D. No. (Civ. No. 2295, August 30, 1973), *CCH M&M* ¶26,756.

P.L. 92-603 (H.R.1), which redefined skilled nursing services, conforming the definitions in Medicare and Medicaid [§247, P.L. 92-603; §§1814(a)(2)(C), 1905(f); 42 USC §§1395f(a)(2)(C), 1396d(f)] codified by effect the "total patient condition" test. The provision says that

"skilled nursing facility services" means those which are or were required to be given an individual who needs or needed on a daily basis skilled nursing care ... or other skilled rehabilitation services which, *as a practical matter* can only be provided in a skilled nursing facility on an inpatient basis.
(Emphasis added.)

The legislative history specifically says, "skilled nursing services include: *assessment of the total needs of the patient* ...." (Emphasis added.) *Sen. Fin. Comm. Rpt.* at 283. Although, of nursing services, Medicare covers only skilled nursing care [§§1812(a)(2),(3), 1861(h),(i),(j); 42 USC §1395d(a)(2),(3), §1395x(h),(i),(j)], Medicaid does cover intermediate care as well [§1905(a)(15); 42 USC §1396d(a)(15)], despite the new conformity of labels. The legislative history says that payment would be made commensurate with the level of service required. "The [Senate Finance] Committee expects that the [PSROs] . . . would provide scrutiny over whether appropriate patient placement was being made . . . ." *Sen. Fin. Comm. Rpt.* at 285. The provisions apply to services provided after January 1, 1973.

One recent case has specifically rejected the "course of treatment" approach. *Hamon v. Weinberger*, S.D.W.Va. (Civ. No. 72–283–CH, February 20, 1974), *CCH M&M* ¶26,923.

4. *Physician's Opinion vs. Substantial Evidence:* The final test which has been used takes into account the physician's opinion and then considers whether the Secretary has substantial evidence to over come it. Several cases have found for the beneficiary using this test. See *Weber v. Weinberger*, E.D. Wisc. (Civ. No. 72–C–672, March 21, 1974), *CCH M&M* ¶26,969. In *Lee v. Weinberger*, D. Neb. (Civ. No. 72–0–126, May 5, 1973), *CCH M&M* ¶26,679, the court found for the patient because there had been no medical advisor at the hearing. In *Stephens v. Weinberger*, N.D. Ohio (Civ. No. C72–1330y, August 23, 1973), *CCH M&M* ¶26,673, the court found for the recipient, in part, because the physician and utilization review committee did not support the fiscal intermediary's medical advisor's opinion. In cases where a fiscal intermediary's medical advisor only examines the records in the case, and never sees the patient, the patient's attorney sometimes has been successful by emphasizing the attending physician's immediate and intimate knowledge of the case. But see, *contra, Richardson v. Perales*, 402 US 389 (1971), where written hearsay evidence of experts was upheld as the sole basis for denying a claim.

84. See *Roe v. Wade*, 410 US 113 (1973); *Doe v. Bolton*, 410 US 179 (1973); *Doe v. Rampton*, 366 F. Supp. 189 (C.D. Utah 1973).

   See also *Word v. Poelker*, a decision by the US Court of Appeals in the 8th Circuit, relying even more heavily on the fact that the decision to abort is a medical decision, the basic responsibility for which must rest with the physician. 495 F. 2d 1349 (8th Cir., 1974).

85. 397 US 254,261 (1970), quoting from *Kelly v. Wyman*, 294 F. Supp. 893,899,900 (1968).

86. Although most of the cases establishing prior hearings on the basis of *Goldberg* involve revocations of benefits to which a right has been established, due process rights can attach where there is a denial of benefits in the first instance, before any right to benefits has been established. See *Holmes v. New York City Housing Authority*, 398 F. 2d 262 (2d. Cir., 1968).

   An absolute right to a benefit need not be established for courts to require due process; nor will characterization of the benefit as a "privilege" in itself preclude or extinguish due process rights. See *New York City Housing Authority v. Escalera*, 425 F. 2d 853 (2d Cir., 1970); and *dictum* in *DeRodulfa v. US*, 461 F. 2d. 1240, 1256(1972).

87. No. 1989 (D.N.M., October 21, 1971), *CCH Pov. L. Rpt.* ¶14,406.

88. See Chapter Two at 42 *supra.*
89. 472 F. 2d 112 (10th Cir., 1973).
90. 45 CFR §205.10(a)(4)(ii)(D),(H).
91. 45 CFR §205.10(a)(4)(i)(A).
92. 45 CFR §205.10(a)(4)(ii).
93. 45 CFR §205.10(a)(4)(ii)(D).
94. 45 CFR §205.10(a)(4)(ii)(H).
95. See this chapter at 149 *supra.*
96. HEW Medical Assistance Manual (MSA-PRG 12) §5–30–00, p. 1.
97. *Id.* at 4.
98. An additional remedy may exist in the form of a suit alleging denial of due process, seeking two possible forms of relief: (1) withdrawal of the Secretary's agreement from the offending PSRO or withdrawal of delegated review from the offending utilization review committee, and (2) compensatory damages where appropriate.
99. See, for example, *Turner* v. *Wohlgemuth,* No. 74–1680, (E.D. Pa., filed July 4, 1974), (reported at ¶13116, 8 *Clearinghouse Rev.* 371 (September 1974), where the patient, suffering from severe coronary and respiratory disease, was discharged from a Philadelphia hospital where he was receiving oxygen. The hospital discharged him notwithstanding that it knew a request for a prior authorization for oxygen at home had been filed a month earlier, but had not been processed. He died two days after his discharge. The approval was given the day he died. Two other plaintiffs in the action waited nine and twelve months respectively for approvals for dentures during which time they had to restrict their diets to soft foods.
100. §1155(a)(6); 42 USC §1320c–4(a)(6).
101. 397 US 254, 270 (1970).
102. See this chapter at 149 *supra.*
103. §1161; 42 USC §1320c–10.
104. 397 US 254, 269 (1970).
105. Other considerations would be necessary in the creation of such a scheme. For example, it might prove unnecessary to have one advocate for every institution (particularly in underserved areas or where the need otherwise is not great), in which case advocates could "ride circuit," serving several institutions with frequent and regular visits. Because timeliness is so important in the review process, sufficient resources would have to be devoted to staffing such a corps to prevent the emergence of another level of time-wasting bureaucracy piled on top of the maze already created by this statute. The purpose of patient advocates would not be to insulate patients from the processes to which they are entitled, but to facilitate their access by virtue of special help from a specialist with knowledge to cut through the administrative labryinth a patient or even a patient's attorney might encounter.
   Funding for such a program would, of course, be a problem. Because intermediaries and PSROs attempt to minimize costs,

funding through intermediaries or PSROs would present conflicts of interest where advocates sought to establish coverage. Institutions seeking review of some cases may feel it too costly to pursue others, leaving the debt for uncovered care to be absorbed by the patient. In such cases, the institutional interest would conflict with the patients'. For those reasons, and to ensure accountability of patient advocates to the populations they serve, funding for them should come from an independent source with ties to the type of patients the advocates would represent. The new Title XX of the Social Security Act, providing federal moneys to the states to encourage the provision of wide-ranging social services, would be an appropriate funding source.

106. It may not always be in the patient's interest to have coverage approved. For example, unnecessary procedures sought without valid reasons by physicians are probably better not performed. Also, in the PSRO structure, negotiations between the PSRO and the requesting physician should ordinarily persuade physicians to forgo unnecessary treatment. The physician would then communicate with the patient. If he or she remained unconvinced, and he cared strongly, he would probably seek to press an appeal on behalf of the patient. A patient advocate would not then be needed to act in the physician's stead. Presumably, patient advocates would contribute to better communication, not the disruption of existing rapport.

107. Simple handbooks distributed to patients whose care is reviewed by PSROs would be one obvious means of conveying the necessary basic information. Other educational programs could also be employed (e.g., classes at Social Security offices or by consumer groups themselves, or seminars run by local hospitals or nursing homes).

108. *Sen. Fin. Comm. Rpt.* at 266.

109. Should a state Medicaid agency be given the responsibility to act as a PSRO, a state role would exist. State action arguments would then be relevant. In that case the Fourteenth Amendment would apply instead of the Fifth. See n. 113 *infra*. The governors of states where Statewide Councils are to exist are given the responsibility to appoint at least two or the members of the Statewide Council.

110. Early discussions by the AMA of the contract process considered ways to undermine the Secretary's authority in the process. One suggestion urged that contracts be of a tripartite nature, in which state, county, and federal organizations were joint—and equal—parties, undercutting the Secretary's paramount role and increasing the AMA's. Another recommendation was that the AMA be a prime party to all PSRO contracts, in order to "guard against . . . the government's penchant for 'picking off groups of MDS one by one.' " See "PSRO issues: 'quality', norms jurisdiction," *American Medical News,* April 23, 1973 at 6.

111. *Hannah* v. *Larche,* 363 US 420 (1960).

112. There may also be equal protection claims because of the discrimination between the sick (those needing services worth more than $100 and $1000) and the healthier patients unable to meet the jurisdictional amount requirements. Although there is no equal protection clause in the Fifth Amendment (only in the Fourteenth), ". . . the concepts of equal protection and due process, both stemming from our American ideal of fairness, are not mutually exclusive." *Bolling* v. *Sharpe,* 347 US 497 (1954).

113. Although constitutional analysis requires the presence of "state action" before constitutional standards can be applied to activities by state governments, the concept as required under the Fourteenth amendment is irrelevant to PSROs. The PSRO does not, itself, engage in state action, although as a nonprofit corporation it may be subject to state laws. "State action" only applies where state law or activity is involved. The PSRO law is federal law.

Reliance on the concept of "state action" and the Fourteenth Amendment's due process clause may be dangerous for the consumer advocate as well as unnecessary. On health related issues, the federal circuits are split in their decisions on when a *private* entity becomes sufficiently entangled with the state to become involved in "state action." In *Barrett* v. *United Hospital,* 42 USLW 2631 (May 23, 1974), tax exemptions and state regulation of private hospitals were not sufficient to create state action in the hospital's refusal to restore staff privileges to a dismissed physician. See also, *Watkins* v. *Mercy Medical Center,* 364 F. Supp. 799 (1973), where tax exemptions and receipt of federal construction funds were insufficient involvement with the state either to compel a Catholic hospital to make its facilities available for abortions or to require it to grant staff privileges to a physician insisting on his right to perform them. Similarly, in *Doe* v. *Bellin Memorial Hospital,* 479 F. 2d 756 (7th Cir., 1973), Hill-Burton hospital construction moneys were not sufficient to create state action in a private hospital refusing to perform abortions. The cases do hold that *public* institutions are engaged in state action, and may not, therefore, violate due process requirements nor condition constitutionally protected rights. See, for example, *McCabe* v. *Nassau County Medical Center,* 453 F 2d. 698 (2d. Cir., 1971), *Nyberg* v. *City of Virginia,* 361 F. Supp. 932 (D. Minn., 1973), *aff'd.* No. 73–1686 (8th Cir., February 19, 1974). PSROs are distinctly private entities. ("Employees of the PSRO would be selected by the organization and would not be government employees." *Sen. Fin. Comm. Rpt.* at 266.) While one might argue that they are engaged in governmental activities, the recent trends in "state action" cases seem to oppose the assertion that they are engaged in "state action."

There are cases which have found state action in *private* health related institutions. Unfortunately, most of them follow a line of reasoning stemming from racial discrimination issues. Race discrimination is subject to "strict scrutiny" by courts and raises more compelling political issues for "state action" purposes than those involving substantive due process. See *Simkins* v. *Moses H. Cone Memorial Hospital*, 365 US 715 (1961); *Sams* v. *Ohio Valley General Hospital Association*, 413 F. 2d. 826 (4th Cir., 1969); *Eaton* v. *Grubbs*, 329 F. 2d. 710 (1964). For recent discussions on these issues see, "Recent Developments—Constitutional Law—Abortion—Private Hospital May Refuse to Perform Abortion," 18 *St. Louis U. L. Rev.* 440 (1974); and Elkind, "State Action: Theories for Applying Constitutional Restrictions to Private Activity," 74 *Columbia L. Rev.* 656 (1974).

The author would like to thank Edward F. Shay for his observations on these points.

114. Aggregation of claims (retrospective and prospective) is one possible technique. An assertion that the actual value of the services to the patient is incalculably high is another possibility. But, see *Hamilton* v. *Blue Cross of No. Dakota*, (D. No. Dal., Civ. No. 4885, May 23, 1974), *CCH M&M* ¶27,013, for a case where the claim was for $690.55 and the case was dismissed.

115. *Boddie* v. *Connecticut*, 401, US 371, 376 (1970).

116. *Id.*

117. See n. 113 *supra.*

118. *Bolling v. Sharpe*, 347 US 497 (1954).

119. 409 US 434 (1972).

120. *Id.* at 438.

121. *Id.*

122. This argument is similar to the "brutal need" argument made earlier in the context of administrative review. See this chapter at 150 *supra.*

123. *Boddie, supra* n. 115, at 374.

124. 428 P. 2d. 757 (1972), 410 US 656 (1973) *r'h'g den.* 411 US 922 (1973), *CCH Pov. L. Rpt.* ¶¶16,157, 16,759.

125. For further consideration of issues in access by indigents to judicial review, see the following articles: "Constitutionality of Cost and Fee Barriers for Indigent Litigants: Searching for the Remains of Boddie after a Kras Landing," 48 *Ind. L.J.* 452 (Spring, 1973); "*Boddie v. Connecticut*: Whither the Indigent Civil Litigant?", 22 *Catholic U. L. Rev.* 427 (Winter 1973).

126. See this chapter at 149 *supra.*

Chapter Six

Accountability

The notion of "accountability" is one which frequently surfaces in consumer-oriented analyses. Rarely are attempts made to define the concept and explain why it is an essential element of a properly functioning social program. Yet accountability is the sine qua non of a consumer-responsive analysis, because its recognition establishes that attention to the consumer's interests is necessary and legitimate. The underlying theme in this book is that the PSRO program will not work effectively unless consumer-accountable mechanisms are an integral part of the program's structure and are, therefore, included among the techniques the program will use to achieve its professed goals—cost control and quality assurance.

There are varying types of accountability. Some have already been discussed. Administrative accountability is embodied in the requirements that HEW monitor paying agents and PSROs; it is the sanction and enforcement tool which guarantees the existence and integrity of the components of a program to the program itself.[1] Governmental accountability exists in the system of checks and balances by which one branch of government oversees and limits the activities of another branch. In the PSRO program this is represented by the requirement that the National PSR Council issue annual reports to Congress detailing for each year the activities and accomplishments of the program.[2] Taxpayer accountability (often called "public" accountability) requires cost accounting and consequent control measures and was present in the drafting of the PSRO law, through the emphasis on reducing costs of Medicare and Medicaid to taxpayers.[3] Each of these types of accountability responds to the different, sometimes antagonistic, interests represented in the operation of any social program. Consumer accountability requires inclusion of a still different, and still sometimes conflicting, set of interests.

Throughout this book particular potential obstacles to consumer accountability have been pointed out, and specific techniques for making the program more responsive to consumer needs and interests have been presented. This chapter examines the consumer accountability of the PSRO system as a whole, on the basis of a theory of accountability (set forth below), and concludes that the system has not been made consumer-accountable under the law. But, based on the theory, this chapter goes further, to discuss mechanisms both necessary and achievable which would lead to a more effective and responsive PSRO system.

THE THEORY

Consumer accountability in any social program is the factor which permits the system both to adapt to and to incorporate the views of the people it serves. Who is "served" by the PSRO process is a question which is often answered differently depending on who is asked. Senator Bennett believed that the taxpayers were served by PSROs, as they will be if cost control results from PSRO review. Some health care professionals see themselves as served by the program because it provides a mechanism for education and improved care. They are served by the program, but will also serve it themselves by participating in its activities and altering their behavior according to its dictates. But practitioners are not, because of that, the PSRO program's consumers. No one in fact "consumes" PSRO services; yet to the extent that the program will have impact on the health care and financial responsibilities of the patients whose cases it reviews, the PSRO system serves or disserves the patients. Health care professionals may choose whether or not to participate at all in PSRO activities; and their financial interests are derivative through the patients they treat. In the last analysis, PSROs cannot intrinsically affect the behavior of any one practitioner. The only group whose interests are necessarily, inherently, affected by PSRO activities are the patients. Despite the fact that they have no choice of participating in the program, and therefore no choice of whether to exercise their "consuming" power in the PSRO marketplace—if they need health care services they must submit to PSRO review—they are the only group which can be considered the PSRO program's consumers. They are also the only group whose interests have not been balanced with the others' in the design of the system.

A consumer-accountable system responds to consumer input before it acts, and is held responsible or answerable to consumers for actions taken on its own initiative (or the initiative of its components). The importance of consumer accountability lies in its ability to enhance the effectiveness of the program. The PSRO program's success will depend, in part, on the extent of its responsiveness to consumers, because that will in turn determine the credibility and acceptance the system enjoys among those segments of the community whose lives it directly affects. The program cannot be maximally effective if those who must use it, suspect it. Suspicion leads to cynicism, avoidance, and, ultimately, abuse, and, therefore, to a weakening of the program.

In the ideal process of designing a social program, all interests which are affected by it, through compromise, come to agree on the goals of the system, and therefore work within the system and for it when they must come in contact with it. Toward that end, and to make the program credible, the law creating it must include an enforceable obligation for the program's structure to interact with the people who will be affected by it. Without the legal obligation to seek out, respond to, and incorporate the views and values of the program's consumers, the program's credibility and responsiveness will depend solely on the good will of particular individuals. Without the legal obligation for consumer accountability, if the "wrong" group of individuals were to capture control of the program, nothing could be done to prevent them from destroying any prior steps to insure the integrity of the system.

This book continually refers to diverse interests and values reflected in the PSRO statute and its implementation. In a democratic society, a basic premise is that diverse interests are recognized in government operation. Elected officials are chosen because of their stated choice of values, and support of interests, among different options. Lobbyists exist and are subsidized for the sole purpose of influencing government activites so they will recognize and respond to particular interests. In the PSRO program some of these diverse interest groups are physicians, hospitals, medical schools, health insurers, health planners, ancillary care practitioners, Congress, the HEW bureaucracy and its subdivisions, and taxpayers. Because these interests often conflict, equity requires that they all be fairly represented in the program's structure and considered in the policymaking process which will determine how it functions. Because the PSRO system, through its medical care determinations, will allocate scarce resources (Medicare and Medicaid funds), some of its determinations will necessarily meet one group's needs and deny another's. How should those critical choices be made?[4] To exclude consumers is to thwart the democratic process. One PSRO commentator has chosen the social contract theory to argue the general need for PSRO interaction with those outside the medical profession. "[P] hysicians, hospitals, and other providers derive their authority from society at large, under a social contract that has been formalized through such legal mechanisms as licensure."[5] In formulating a contract, bargaining and compromise among those whose interests are determined under the contract is necessary. Furthermore, traditional legal theory holds that inequality of bargaining power between the parties to a contract renders the contract void. The analogy demonstrates the need for equitable representation in policymaking and other decisionmaking processes in the PSRO program.

In analyzing which interests are to be represented, it is critical to distinguish between consumers, the "public," and other so-called impartial participants. In health care, there is no such thing as an impartial or public representative; and the same person may reflect different interests at different times. A physician treating a patient usually identifies with other physicians in the same position and reflects their common values and interests. When that same physician becomes ill and is himself a patient, he often responds as a patient, but rarely abandons his parallel identification with his colleagues. (This may be the reason why common health care mythology holds that "doctors make the worst patients.") In choosing consumer representatives, or including consumer values in program design, it would be improper to rely on the physician-as-patient as typical of health care consumers.

One self-proclaimed "consumer spokesman"[6] suggests that public accountability requires the presence, among others, of "public representatives ... individual[s] who may be health care consumer[s] or providers[s] but, in either case, [have] distinguished [themselves] by objective scholarship and/or leadership in the health field or a related field and [are] not identified with a single-interest point of view."[7] It is unclear whether Somers means are not self-identified or are not publicly identified with single-interest points of view. Like reportorial objectivity in journalism, there is no such thing as objectivity in health care analysis, precisely because to choose one set of values necessarily excludes others. For that reason, there can be no "impartial" public representatives because there is no single identifiable "public interest." It may in fact be easier to identify an advocate or representative by the set of values he does not subscribe to, rather than to try to classify what may be differing values in his one point of view. As Ms. Somers suggests, her definition of "public representative" is expansive and would consider as a public representative someone who holds some views which may be identified with one or more interests. To do otherwise, she suggests "could get to the point that no one could represent the public except people who know nothing about health care. This would obviously be self-defeating."[8] The issue in consumer accountability (or any other recognition of diverse interests) is not to find someone who is impartial, but to find people who are so strongly identified with single interests that they can be proper advocates for them in the debates leading to compromise on program design, implementation, and operation.

It may be instructive to look to the jury system as an example of this process. Although popular teachings and civics book analysis would lead one to believe that a jury is supposed to be "impartial," the law establishes a jury selection process which in fact encourages the opposing attorneys to select as jurors those people whom they believe are strongly supportive of their clients' interests. The opposing attorneys recognize that every prospective juror brings with him or her a set of inherent prejudices and biases, which, although not immediately related to the case under litigation, will necessarily influence the decisions with regard to the case. The attorneys then attempt to select from the prospective jurors those people whose prejudices most closely correspond to their clients' interests in the trial. As in the trial analogy, fair representation in the PSRO system implies that there must be a representative or typical quality to the person who represents. The concept clearly demands the inclusion of the panoply of relevant interests through well-identified advocates throughout the system.

Consumer accountability can be of two kinds, systemic and individual. Measurement of systemic accountability entails an examination of the interaction of the structure of the whole program with the consumers as a group. For systemic accountability to exist, there must be specific legal requirements for intersection between the two spheres under consideration—the system and the patients. Including consumers in the various councils of the PSRO program would have been one example of systemic accountability. There are, however, no true examples of systemic accountability to consumers in the PSRO program. The only possible example is the Statewide Councils, which must include among their members four people "knowledgeable in health care."[9] Because the law imposes no other conditions on these members, they could be consumers, but nothing *requires* that consumers be appointed.

Individual accountability exists to the extent the system accommodates individual complaints in a responsive manner. For example, when a patient is held liable for uncovered services, and he or she disagrees with the determination, the hearing process affords a means for bringing a complaint.[10] The law provides for a mandatory process of appeals when such dissatisfaction occurs. By this process, the system is made accountable to the individual with the complaint. In examining systemic and individual accountability, a critical question to ask about the hearing process is whether individual accountability can create systemic accountability as well. If each successive review authority in the hearings process strictly scrutinizes the case and the determination eventually is changed to conform to the patient's interests, then the PSRO has been held answerable to an individual outside its own ranks. In a truly accountable system, that process of adjustment and response on an individual basis will lead both to a general evaluation of the hearing process and to examination of other elements of the system implicated by the complaint, with commensurate response and improvements diffusing throughout the system.

According to this general theory of consumer accountability, PSROs fail the test. There are no legal obligations requiring PSROs to seek out or respond to consumer interests either in the design, operation, or implementation of the program. The statute does include enforcement techniques[11] which impose sanctions on individual physicians for failure to comply with PSRO guidelines. But enforcement makes physicians and other participants internally accountable to the program itself. It does nothing to govern the relationships between the program and those outside of its operations. Other statutory provisions, if utilized by responsible, consumer-oriented parties, may expand the accountability of the program; but there is nothing that requires such interpretation, nor any indication that those provisions were created for that purpose.[12] Finally, the provisions of the statute which restrict the availability of information outside the system[13] may specifically impede, if not preclude altogether, the single most important element of consumer accountability—open and widespread dissemination of information.

This discussion of the theory of accountability raises the question of whether there has ever been such a consumer-accountable program. There probably never has been an ideal program. Because of the power of vested interests and the nature of the legislative process, combined with the vicissitudes of administrative implementation, an ideal process may be unattainable. But there are and have been programs very much more responsive to their consumers[14] than PSROs; and there is no reason that PSROs cannot be made more so. There are two reasons to undertake such efforts: (1) PSROs represent a change of gears in health care delivery. Because so many aspects of health care will be reevaluated in light of PSROs' statutory duties and their implications, it is possible to use the reevaluation process to create mechanisms to improve the effectiveness of the program. (2) PSROs will have tremendous, incalculable effects on health care delivery—costs, quality, and planning. If a national health insurance program is passed in the near future, the impact of PSROs will go even further than the system's present design. The body of consumers will be significantly enlarged and, therefore, more powerful. Unless the program responds to their needs it will be dominated by the smaller but more powerful blocs of vested health care interests. With or without national health insurance, cost containment will continue to be an increasing concern in all social programs. PSROs will be the model for future systems to allocate scarce resources and funds. With an eye to the future, the process of breaking the barriers to a democratic system can begin now and will be much easier before the PSRO structure is fully operational and in place. Despite the initial failure to recognize the legitimacy of consumer interests in the creation of the program, there are still many opportunities for change. But it is better and easier to take advantage of them as early as possible, rather than after the vested interests are entrenched and better able to resist pressure to include the entry of others.

The discussion below focuses primarily on problems of systemic accountability in the PSRO program. Beginning with the legislative process, this chapter looks at the totality of the system as well as particularly relevant provisions of the statute, to uncover and elucidate the lack of consumer accountability in PSROs. Where a reasonable, achievable method of making the program more responsive is available, it is presented.

LEGISLATIVE AND REGULATORY PROCESS

Many interests were considered during the legislative process creating PSROs. Consumers were not among them. In 1970, Senator Wallace Bennett (R–Utah) introduced the forerunner to the final PSRO amendment as part of the Social Security Amendments of 1970 (H.R. 17550). The amendment (no. 823) failed to pass in 1970 and was reintroduced on January 25, 1972 as part of the Social Security Amendments of 1971 (H.R.1).[15] The Senate Finance Committee conducted its hearings for administration witnesses on H.R.1 in late July and early August 1971. None of them was a consumer, by definition, nor, because of the timing, could they speak to the issue of PSROs as reproposed.

Additional hearings for public witnesses were conducted at the end of January and through early February 1972,[16] but included almost no discussion of PSROs. Since the bill had only been introduced at the end of January, when some of the public witnesses had already testified, it is not surprising that PSROs were not a prime topic. Of those who did testify about PSROs, none was a consumer, and no one else spoke of the possible significance of the program for patients or taxpayers.[17] One law professor, Clark C. Havighurst of Duke University, speaking about PSROs and their relations with health maintenance organizations (HMOs), indicated he thought PSROs would stifle HMO growth.[18] Governor Richard Ogilvie of Illinois, prompted by Senator Bennett, spoke of Illinois' peer review program (Hospital Admission and Surveillance Program [HASP]); but the Illinois program had, at that time, been in effect for only a few days.[19] Among those who spoke directly to the issue of PSROs were representatives of the following groups: the American Hospital Association;[20] Group Health Association of America[21] (a group which promotes HMOs); the American Dental Association[22] (by written submission only); the American Medical Association[23] (by written submission only); the American Nurses Association;[24] the American Association of Foundations for Medical Care;[25] the American Nursing Home Association of the Medicare and Medicaid Programs;[26] the American Association of Physicians and Surgeons;[27] Health Insurance Association of America;[28] National Association of Blue Shield Plans;[29] Blue Cross Association;[30] and some local affiliates of these or other similar organizations. Some referred to testimony they had offered previously on H.R. 17550.

All of the 14 groups indicated above are providers or practitioners and, therefore, incompetent to speak for consumers. The American Public Health Association's (APHA) written testimony included some analysis of PSROs specifically;[31] but as the largest public health organization in the world[32] the group does not purport to, nor can it, speak for consumers. Yet the groups mentioned were the only witnesses testifying on the proposed PSRO amendment.[33] The striking absence of any consumers from that list demonstrates both where interest in the PSRO program has been strongest and who has the ability (financial, professional, economical, and social) to present testimony on short notice on an issue as important as this one.[34] Review of the *Hearings* reveals the pattern that consumers and consumer-oriented groups who did testify spoke primarily to the substantive issues of eligibility, hearing rights, and coverage under Medicare, Medicaid, and the several welfare titles of the Social Security Act. Of those who did testify, many did not have the opportunity to speak on Senator Bennett's bill because he had introduced it after they testified. There were no further hearings on the amendments, and the bill became law on October 30, 1972.[35]

That the professional groups noted above could not and did not speak for consumers is unquestionable. Neither could they have spoken for the taxpayers' interests. As participants in the proposed program, all had a stake in the outcome of the bill in addition to any "public" interest they might profess. Many spoke on general problems of peer review. A major specific theme in the testimony by practitioner groups was that practitioners must be reviewed by members of their own profession only—for example, dentists, psychologists, nurses, and podiatrists could not be appropriately reviewed by physicians.[36] This adherence to parochial concepts of professionalism is directly antithetical to consumer accountability. It is true that consumers are unable and incompetent to challenge practitioners on technical issues of expertise, but as this book has discussed many of the determinations PSROs will make are not technical or medical.[37]

The legislative process, then, did nothing for consumer accountability. Statutory interpretation—developing regulations that will mold the actual functioning of PSROs—is a critical process for establishment of a more responsive system. Many changes in the law can be wrought through regulations, as long as the statute does not specifically exclude a particular course of action. Administrative activity will be the principle avenue for improving the program as it was initially designed. That the mechanism of regulatory development is available to further consumer accountability is amply demonstrated by its use to defeat their interests.

A critical demonstration of total disregard for consumer interests in the regulatory process was the creation of "Statewide Support Centers." Nothing in the legislation gave specific authority for them. Many state medical societies were opposed to the local control PSROs would give to local medical societies; and state societies, particularly in Texas, Georgia, and Indiana, sought designation as the single PSRO for their entire state. Although both Senator Bennett and the Senate Finance Committee opposed single PSRO designations in populous states, and consistently and publicly emphasized the local orientation of the program, the AMA fought vigorously for state society control. Organized medicine's response to proposed regulations designating PSRO areas was so vigorous that the period for commenting on the proposals was extended. When final area designations appeared in the Federal Register, the usual prefatory comments suddenly gave the Secretary authority to contract with and financially assist Statewide PSRO Support Centers. State medical societies may serve as Support Centers. The comments went further.

> The designation of multiple areas in various large heavily populated states has however caused concern that Statewide organizations would be precluded from participation in the PSRO program. Such designations are not intended to exclude experienced State organizations.... Within the framework of the Secretary's policies and guidelines, a Support Center could carry out a number of functions such as general assistance to local PSROs, upon request, in all phases of professional and technical activity. Finally, a Support Center under appropriate arrangements could provide assistance to State PSRO [*sic*] Councils in the accomplishment of their responsibilities under the Statute.[38]

A liberal interpretation would permit Support Centers to participate in review. Given such an interpretation, their designation, then, differs little from the statewide PSROs the state medical societies had sought. Depending on the extent and substance of the responsibilities they assume, Support Centers, like inappropriate single statewide PSROs, would be inimical to consumers for the following reasons:[39]

(1) Because the PSRO program does not require affirmative action by PSROs to seek consumer input, it is imperative that the program be structured so that consumers can at least gain access to it. The poor and aged people who are the consumers do not have the resources to involve themselves in an organization whose center of activity may be geographically and financially inaccessible to them. In addition, the nature of the issues over which PSROs have jurisdiction is essentially local—the effectiveness of a hospital review system, the payment of an individual's bill. Consumer activity around PSROs would be severely curtailed by statewide designations or centralized Support Center responsibility for ongoing operational responsibilities. Efforts to focus power at the state level perhaps should be seen as another attempt to minimize consumer impact on the program.[40]

(2) PSROs have the duty to conduct primary determinations and hearings on review of determinations with which beneficiaries are dissatisfied.[41] The mechanics of the hearing process—mustering an argument, gaining access to information necessary to the case, marshaling support from providers or practitioners, effective presentation of the case—are complicated and difficult. To centralize the review process at the state level (in a Support Center or a single statewide PSRO) can abrogate the few consumer rights the statute guarantees. It would place an unjust burden on Medicaid and Medicare beneficiaries, who would be forced to travel long distances in order to present their cases effectively. Making the process inaccessible by virtue of a state focus would again thwart attempts by consumers to avail themselves of their rights.

(3) If PSRO review will improve the quality of medical care through an educational process involving substantial numbers of physicians actively

participating in day to day review, locating the review authority in a Support Center or statewide PSRO will attentuate the process and weaken its value. A larger number of physicians in each review entity will mean that participation by any one of them will be occasional and sporadic as attempts are made to include everyone. If the educational value of review is real, frequent participation can only enhance its positive effects and is therefore in the consumers' interests.

The injustices just noted which could occur if the basic PSRO responsibilities were centralized in each state are unlikely. But as each Support Center assumes a greater role in PSRO activities and expands its influence over local PSROs, consumer interests may be threatened. The regulatory process which created Support Centers did not permit fair compromises among the parties who would be affected by the creation of these nonstatutory bodies. Only a few of the interest groups so affected participated in the negotiated compromise, in isolation from consumer scrutiny, despite the fact that the regulatory changes introduced a potentially critical element which could reorient the focus of the PSRO program.

The regulatory process must seek out consumer groups for comment, criticism, and discussion if the program is to improve its consumer accountability quotient. Notice of meetings of the National Advisory Council are supposed to be open. As a practical matter, notice of them has been restricted to publication in the Federal Register, professional journals, and specialized newsletters. Although the policy has been changed, initially National Advisory Council meetings excluded the few consumer-oriented advocates who had sought access to them. Federal law requires that the Council publish timely notice of meetings in the Federal Register and "other types of public notice to insure that all interested persons are notified of such meeting prior thereto."[42] On one occasion, notice of a meeting was published only three days before it was to take place; and two consumer representatives were forced to leave an "executive session" of the same meeting under a possibly spurious assertion of the Freedom of Information Act.[43]

These episodes and developments indicate at least that the initial reaction of program implementers, when faced with an obvious policy choice, is to opt for the one which denies a significant consumer orientation or role in the program.

MAKING THE SYSTEM MORE RESPONSIVE

Release of Information

PSROs will absorb and generate enormous quantities of information about the health care delivery system across the nation. Getting that information to consumers is the simplest and most basic step toward systemic accountability. The need to disseminate information about health care delivery, technology, and its results exists because of several factors. Tancredi and Barsky [44] suggest that society's informed consent to the policy choices made in providing health care technology to large groups of people requires adequate information on which to base the consent.

> Consumers of health care and society at large have not had access to requisite information for intelligent and rational determinations on the development of technologies.... Some mechanism must be established for ferreting out relevant social, economic, and ethical considerations and disclosing these to the public or appropriate representative bodies so that decisions can be made by the existing political structure, at the same time, providing a milieu for maximum flexibility in the development of potentially useful technologies. [45]

Discussing how to make decisions of where and when to supply kidney dialysis units to individuals and communities, they say:

> ...introduction of costly medical technology has produced political changes, particularly on the national constituency–federal government level. We believe the only way to monitor, and perhaps alter if necessary this process is through political, not technological institutions. And, we suggest this should be done through the systemic collection, processing, and relaying of information gathered by the participants in the decision to evaluate, develop, employ or purchase a new technology. [46]

The analysis is directly applicable to PSROs and their decisions to allocate scarce monetary resources.

Dissemination of information to consumers will provide other salutary effects. It will contribute to consumer education and better informed health service consumption generally. [47] Improved consumer participation in those aspects of health care delivery in which they are permitted to be involved would result from their access to better information on which to base their decisions. Effective evaluation of the PSRO program in general and of its individual components—local PSROs, Statewide Councils, Advisory Groups— cannot proceed without affirmative action by those who control information to make known the program's functions and activities. [48]

If consumers are to understand what PSROs can and will do, and the extent to which the program will affect their lives, they must have full access to a wide array of information. This process has been additionally hampered by the fact that basic information about the program has not been widely circulated. [49] Other participants, most significantly the physicians on whom the program depends, have also been uninformed about PSROs.[50] Release of information has been a subject of some controversy in the development of the program. It is, however, vital to the effective operation of the PSRO program.[51]

Sources and Uses of Information. PSROs will collect as well as generate data. Considerable reliance on existing information systems will be the foundation of the PSRO information network.

> The data collection and processing system is structured in accordance with guidelines developed by the Secretary in consultation with the National PSR Council, with a view toward assuring maximum efficiency, economy, and coordination in all data-gathering efforts and the compatibility of data across different geographic areas. Data flowing from the Medicare and Medicaid claims process is to be utilized to the maximum extent possible.[52]

Both the variety of existing health care–related information systems and their relative adaptability to PSRO purposes are extensive. Government systems exist at all levels.[53] HEW alone maintains so many banks of data that at one time the federal government was reported to have published a "Guidebook to U.S. Department of HEW Computer Data Files." (Recent inquiries revealed the book was never produced.[54]) Moreover, in addition to government sources, large numbers of private systems under varying sponsorship[55] develop and publish, for hospitals and other buyers, data on health care delivery. Individual computer systems maintained by some hospitals will further complicate integration of data systems.[56] Yet, despite the plethora of available data sources, PSROs will find some areas where no data exists. For example, "PSROs looking at the utilization of other institutions like nursing homes will find no base-line national information to guide them at present."[57]

The importance to the PSRO system of the data gathering and processing functions is seen in the fierce competition to capture control of those activities. Blue Cross and Blue Shield have mounted large efforts to secure their positions at the forefront of the data source fight.[58] Not to be outdone, the private data systems have conducted "continuing education programs" designed to demonstrate their value as a data source in the PSRO system;[59] and foundations for medical care have emphasized the advantages they offer as clinical managers of data contrasted with "the Blues" orientation toward fiscal management and cost control.[60] Some commentators have expressed fears that the existing systems will not share information freely with PSROs,[61] while others focus on the government's need to get accurate information from reporting systems as an inherent aspect of "public accountability."[62]

The statute itself provides the initial clue to the varieties of information which will be developed during PSRO processes and therefore available for dissemination.[63] The following discussion elaborates on what those basic types of data will be and their use and importance to consumers.

Norms and regional variations from them are the most fundamental pieces of information that will pass between the National Council and local PSROs.[64] In addition, initially established norms will be changed, although the statute does not specifically require such changes. It merely says "...data concerning norms shall be reviewed from time to time."[65] The *Program Manual* provides for modifications and specifies that they be made available to practitioners and hospitals.[66] Because norms will set the range of services that will be covered by government benefits, consumers must know what they are and how they have been modified in order to make informed decisions regarding their own care. To consent to medical care, patients will want to know whether they can reasonably anticipate coverage for the proposed services. Knowledge of the applicable norms is essential for their proper consent. Regional variations will statistically demonstrate which areas are medically underserved.

The statute requires PSROs to publicize which types of services or conditions will be subject to advance determinations.[67] While no specific restrictions or requirements have been placed on who shall have access to the material, most of the information mentioned in the *Program Manual* is mandated for publication only to hospitals and practitioners.[68] Because consumers will be most directly affected by the financial results of PSRO determinations, they must know which types of care can be reviewed prospectively in order to assure themselves that coverage will be available.

Profiles of practitioners and providers (and patients) will be continually generated by PSROs.[69] These profiles can reveal much about the practice of medicine in general. Among other things, they will demonstrate which types of practitioners most often perform selected procedures—whether, for example, otolaryngologists (ear, nose, and throat specialists) perform more tonsillectomies than pediatricians. This type of information can be important to a consumer who is trying to decide whether to undergo surgery. Based on profiles, he can evaluate his case in the context of others. A patient may decide, for example, that general surgeons, such as the one he has consulted, do not perform enough pacemaker insertions to be optimally competent. He may then choose a cardiothoracic surgeon who specializes in pacemaker insertions. On the other hand, a hypertensive patient for whom a vascular surgeon prescribes surgery might choose to consult an internist instead, if from profiles he knows that vascular surgeons generally treat hypertension with surgical intervention, while an internist would be more likely to treat high blood pressure with drugs. Profiles of institutions can give consumers basic information on existing quality of care as well as trends toward improvement or degeneration of institutional practices. If an institution's profile indicates a high rate of compliance with PSRO norms and guidelines, a patient can expect a better rate of coverage for services delivered there as compared with an institution with a high rate of PSRO disallowances.

"In carrying out its responsibilities, the PSRO would be required to regularly review provider and practitioner profiles of care and service (that is, the patterns of services delivered to Medicare and Medicaid beneficiaries by individual health care practitioners and institutions) and other data to evaluate the necessity, quality, and appropriateness of services for which payment may be made under the medicare and medicaid programs."[70] Since case by case determinations of coverage will be made through an individual case review process, the Senate Finance Committee can only have meant that information developed from PSRO review of patterns of care already rendered will be used as a basis for modification or reform in the basic benefits offered under the Medicare and Medicaid programs. For that reason, practitioner and provider profiles will shape the entire Medicare and Medicaid programs in the future. For consumers to participate meaningfully in the process by which their health benefits will be changed, they must have available to them the information on which such changes will be based. Beyond this, "PSRO[s] would be expected to analyze the pattern of services rendered or ordered by individual practitioners and providers and to concentrate [their] attention on situations in which unnecessary, substandard or inappropriate services seem most likely to exist or occur."[71] Divulgence of these demonstrations of poor quality care are important to consumers who seek to shop wisely for their health care services. Knowing that substandard care exists without revealing that fact to the people whose lives will be directly affected by that care is unconscionable.

The hearings and review process conducted under PSRO aegis will produce material on complaints about PSRO activities and individual participants' behavior in delivering health care services. Data on the propriety of initial PSRO determinations will also be created in the course of hearings and appeals. Access to that data can help a consumer who is considering whether to appeal an unsatisfactory determination. Just as a lawyer evaluates his prospects for success on appeal according to the precedents on that issue and the record of the lower court on appeals, a consumer will need to know the likelihood of success with a higher review authority in the PSRO system. Furthermore, as indicated earlier in this discussion,[72] patterns of complaints that will emerge from the hearings and review mechanism should be used in systemic evaluations of the effectiveness of the PSRO system. Consumers must have access to that information in order to participate effectively in efforts to improve the program, should they arise.

The variety of information just catalogued is the most basic material which PSROs will have at their disposal. As the system gains more experience, additional information and uses for it will undoubtedly be developed. For example, PSROs have authority to "examine the pertinent records of any practitioner or provider of health services" with regard to services over which they have review responsibility.[73] They also have the authority to "inspect the facilities in which care is rendered or services provided ... of any practitioner or provider" operating in their areas.[74] Access to files and other compilations of data, including analysis of raw data, will be actively sought not only by consumers, but also by individual practitioners, provider institutions, paying agents, state Medicaid agencies, and the many administrative divisions in HEW which have something to do with the PSRO program or other aspects of public health care delivery. The degree to which the PSRO system seeks to maintain exclusive control over the information it generates will be a subject of continuing controversy throughout the program's existence.

Statutory Provisions on Dissemination of Information. The PSRO statute requires that certain categories of information be transmitted from one element of the program to another. Reports on possible provider and practitioner violations of legal obligations must be submitted by the local PSRO to the appropriate Statewide Council.[75] The Statewide Council, in turn, must forward those reports, with their recommendations, to the Secretary of HEW.[76]

The local PSRO is charged with an affirmative obligation to provide information about itself by "utilizing, whenever appropriate, medical periodicals and similar publications to publicize the functions and activities of Professional Standards Review Organizations."[77] Such publication, however, is intended to familiarize physicians with PSRO activities in order to encourage their participation in the program. Nowhere is there a requirement that such information from PSROs be directed at consumers in order to familiarize them with PSRO activities and functions.

The National Council has the obligation to "make or arrange for the making of studies and investigations with a view to developing and recommending to the Secretary and Congress measures designed more effectively to accomplish the purposes and objectives" of the PSRO program.[78] Further, it must submit a report, "not less often than annually," to the Secretary and Congress on the findings of its studies and investigations and its recommendations for improving the program.[79] The report must also contain comparative data on the results of PSRO review activities in each state and each area in it.[80] Although some analysts believe the provision is sufficient to ensure consumers' access to the report,[81] there is no specific requirement that the report be made available to them.

The PSRO statute specifically prohibits disclosure of information outside the system.

> Any data or information acquired by any Professional Standards Review Organization, in the exercise of its duties and functions, shall be held in confidence and shall not be disclosed to any person except (1) to the extent that may be necessary to carry out the purposes of this part or (2) in such cases and under such circumstances as the Secretary shall by regulations provide to assure the adequate protection of the rights and interests of patients, health care practitioners, or providers of health care.[82]

Penalties for violating that provision include a fine of up to $1000, imprisonment for up to six months, or both, with the costs of prosecution.[83] The two possible situations where the law would allow disclosure of information give great discretion to both local PSROs and the Secretary. Disclosure as "necessary to carry out the purposes" of the program could permit a local PSRO, concerned about quality of health care services in its area, to publish a broad range of information, if it construes such release as necessary to its carrying out its statutory duties.

All of the information alluded to above pertains to the nature and quality of health care services delivered to the Medicare and Medicaid populations. The importance of making known that type of information was recognized by the Senate Finance Committee.

> Physicians and the public are currently unaware as to which hospitals, extended care facilities, skilled nursing homes and inter- mediate care facilities have deficiencies and which facilities fully meet the statutory and regulatory requirements. This operates to discourage the direction of physician, patient, and public concern toward deficient facilities which might encourage them to upgrade the quality of care they provide to proper levels.[84]

While the statement was made with regard to a new provision in the Social Security law requiring the Secretary "to make public in readily available form and place" reports on compliance by providers with conditions of participation in the Medicare program,[85] the value in disclosing PSRO information is similar.[86]

Beyond the benefits from releasing information, it should be noted that all the information produced by the program is only as valuable substantively as the process which created it is reliable. Unless PSRO information can be reviewed, a major element of the program's effectiveness will be shielded from open scrutiny, thereby hampering accountability of all kinds. As one commentator has noted, the issue is not really whether information should be released, but how to present it so it is accurate and useful.

> It would be far better for the public to be given data that have been collected properly and analyzed carefully and equitably. We do not have a choice between making some information or no information available to the public. Our only choice is between incomplete and misleading information on the one hand, and information that has been properly assembled and analyzed on the other.[87]

Effects of Nondisclosure. Besides the policy arguments for disclos- ing to consumer groups any PSRO information which is not confidential, there are additional reasons to disclose information in individual cases. To deny access to information in certain individual cases can seriously affect individual consumers.

1. The Secretary, with advice from Statewide Councils and PSROs, has the authority to deny the right to participate in the Medicare and Medicaid programs to practitioners who flagrantly abuse the system, consistently fall below PSRO standards, or otherwise violate their legal obligations.[88] Once the Secretary determines that the sanction should apply, the law requires that the public know who those practitioners are in order to preclude their becoming liable for services rendered by a disqualified practitioner from whom they have unwittingly sought care.[89] Some practitioners' advocates would argue that it is unfair to penalize someone whose substandard behavior has not been conclusively established. But when a practitioner's name has been passed from the PSRO to the Statewide Council, it is likely his abuses are sufficiently obvious that a patient patronizing that practitioner runs a high risk that coverage for those services will be disallowed, as well as a risk of poor quality medical care. Just as disclosure of reports on providers is intended to help them improve their services, so such disclosure on practitioners seriously suspected of abusing the system would help them improve.[90] With disclosure, patients would not be penalized with poor quality care because they unknowingly sought services from a poor practitioner. But considering the questionable reliability of many of the existing information systems,[91] it seems only fair that, before profiles or other reports on an individual practitioner are distributed, the individual practitioner should be given the opportunity to add any written rebuttal, explanation, or other comment to the material that will be distributed.

2. Similarly, if PSRO analyses of patterns of services uncover cases of unnecessary, substandard, or inappropriate medical care, consumers have the right to know that. Traditionally, discovery of substandard practices is publicized only in the context of a malpractice lawsuit. Even then, the harm to the plaintiff has already occurred and other potential patients learn of substandard care only to the extent that the litigation itself is publicized. This tendency is exacerbated in the PSRO context because of a statutory malpractice exemption.[92]

But, in addition to the right to know where substandard care is delivered in order to avoid it, consumers should also be given access to information which names practitioners and providers who consistently render the highest quality care—have the fewest services disallowed, or have the lowest incidence of overturned utilization review committee decisions. Even those analysts and practitioners who most favor a free market for health care with minimal, if any, government regulation must recognize that a free market entails competition. Unless consumers have the ability to affect that competition by exercising choice among providers based on relevant information, there can be no free market.

3. Individual consumers must also know which norms are applied in their areas in order to assert effectively their rights as Medicare and Medicaid patients. Where an advance approval is given, there is a presumption of

appropriateness of the services subsequently rendered, and, therefore, the patient may be entitled to all the services the norm would have covered, even if they were not all rendered.[93] In that case a patient must know to what he or she was entitled in the first instance when a question arises subsequently about the initial presumption of coverage. Similarly, in all situations where a dispute arises over a PSRO's determination, a patient who is ignorant of the appropriate norms is unable to challenge the determination effectively. If the system is to curb retroactive denials of benefits, the beneficiary should have available to him the appropriate norm for his condition in order to consent to any stay beyond the norms, since the extension might place the ultimate burden for payment on him.[94]

       4. Nondisclosure of information could infringe on a patient's right to discovery in litigation. Discovery is the process in litigation where each party gains access to the information available to the other party. The process is governed by law. If a PSRO determines on a retrospective basis that hospital or nursing home care was medically unnecessary, government payment for these services would be denied. The institution might then sue the patient to recover the costs of the services already rendered.[95] In the defense of such a lawsuit, the following information might be relevant and useful: (a) how effective the provider's own utilization review is, including the committee's consideration of the amount and duration of services rendered to the patient; (b) whether and to what extent the provider sought to justify to the PSRO its deviation from PSRO norms; and (c) whether the provider attempted to negotiate a settlement with the PSRO. A restrictive reading of the confidentiality provision would preclude discovery by the defendant-patient.[96]

       5. Although the legislative history clearly states that a PSRO may not itself force the discharge of a patient because of its determination of no medical necessity,[97] abuses may arise where a physician fails to understand the legal significance of a PSRO determination. In such a case, if the physician said to the patient, "You must leave; the PSRO has disapproved your continued stay in the hospital," the patient might then feel the PSRO had forced his discharge. If that patient suffered an injury as a result of his leaving the hospital, he might choose to sue the PSRO. (This is not to imply he would necessarily be successful.) In litigation, the patient would have the right to discover a variety of information from the PSRO about its activities, but could be denied his rights under a restrictive interpretation of the PSRO statute. Although no individual working for a PSRO who has exercised due care in performing his statutory responsibilities may be held liable for the consequences of his acts, the statute does not exempt the PSRO as an entity from liability, and its collective determination and the consequences of them may be actionable.

       In examining disclosure policies it is significant to note that past attempts to obtain information from HEW under the Medicare statute have met with substantial resistance. For example, U.S. Congressman Ronald W. Dellums

(D–Calif.); James Ridgeway, an editor of *Ramparts* magazine; and the Health Law Project of the University of Pennsylvania requested from the Social Security Administration many different types of information, including manuals governing the operation of the Medicare program, reports of findings derived from investigations of the operations of fiscal intermediaries, and data relating to prevailing doctors' fees in Pennsylvania. After several months' delay, HEW rejected almost all of the requests (the manuals were given) and the three parties joined in a suit under the Freedom of Information Act[98] to gain access to the intermediary performance reports and the data on doctors' fees. Because most of the materials were subsequently provided (in large part because of the 1972 Amendments to the Social Security Act and internal changes at HEW), the case finally concerned only access to physician fee data. The District Court ultimately held that HEW should disclose the documents;[99] but a Freedom of Information Act case can, at best, create only a limited obligation to disclose. A decision that material is disclosable does not create a requirement that it be distributed.

Confidentiality. The confidentiality of information which passes between patient and physician in the course of medical care has been honored since at least the time of the Hippocratic Oath.[100] It has been codified in the form of physician-patient privileges in rules of evidence which prohibit revealing in a courtroom the contents of exchanges between patients and their doctors unless the patient waives that right.[101] Tort law has also made breaches of confidence outside the courtroom actionable. [102]

The need for confidentiality is rooted in the physician's need to know anything and everything which may be relevant to the patient's medical treatment. Because the patient will many times not know what factors bear on his condition, an atmosphere of total candor is essential to the delivery of high quality care. Fear of disclosure to parties outside the doctor-patient relationship might prevent a patient's revealing information critical to his treatment. While every member of the health care delivery system must strictly honor the right to confidentiality above other administrative concerns [103] (if the goal of high quality medical care is to be achieved), the prerogative to assert that right is the patient's alone. For example, where physician-patient privileges exist the law does not give the physician the right to refuse to disclose information in the courtroom; only the patient may justifiably assert the right. Further, it is important that confidentiality extend only to information which is, in fact, of a confidential nature. Norms and profiles of practitioners and providers, for example, are not confidential. They are not part of physician-patient interchanges made in the course of medical treatment. Although they have an ethical obligation to respect their patients' rights, physicians (and administrators) properly cannot seek to assert the right to confidentiality on behalf of their patients; nor should such an assertion be permitted to be invoked as a shield to prevent appropriate disclosure of information which would ultimately serve the needs of patients in the medical care system.

In the implementation of the PSRO program, confidentiality of medical records has been a major focus of controversy. The subject was discussed at considerable length in the *PSRO Oversight Hearings*. [104] Opponents of the program have looked to the issue of confidentiality as a means to thwart its implementation. [105]

The potential for abuse of patients' rights to confidentiality is created in the system through its vast information gathering and distribution potential. In addition to reviewing cases to determine if they will be covered by government reimbursement, PSROs are authorized to examine individual records of individual practitioners where pertinent. [106] The fears that agencies will seek more information than is necessary is not unfounded. Past President of the AMA Malcolm C. Todd warned his fellow physicians that in the societal atmosphere which rationalizes bugging and other intrusions into civil rights, "people are being compelled to make disclosures about themselves that serve no legitimate purpose, or the information is obtained from others without the informed consent of the subjects." [107] In examining the problem of giving information to health insurers, Todd has said,

> To give them what they genuinely needed . . . the most common practice used to be hand-copying merely those items in a medical record that had specific bearing on the issue in question. Now some physicians find it less expensive and time consuming to let an office assistant photocopy an entire record and mail it off. Some third parties are actually sending representatives to physicians' offices to do the copying themselves. Even when the patient consents to disclosure, he may not be aware of what or how much he's authorizing. [108]

In addition to abuse by physicians indiscriminately delivering information into the hands of third parties, abuses can occur when the electronic system storing computerized information is sabotaged. [109]

The potential for abuse should not be used to preclude proper gathering and disclosure of medical information. Indeed, the right to know and the right to privacy are not necessarily mutually exclusive. Although the right to confidentiality of medical records has been a strongly protected one, no right to privacy in this society has ever been absolute. [110] Courts, for example, have upheld physician revelation to third party payers of otherwise privileged information. [111] The medical system as it now operates permits disclosure of many types of information in order to create a functional delivery mechanism. [112] The two critical questions to ask in balancing the right to privacy and the need to know in the design of PSRO data systems are (1) is there a change in the type of information kept, the means of collecting and storing it, and the means of disseminating it which will require new administrative mechanisms to adequately safeguard privacy; and (2) what types of administrative measures will serve to improve the chances that abuses will not occur. Studies have demonstrated that in the most sophisticated medical information systems today there has been very little change in the types of information stored from that which was traditionally tabulated and recorded manually.[113] PSROs are not gathering different information; rather, they have the potential to centralize the information, analyze it for new purposes, and use it in constructive ways. There is no new body of information which PSROs will ask for to perform review that has not been given before for reimbursement purposes in the Medicare and Medicaid programs.

When a system gathers only that information which is directly applicable and necessary to effective administration, the potential for abuse is restricted. Carefully framed forms and inquiries increase efficiency and better serve both the program's needs and those of consumers and others seeking information. In examining Medicare data administration practices specifically, one analyst has said,

> ... [O]nly that information should be collected routinely that is needed for the day-to-day operation of the system. Medicare is primarily a bill paying mechanism. . . . It follows that the bills submitted must have sufficient information to make a decision on eligibility for payment and on the amount of payment under the rules of the game. . . .[114]
>
> Unless there are overwhelming, compelling reasons all other information not directly required to operate the program should be obtained through special studies. . . .[115]

Once information needs have been determined, the use of collected data should be similarly conditioned. The Medicaid program restricts the use of information. The statute requires that each state with a Medicaid plan "provide safeguards which restrict the use or disclosure of information concerning applicants and recipients to purposes directly connected with the administration of the plan."[116] In contrast with the PSRO statute, the Medicaid provision applies to *applicants* and *recipients*, not to all participants in the program, such as physicians or hospital fiscal agents. The regulations under that provision take the broadly phrased, but clear directive to honor confidentiality, and supply technical details, including a specific mandate that medical data be safeguard.[117] In the Multi-State Information System for Psychiatric Patient Records (MSIS) extensive consideration was devoted to ensuring the protection of patient records in a computerized system which compiled data from several states. By preventing access by any institution to any information not generated directly by itself, reports indicate there has been no transfer of information between states or between facilities. By eliminating any individual patient identifiers, confidentiality has been maintained. To date, despite significant concern by practitioners about the potential for abuse of confidentiality, there have not been any significant reported problems with the program.[118]

But establishment of legal safeguards for confidential material as part of program design is not a sufficient answer to meet the need for protecting patient information. Monitoring information use will be essential to continued guarantees of adequate security. Recently a coalition of physicians, patients, and public health representatives called for the formation of a national commission for the preservation of confidentiality of health records, to be created without participation from federal government representatives.[119] Such private monitoring efforts will undoubtedly flourish with expanded health data networks and programs; and consumers, whose rights such groups will assure, will want to be directly involved in those activities.

Two additional factors must be considered for development of an appropriate system balancing the right to privacy and the right to information: (1) specific problems created by the electronic nature of information collection and storage systems; and (2) potential problems arising from existing statutes authorizing information release.

Computerized data banks compile vast varieties of information and often exchange or sell the data they have stored. The growth of these stores of information has been attributed to diverse factors including,

> "[t]he complexity of the policy decisions that have been explored in recent years and the increasing availability of new technologies for collecting, transmitting and processing information [leading to] an increased demand by government, university and private sectors for more efficient access to information about multitudinous aspects of the lives of individuals.[120]

In case by case review[121] and compilation of profiles, PSROs will depend heavily on computers. Blue Cross and Blue Shield are cited by the Senate Finance Committee as organizations specifically suited to perform data collection and sharing functions in the PSRO system.[122] Although considerable attention has been devoted to legal protection of the right to privacy in the face of burgeoning data banks, optimal safeguards remain elusive.[123] Patient-identified information at least should be the first priority in PSRO policy decisions establishing the parameters for use of information.

There are some laws which permit some public access to information in government data banks. The Freedom of Information Act,[124] for example, permits some access to government agency materials without the consent of (or even notice to) the person about whom information has been compiled. Medical files, however, are exempt from disclosure.[125] Other statutes attempt to limit the government's power to collect information. The Federal Reports Act,[126] aimed primarily at mitigating the burden on business enterprises to produce information for government agencies, interposes prior approval by the Office of Management and Budget when a federal agency seeks to collect identical information from 10 or more persons.[127] Other conditions are imposed on sharing with other federal agencies material collected under the act.[128] The Fair Credit Reporting Act[129] attempts to regulate the activities of consumer reporting agencies (e.g., credit bureaus, investigative reporting companies) by holding these agencies to standards of accuracy, limited use, and notice to individuals. Under the law, individuals must be given access to all data collected, except medical information.[130] Through the use of these statutes, consumers, or anyone else, could gain access to information stored in various banks.

Although these laws do not apply to PSROs, they do exist as examples of previous efforts to confront and resolve some of these issues. The PSRO statute as it stands is phrased too broadly to condition inherently either the collection or use of data. The statute recognizes equal "rights" to confidentiality among all participants in the health care system, without giving paramount consideration to patients.[131] Minimally, the PSRO system must provide for strictly conditioned uses of patient-identified information. Any information which is disseminated should be subject to (1) prior consent to the transfer of information by the person about whom the information is collected (if he can be identified from the information); (2) an opportunity for that individual to look at the material and add to it anything he might think is relevant, and (3) limitations on the amount of time during which information may be stored.[132]

Regulations on confidentiality and dissemination of PSRO information will undoubtedly change with the experience of the program. Some of the issues that are being addressed include the following: (1) appropriate use of a personal identifier, including designation of those documents, forms, and printouts which will and will not require personal identification; (2) control of the acquisition of data needed for PSRO purposes, including those data acquired through the claims process and by the PSRO itself; (3) procedures for the handling of data by PSRO personnel and other data processing personnel; (4) procedures for training PSRO personnel, including guidelines for the use of printed materials and on-site training sessions; (5) procedures for maintaining physical security of both PSRO and data processing facilities; (6) mechanisms for data verification by physicians, patients, and the PSROs; (7) procedures for determining that unauthorized disclosure of information has occurred, including a specific interpretation of what constitutes authorized disclosure and to whom information may be disclosed; (8) provisions for purging files that are (a) inaccurate or (b) no longer necessary for PSRO purposes (including definitive points in time when files must be purged) and procedures for permitting verification of data maintained by PSROs; (9) procedures for maintaining records of access to or the use made of information in the PSRO review system.[133]

Conditional Status and Final Designation

One of the primary aspects of accountability is the requirement of adaptability and change on the basis of input from outside the program. Enlightened information dissemination policies are the first step toward that process. Consumer accountability may be considerably enhanced if the process of "conditional" and "final designation" of PSROs is used to further assure the program's accountability.

If a conditional PSRO is deemed to be unsatisfactory it may not be finally designated as the PSRO for that area. An unsatisfactory PSRO, theoretically, would then be eliminated in favor of a more effective entity. The provisions of the statute on this, however, are essentially value neutral and, if subject to improper manipulation, could equally well result in the elimination of those PSROs most oriented toward principles of consumer accountability.

Because each PSRO must face a review and possible exclusion from the program before the final designation can be granted, each one will be held to some standard of performance. Moreover, initial designations are to be made with a view toward "determining the capacity of [each] organization to perform the duties and functions" imposed by the statute. [134] The initial designation may not extend beyond 24 months. [135] During that trial period, a PSRO may undertake review activities only to the extent that the Secretary believes it is capable of performing them satisfactorily. It is expected that initially assigned responsibilities will be gradually increased in number and type "so that by the end of the period, [the] organization shall be considered a qualified organization only if the Secretary finds that it is substantially carrying out in a satisfactory manner" the activities it must perform as a PSRO. [136] A fall-back provision has been written into the statute as well, so that during the phase-in period and "pending a demonstration of capacity for improved review effort with respect to matters involving the provision of health care services in the area" [137] any duties for which the PSRO does not have full responsibility will be charged to other existing mechanisms. [138]

The statute does not specify on what evidence the Secretary must base his evaluation of a PSRO's performance. Initial designation itself is contingent on approval of a written plan submitted by the applicant organization "as well as on the basis of other relevant data and information." [139] According to the Senate Finance Committee, "once an organization is accepted as a PSRO, the Secretary would regularly evaluate its performance using statistical comparisons and other means of evaluation including the findings and recommendations of the statewide and national professional standards review councils established under the amendment." [140] The *Program Manual* does require the PSRO to transmit reports on its activities to the Secretary. [141] Nothing in either document explicitly precludes consideration of consumer evaluation as a measure or determinant of performance; and inclusion of evidence on consumers' perspectives should be sought in the final designation process.

A particularly useful technique for seeking out and bringing into consideration the views of consumers would be open hearings by the Secretary prior to final designation of each PSRO. Hearings will not only provide an organized, open forum to receive such relevant information, but also will rectify some of the problems that will arise because of the absence of specific standards for evaluating each PSRO's performance. Presently, hearings are required only where there is termination for cause, by the Secretary, of the agreement with a finally designated but recalcitrant PSRO.[142] As the Finance Committee noted, "once an organization is accepted as a PSRO ... [w]here performance ... was determined to be unsatisfactory, and timely efforts to bring about its improvement failed, the Secretary could terminate its participation after appropriate notice and opportunity for administrative hearing."[143] Although conditional designations are subject to comment [144] through the requirement that notice of them be published in the Federal Register,[145] comments are sought only from physicians practicing in the area to be served by the proposed PSRO;[146] and no hearing is required to determine the capabilities of each or any of the organizations seeking designation.[147]

An open hearing, held locally, prior to final designation, would both encourage and accommodate comments from consumers who might otherwise have no opporutnity to give their evaluation of the local PSRO's performance. The solicitation and considerations of such comments are necessary to ensuring the credibility of the program, and, therefore, its effectiveness. Without such a requirement, evaluations of each PSRO's performance will be made purely at the discretion of the Secretary on the basis of evidence submitted to him only by the PSRO itself and, where it exists, the Statewide Council.[148] Without an affirmative requirement to solicit evidence from sources outside the program, the information available to the Secretary can reflect only the needs of the PSRO program as a government bureaucracy. Because of the peer review nature of the program and its direct impact on individual patients, the views of consumers are essential to a meaningful evaluation of each PSRO before final designation. There is ample legal authority for the creation of such a hearing requirement through resort either to the Administrative Procedure Act (APA) [149] or administrative common law principles, or both.

Under the APA, a "license" includes the "whole or a part of an agency permit, certificate, *approval*, registration, charter membership, statutory exemption or other form of permission." [150] The APA defines "licensing" as "agency process respecting the grant, renewal, denial, revocation, suspension, annulment, withdrawal, limitation, amendment, modification or conditioning of a license."[151] Applying either or both definitions, the Secretary's act of final designation through agreement is, in effect and functionally, a "license" to the

PSRO under consideration to perform as a fully operational entity. The importance of so viewing the final designation process lies in the procedural requirements (due process) which the APA imposes on the licensing activity of agencies subject to it. The act requires that a hearing which meets specific statutory standards [152] be held "when an application is made for a license required by law" [153] (unless other specific statutory requirements exist). Furthermore, the hearing must be conducted "with due regard for the rights and privileges of all the interested parties or adversely affected persons." [154]

Under the PSRO scheme, there is no formal application process required of the PSRO prior to final designation. The conditional designation is limited to 24 months, by which time the PSRO "shall be considered a qualified organization only if the Secretary" finds it to be performing properly. [155] There is no specific point in time when final designation takes place. The execution of the agreement between the Secretary and the PSRO includes the final designation.

> If, on the basis of its performance during such period of conditional designation, the Secretary determines that such organization is capable of fulfilling, in a satisfactory manner, the obligations and requirements for a [PSRO] . . . he shall enter into an agreement with such organization designating it as the [PSRO] for such area. [156]

The agreement [157] by which the PSRO is designated is, then, the license to perform as the only PSRO in that area. For purposes of the APA argument, the initial application for conditional status continues in effect as an application for final designation, to be considered when sufficient and appropriate evidence about the PSRO has been gathered. It is significant for the argument that the format of the printed statute differentiates between PSRO "Trial Periods" [158] (conditions on initial designations) and final designation itself. [159] Although the activities of a conditional PSRO, at least initially, may vary quite substantially from those of a finally designated PSRO, [160] the statute requires that each PSRO submit only one written plan in petitioning to be considered a "qualified organization" by the Secretary. [161] That plan, then, must be considered the application of the PSRO for the license to serve as a qualified organization, unless and until other requirements are specified in the later stages of implementation of the program.

Once the hearing requirement is established, the issue becomes how to facilitate consumer participation. The right of public (extraparty) intervention in agency process has been recently recognized and expanded by some courts. In surveying these cases and the arguments supporting public and consumer participation in administrative hearings, one commentator [162] cites among the criteria for permitting intervention the intervenor's interest in the outcome of the proceeding. [163] Among other cases, he cites *National Welfare*

Rights Organization v. *Finch,* [164] where a group of welfare recipients sought to intervene in a welfare conformity hearing by the federal government against a state. The court held there that the recipients did have the right to intervene in a hearing, but they had no right to intervene in any of HEW's informal measures to bring about compliance. Professor Gellhorn notes that "[t]he welfare recipients's viewpoint is also important because it is likely to be distinct from that of the state or of HEW, and in reaching a sound decision these views should not be ignored." [165] The analogy of the decision and Gellhorn's comment to PSRO compliance determinations for purposes of final designation is inescapable. Medicare and Medicaid beneficiaries have a clear and direct interest in the proper functioning of the PSRO which oversees the quality of their health care; their interest is certainly no less critical than that of the welfare recipients in *NWRO* v. *Finch.* [166]

One of the principle reasons for holding hearings in the "licensing" situation has been recognized in the "Ashbacker doctrine" from the case of *Ashbacker Radio Co.* v. *F.C.C.* [167] The statute at issue there in effect provided that applicants for broadcast licenses had the right to a hearing before applications were denied. Two applications which were mutually exclusive were pending. In holding that the FCC could not grant a license to one applicant without a hearing on the other, the Supreme Court said, "[I]f one grant effectively precludes the other, the statutory right to a hearing which Congress has accorded applicants before a denial of their application becomes an empty thing." [168] Although the PSRO statute does not now provide a statutory right to a hearing, failure to provide a hearing prior to final designation forecloses to an insurgent PSRO a formal mechanism through which it can challenge the conditional PSRO's right to a final designation. As in *Ashbacker,* [169] the final designation of one PSRO is exclusive for that area. An organization seeking to challenge the conditional PSRO should be afforded a meaningful opportunity to present the case against the conditional PSRO and evidence supporting its own designation. Of course, a provision for hearings might be disadvantageous to a consumer-oriented PSRO in those instances where a non-consumer-responsive PSRO, which may be financially stronger and politically more powerful, gains, through the hearing requirement, otherwise nonexistent rights. But the APA does safeguard the rights of conditional PSROs in some respects. Withdrawal, suspension, revocation, or annulment of a license is lawful only if, before the hearing is instituted, the applicant is given notice "in writing, of the facts or conduct which may warrant the action" [170] and it is given an "opportunity to demonstrate or achieve compliance with all lawful requirements." [171] The Senate Finance Committee contemplated this precise approach when it provided for termination midterm by the Secretary if a PSRO had been deemed unsatisfactory and "timely efforts to bring about its improvement failed." [172] Because the law would protect the interests of the conditional PSRO, there is no reason to exclude evidence from outside parties on the issue of the performance of the PSRO.[173]

Regulations requiring such a hearing may be issued without specific statutory authority. Some of the reasons for holding a hearing, on the record, with a decision enunciating findings and reasons, have been recognized by the courts. The requirement that a hearing determination be based on standards is linked to the reasons for holding the hearing in the first place:[174] It (1) facilitates judicial review; (2) encourages more careful administrative consideration; (3) assures the agency does not exceed its jurisdiction; and (4) helps the parties plan for rehearings and judicial review.[175] Unless administrative hearing officers are forced to explain their actions according to established standards, the potential for unexplainable actions will persist.[176]

There are no specific standards in the statute for measuring the performance of a PSRO seeking final designation. Unless the Secretary is required, in each case, to state the standards used and his conclusions based on them, there will be no method for holding him accountable in any way for his final designations.

CONSUMER PARTICIPATION

Consumer participation as an aspect of consumer accountability has not been included under "Making the System More Responsive" because the statute implicitly and effectively excludes consumers from direct participation in the structure of the PSRO program. PSROs are "peer review" entities, meaning that only physicians will review the work of other physicians. Were consumer participation an integral part of the PSRO system, it would create systemic accountability by bringing the consumer point of view directly into the program. In the same way that liberal policies on release of information bring the program to consumers, consumer participation channels the flow of interaction in the other direction.

To create a PSRO program embodying significant consumer partici- pation would entail a comprehensive change in the law and its orientation. Those recommendations are beyond the scope of this work. Although the theory of consumer accountability set forth in this chapter posits that such change would create a more effective, more democratic, and, therefore, better program, the changes that would be necessary to incorporate those principles would be so great in degree as to become changes in kind. The PSRO system is not consumer-accountable and if made so would be something so fundamentally different from PSROs that it could no longer appropriately be called Professional Standards Review Organizations.

This section accepts the PSRO program as created under law. Examining each level of the PSRO hierarchy, the possibilities and reasonable roles for consumers are analyzed and set forth. There are roles for consumers in the program, as this book has demonstrated throughout.[177] But in some cases, as this section will demonstrate, those roles have been ignored, and decisions to exclude consumers, their representatives, and their interests have prevailed. The following catalogue of possible consumer roles in the program is just that—a catalogue. There may be instances where the costs of involving consumers, in time, effort, and organizational skills, may outweigh the benefits to be gained from their participation, because their activities and authority have been so circumscribed by existing law. But, returning to the theory of accountability, that decision must belong to the consumers themselves; and decisions by nonconsumers—bureaucratic policymakers, representatives of other interests—to exclude them based on a cost-benefit analysis would be at least inappropriate if not lacking in fundamental fairness.

Under the statute, the National Professional Standards Review Council's membership is prescribed. It

> shall consist of physicians of recognized standing in the appraisal of medical practice. A majority of such members shall be physicians who have been recommended by [sic, to] the Secretary to serve on the Council by national organizations recognized by the Secretary as representing practicing physicians. The membership of the Council shall include physicians who have been recommended for membership on the council by consumer groups and other health care interests.[178]

The Senate Finance Committee report provides virtually the same information, with the added clarification that "other health interests" shall include hospitals.[179]

The Council has been named.[180] Reports on the selection process differ. One story reported that

> [m]embers of the Council were selected from among 200 physicians nominated by national organizations representing practicing physicians and by consumer groups and other health care interests. . . . [E]very effort had been made to achieve a balanced representation on the Council of those in the field of health care most involved in, and affected by PSROs including providers of care, medical insurance organizations and consumers.[181]

Another report stated that suggestions for participants on the council came from 15 to 20 organizations, including consumers and hospitals.[182] A third report said nominations were submitted by about 50 organizations.[183] Although there has been little discussion of who had nominated which members, later reports indicated the following break-down among the Council's members: a nominee each from the American Hospital Association, the American Public Health

Association, HEW itself, the National Medical Association, the National Urban Coalition Health Project, the Senate Finance Committee, the AMA, and the House HEW Appropriations Subcommittee. In addition, a physician who had helped develop a PSRO prototype in Utah, an osteopath, and the President of the Group Health Association of America were also appointed.[184] These members closely parallel the interests represented at the Senate Finance Committee *Hearings* on H.R.1, and at the subsequent *PSRO Oversight Hearings.*[185]

The Council's powers are basically advisory,[186] but all regulations may be issued only after National Council comment on them. With regard to norms, the Council itself has direct approval authority.[187] In addition, it advises and assists Statewide Councils and local PSROs by developing and distributing information and data. It is given authority to review, evaluate, and compare performance among PSROs and Statewide Councils "with a view toward determining [their] effectiveness";[188] and to initiate or arrange with others to undertake studies and investigations with a view to making recommendations to the Secretary and Congress on ways to improve the program.

The National Council is, then, the primary policymaking body within the PSRO system. One of its members, formerly HEW Assistant Secretary for Health Affairs is reported to have said the Council was "intentionally created by the Congress to represent the concern and interests of the private practicing physician, giving him, in effect, direct access to the HEW Secretary and assuring him constant input on PSRO policy development and implementation."[189] If the statement is a correct reflection of the regard in which the Secretary holds the Council, then its activities can and will shape the functioning of every PSRO accordingly to the interests of physicians alone. Although some of its members may be receptive to consumer-oriented positions,[190] they are chosen because of the physician interests they represent. The statute does allow the Council to utilize "such technical and professional consultative assistance" as it may need.[191] Advice from consumer advocates could appropriately be sought by the Council, if it so chooses, under that provision. At this writing that effort has not been prominent.

Statewide Councils perform operational, substantive tasks in the program. Unlike the National Council, their authority is more than advisory. They participate in the processes which review appeals from initial PSRO determinations,[192] levy sanctions against PSRO participants who violate their legal obligations,[193] coordinate activity among PSROs,[194] and evaluate PSROs in order to advise the Secretary when replacement is necessary.[195] The statutory provision directing their composition appears to offer the greatest opportunity for participation by consumer representatives within the PSRO structure.

The Councils are to include one representative from each PSRO in the state, designated by each; four physicians, two of whom may be designated by the state medical society and two of whom may be designated by the state hospital association; and four persons "knowledgeable in health care from each state whom the Secretary shall have selected as representatives of the public in such State (at least two of whom shall have been recommended for membership on the Council by the Governor or such state)." [196] The Senate Finance Committee characterizes such representatives as "public representatives." [197] Although there is, in these provisions, no explicit recognition of the legitimate interests of consumers, there is nothing which could specifically preclude consumer membership on Statewide Councils. In an effort to win some consumer input into PSRO processes early in the implementation of the program, some activists concentrated their attention on Statewide Council appointments. [198] Their efforts had, at this writing, not reaped significant returns. One report has indicated that an early federal policy decision was made intentionally to exclude consumers.

> Guidelines of the National PSRO office, however, make no mention of informing consumers of openings on Statewide Councils. In fact, the guidelines emphasize that the local Health Administrators should limit the number of solicitations to a reasonable number to minimize the administrative work load. One PSRO official stated that, if the announcements were overly publicized, consumer groups would come out of the woodwork, which would make the administrative proceedings very difficult. [199]

If the report is accurate, it indicates a critical failing in the administration of the program. If the philosophy against consumers actually exists to a significant degree in the federal administration of the PSRO program, it must be changed by applying political pressure on HEW officials responsible for this approach.

An additional group is mandated by law in each state. An Advisory Group of between seven and eleven members is to advise the Statewide Council (or the local PSRO where there is no Statewide Council). [200] The law requires that the group consist of representatives of nonphysician practitioners (more than half), [201] of hospitals, and of other health care facilities. Because there are two types of Advisory Groups—those advising Statewide Councils and those advising local PSROs—there are different functions for the two types of groups. Groups advising Statewide Councils will be selected by those Councils and will help the Statewide Councils assure maximum effective nonphysician health care practitioner involvement in PSROs. [202] Establishment of norms, criteria, and standards for nonphysician health care, development of review mechanisms, and review of such care will be principle areas of concern to them. [203] Advisory Groups also will assist the Statewide Councils in assuring compliance with PSRO requirements through informational and liaison activities, will help the Councils evaluate PSRO performance in their states, and will advise the Statewide Councils on implementation of review in long term care facilities. [204]

Advisory Groups to local PSROs will review the formal plan

developed by the PSRO for HEW with regard to appropriate roles, activites, and implementation efforts of nonphysician practitioners. They will perform liason, information, and support activities for the PSRO, like those their counterparts will perform for Statewide Councils.[205]

Because membership on these Advisory Groups is limited, and will be determined by the Statewide Councils or local PSROs as appropriate, there will be significant efforts by nonphysician practitioner groups to gain a place for their representatives on the committee. Besides the obvious groups of osteopaths and dentists whose care PSROs will review, the personnel performing vital but ancillary medical care services will be represented here. During a recent conference on nonphysician health care practitioners in PSROs, 15 different disciplines and 20 different groups were represented: nurses;[206] nephrology nurses and technicians;[207] pharmacists;[208] social workers;[209] medical technologists;[210] bioanalysts;[211] respiratory therapists;[212] dieticians;[213] radiology technicians;[214] occupational therapists;[215] physical therapists;[216] audiologists and speech therapists;[217] optometrists;[218] and others.[219] Several of these types of practitioners are able to bring to the review process a greater emphasis on the degree to which social factors affect health status and medical care. In states with Statewide Councils they, with the Advisory Groups, will play a critical role in the balance between a cost and quality focus in PSRO review. In states which do not have Statewide Councils, Advisory Groups may be the only vehicle for influencing the work of local PSROs to better meet the needs of consumers. In addition, the guidelines give Advisory Groups the authority to pursue special studies, where there is support for them from the Statewide Council or PSRO.[220] These studies could and should appropriately seek to involve consumers as nonphysicians who will be affected by PSRO review at least as much as nurses, technicians, therapists, and social workers.

At the state level, a third type of entity has been created to participate in PSRO processes. Although there is no statutory authority for them, and their creation may in fact thwart explicit legislative intent, Statewide Support Centers have been interposed between the National Council and local PSROs, regardless of whether a state has a Statewide Council.[221] The Centers can engage in a broad range of activities collateral to local PSROs, from educating physicians about PSROs; developing organizational formats, including by-laws, for PSROs; directly planning for them; and writing conditional designation grant applications;[222] to "provision of common professional and technical services to PSROs, as appropriate,"[223] These centers can also assist Statewide Councils.[224] Support Centers may be used by the PSRO for subcontracted tasks.[225] General principles on PSRO subcontracting would preclude a PSRO subcontracting its basic responsibilities for review, or ongoing management and organization: but, especially during the initial implementation of the program, Support Centers could contract with PSROs to perform tasks otherwise to be performed by PSRO staff.[226]

Because under the guidelines Support Centers may be used to provide substantive technical assistance to both state and local organizations, they have the potential for great influence by injecting their values throughout the system, subject to no accountability constraints whatsoever. To qualify as a Support Center, an organization's membership must be "primarily physicians"; [227] but there is nothing which specifically precludes consumer membership. In fact, the first Support Center grantee has a consumer on its board of directors. [228] Consumer input in Support Center activities will be important to mitigating the otherwise unaccountable nature of these organizations.

At the most local level, direct consumer participation in the review functions of PSROs has been precluded by the statute. [229] This exclusion, however, is not absolute, and there are ways in which consumers can participate in PSRO activites. Although the governing body of a conditional PSRO must be composed primarily of physicians, [230] the *Program Manual* adds that "[c]onsumer representation on the governing body is encouraged." [231] But governing body directors are elected by the PSRO membership, which is open only to physicians. [232] It is likely, therefore, that the only consumers who will succeed in being elected will be those whose perspectives and interests coincide most closely with their physician electors. The circuity of the election process effecitvely weakens the potential for consumer accountability.

Although the *Program Manual* encourages consumer representation in the governing body, which has "the authority to make final determinations on *all the major policies, review considerations, budgetary matters and other significant activities* related to the ongoing operations of the PSRO," [233] the authority of the consumers on that board is conditioned and restricted: "If non-physicians are members of the governing body, the PSRO shall develop procedures to assure that only physicians may vote on issues relating solely to the physician practice of medicine and osteopathy." [234] Considering the scope and effect of PSRO activities, what, then, is open to consumer action? Strict interpretation of the voting exclusion could so limit consumers' authority that they would be cast in an advisory role only. The encouragement professed in the *Program Manual* becomes merely tokenism. True consumer accountability ascribes to consumers more than advisory power. While many programs seek to create accountability through advisory committees, these entities cannot meet accountability demands because there is nothing requiring their advice to be considered when final policy decisions are made. Unless consumers (or others to whom accountability is sought) are given direct participatory roles in program design, implementation, and operation, as mere advisers they will continue to remain outside the real processes determining program functions and, therefore, will remain powerless. Consumers will, then, continue to be able to speak on issues which concern them but will be unable to influence action taken on them.

Accepting the exclusion for purposes of this catalogue of consumer participation activities, consumers will be able to vote on issues relating to nonphysician practitioners, among which whould be norms relating to physical and occupational therapy, social problems, and nursing practices.[235] Consideration of psychosocial and socioeconomic aspects of care as reflected in norms, criteria, and standards, and reconsiderations of determinations based on them, could properly be voted on by consumers. They could also play a part in determining what care should properly be subject to advance determinations, in the development and analysis of profiles of practitioner, providers, and patients (subject to confidentiality restrictions), and in evaluating those services for which payment may be made under Medicare and Medicaid.[236] Dissemination of information from and about PSROs to other consumers is a task which could be most effectively performed only by consumers themselves.

At least two of the PSRO's standing committees suggested by the *Program Manual* would confront issues of immediate concern to consumers: the grievance committee would receive and consider complaints on non-review related matters,[237] and its activities might include patient advocate or ombudsman programs;[238] and the health care guidelines committee would develop or stimulate development of health care criteria and standards and would review them.[239] It would be through the activities of the health care guidelines committee that consumers would appropriately seek to influence the PSRO to review nontechnical, psychosocial, or socioeconomic aspects of care. Two other avenues for consumer participation exist under the *Manual*'s suggested guidelines: (1) The PSRO's governing body has the authority to create study and ad hoc committees,[240] any of which could focus specifically on consumer perspectives on PSROs, quality review, or anything else relevant to PSRO activities. (2) Despite the existence of a Statewide Council and Advisory Group to it, any individual PSRO also has the authority to "formally relate to health care institutions, *organizations*, or health professional associations for advice or assistance in carrying out [its] duties and functions." [241] These groups are eligible for reimbursement subject to HEW approval. Through such arrangements, PSROs could formally employ, consult with, or subcontract with consumer groups interested in health care, seeking their advice on a wide variety of issues.[242]

The PSRO statute offers one final possibility for direct consumer participation in the program. Where physicians groups do not assume PSRO duties, under specific circumstances the law provides for alternate designation of a PSRO formed by "such other public, non-profit, private, or other agency or organization" which the Secretary determines, in accordance with criteria prescribed by him, is of professional competence and otherwise suitable to perform PSRO duties.[243] According to the Senate Finance Committee,

> Physician organizations or groupings would be completely free to undertake or to decline assumption of the responsibilities of organizing a PSRO. If they decline, the Secretary would be

empowered to seek alternative applicants from among other medical organizations, State and local health departments, medical schools, and failing all else carriers and intermediaries or other health insurers.[244]

Designation of an alternative group may not take place "prior to January 1, 1976, nor after such date, unless in such area there is no organization" which qualifies according to the statutory criteria on initial designations.[245]

Although a consumer-oriented and consumer-participatory entity could be designated under this provision, the authority to select an alternate group is strongly conditioned. "In no case, however, could any organization be designated as a PSRO which did not have professional medical competence. And, in no case, could any final adverse determinations by a PSRO with respect to the conduct or provision of care by a physician be made by anyone except another qualified physician." [246] Further, the Secretary's agreement with any alternative organization may not be renewed if he determines there is an organization in existence in that area, not previously designated, but better able to qualify under the statute, willing to accept a designation and having demonstrated professional competence.[247] Finally, the designation of an alternate organization may be made *only* if it is "anticipated to result in substantial *improvement* in the performance of 'PSRO functions and duties'."[248] Although designations before 1976 are subject to approval by physicians in the area,[249] there is no implication in the statute that alternative designations will require such similar approval.

Given the severe limitations on alternate designations, it is unlikely that a consumer-participatory entity would get the chance to qualify. If other anticipated contingencies in the statute failed, an organization combined of consumers and physicians might be able to qualify under the provisions. The most serious obstacle to designating such a group is the requirement of demonstrated professional competence. Unless the demonstrated competence of individual physicians will be sufficient to satisfy this requirement, the condition may be used against other than mainstream groups, because few, if any, have previously been given the chance as review organizations, to perform such activities.[250]

Under the 1972 Social Security Amendments, another set of entities were created which will perform PSRO-related activities.[251] Program Review Teams were created to meet the Secretary's need under the Medicare program "to withhold future payments for services furnished by an institutional provider of services, a physician or other health supplier who abuses the program or endangers the health of beneficiaries." [252] This provision now gives the Secretary authority to terminate payments to someone who defrauded the program through knowingly making false statements in applying for Medicare payments; submitting bills substantially in excess of customary charges or costs; or furnishing services or supplies that were substantially in excess of the patient's needs, or harmful to patients, or of grossly inferior quality.[253] The Secretary's findings in cases of excessive charges or services must be made with the concurrence of a Program Review Team. These teams are to be appointed in each state by the Secretary after consultation with appropriate "State and local professional societies, carriers, intermediaries and *consumer representatives* familiar with the health needs of residents of the State." [254] Membership in each team will consist of "physicians, other professional personnel in the health care field and *consumer representatives*," [255] but only the professional members of the team may review cases of excessive or inferior quality services.[256]

The three basic functions to be performed by Program Review Teams are similar in many ways to some of those to be performed by PSROs: (1) They can review statistical data submitted by the Secretary on program utilization.[257] (2) They can submit periodic reports to the Secretary, making recommendations on the basis of their review.[258] (3) They can submit reports to the Secretary on the basis of their review of individual cases, with analysis and recommendations.[259] Despite the differing membership eligibility for Program Review Teams compared to PSROs, a PSRO may, by law, be used in lieu of a Program Review Team to perform Program Review Team functions.[260] The Senate Finance Committee would recommend that choice: "The committee notes that a ... (PSRO) ... would generally have the personnel and expertise to perform this function and therefore expects the Secretary to utilize the services of a PSRO whenever feasible in lieu of a separate program review team, as PSRO's become operative." [261] The only real distinction between the two entities, for the purpose of Program Review Team responsibilities, is consumer membership. There is no reason given in the legislative history for the PSRO preference. In fact, if consumers were to seek to have Program Review Teams designated wherever possible in addition to PSROs, the political pressure might be sufficient to make it "unfeasible" for the Secretary to choose a PSRO instead. It is interesting to note, as well, that although the Senate Finance Committee has provided that PSROs "not be involved with questions concerning the reasonableness of charges or costs or methods of payment," [262] in those cases where a PSRO acts in lieu of a Program Review Team it would be charged with just that responsibility—determinations of whether charges or costs in specific cases were excessive.

In concluding this chapter on accountability with a discussion of Program Review Teams, there is again clear evidence that, given the choice of endorsing consumer-participatory principles and, therefore, consumer-accountable mechanisms, the consumer-oriented policy response is rarely made. Admittedly, it is generally less desirable to support the proliferation of bureaucratic agencies for similar functions where one entity would be capable of performing; but, in the face of a program which encourages practically no consumer-accountable approaches, such cost-benefit analysis ought to be weighted to sponsor at least minimally accountable entities.

Notes for Chapter Six

1. See Chapter Four at 117 *supra,* and Chapter Seven at 229 *infra.*
2. §1163(f); 42 USC §1320c–12(f).
3. See Chapter One at 9 *supra.*
4. For an especially important consideration of accountability decisions which allocate scarce technological resources, see Tancredi and Barsky, "Technology and Health Care Decision Making—Conceptualizing the Process for Societal Informed Consent," XII *Medical Care* 845 (October 1974).
5. Rogatz, "In light of public scrutiny," 47 *Hospitals, JAHA* 42, 45 (August 16, 1973).
6. "As one who considers herself a consumer spokesman (not all consumers agree that I am!) and with strong ties to two institutions, one public —CMDNJ, one private—Princeton University'. . ." A. Somers, "Role of the Consumer," Joint Meeting of National Professional Standards Review Council and Health Insurance Benefits Advisory Council (OPSR, September 10, 1974), at 23.
7. *Id.* at 19.
8. *Id.* at 20.
9. §1162(a)(3); 42 USC §1320c–11(a)(3). See this chapter at 202 *infra.*
10. See Chapter Five at 145 *supra.*
11. See Chapter Seven at 229 *infra.*
12. The Statewide Professional Standards Review Council provision is one example.
13. §1166; 42 USC §1320c–15. See this chapter at 187 *infra.*
14. Many of these elements exist in programs created during the "War on Poverty," in local boards of education, in health planning legislation and programs, in at least one of the national health insurance proposals, (see Chapter One at 14 *supra*) for example. They have been created through litigation in other health, education, and welfare programs.
15. 118 *Cong. Rec.* S418 (January 25, 1972).
16. January 20, 21, 24, 25, 26, 27, 28, 31, and February 1, 2, 3, 4, 7, 8, 9, 1972. Hearings had been conducted by the Senate Finance Committee on H.R. 17550 (91st Cong., 2d sess.), June 17, July 14, 15, and September 14, 15, 16, 17, 21, 22, 23, 1970.
17. There were many consumer and public witnesses at the hearings. They did not, however, address any remarks to the issue of PSROs.
18. See *Hearings of the Senate Finance Committee on H.R. 1* (92d. Cong., 2d sess.), Social Security Amendments of 1971 (Parts 1–6) [hereinafter cited as *Hearings*], at 2563. The relationship between PSROs and HMOs has been a controversial issue. The PSRO legislation was passed at the same time that incentives to HMOs to serve Medicare and Medicaid recipients were passed. See §1876 of the Social Security Act; 42 USC §1395mm [P.L. 92–603, §226(a)] for Medicare; and §1903(k); 42 USC §1396b(k) [P.L. 92–603, §226 (e)]; and §1902(a)(23); 42 USC §1396a(a)(23); (P.L. 92–603,

§240) for Medicaid. See also Health Maintenance Organization Act of 1973, P.L. 93–222. See Chapter One at 15 *supra,* and Chapter Three at 89 *supra.*

Cohen, "Regulatory Politics: The Case of Medical Care Review and Public Law 92–603" (Paper prepared for delivery at American Political Science Association meeting, New Orleans, September 5, 1973) at 13 cites the *Hearings* at 2390–2408 and 2563–2572 in a discussion of tensions in PSROs between fee for service proponents and HMO proponents.

19. *Hearings* at 1050.
20. *Hearings* at 2282.
21. *Hearings* at 2393.
22. *Hearings* at 2415.
23. *Hearings* at 3252.
24. *Hearings* at 2421.
25. *Hearings* at 2511.
26. By written communication, *Hearings* at 2532.
27. *Hearings* at 2644.
28. By written communication, *Hearings* at 2725.
29. *Hearings* at 2737.
30. *Hearings* at 2744.
31. *Hearings* at 3371.
32. See "Amicus Brief" of APHA in *Cook v. Ochsner,* No. 70– 1969 (E.D. La., May 29, 1973).
33. Some similar groups did discuss the practice of peer review in general in their written submissions. See, for example, testimony of College of American Pathologists (*Hearings* at 2885); Oregon Physician's Service (*Hearings* at 2967); American Podiatry Association (*Hearings* at 3305); and the Coalition of Independent Health Professionals (*Hearings* at 3363).
34. The list of witnesses does not necessarily reveal who was solicited to speak before the Senate Finance Committee on issues in H.R. 1. One group, for example, specifically criticized the Committee for failure to seek a broad spectrum of opinion. See testimony of Planetarium Neighborhood Council (*Hearings* at 3361).

The list of witnesses testifying on PSROs at the hearings on H.R. 1 is very similar to the groups which testified on H.R. 17550. Even fewer consumer groups testified in 1970 and none spoke on PSROs. See n. 16 *supra.* The same problem existed at both hearings—the short time between the introduction of the amendment and the hearings on it. The amendment was first introduced on August 20, 1970. Public witnesses began testifying only three weeks later, on September 14.

Hearings on the implementation of the PSRO program were conducted by the Subcommittee on Health of the Senate Finance Committee, May 8–9, 1974. Of the 24 groups presenting oral testimony, all but one, the National Urban Coalition, represented providers or practitioners. The American Public Health Association also called for consumer accountability. See "Implementation of PSRO Legislation," *Hearings Before the Subcommittee on Health of the Committee on Finance,* U.S. Senate, (93d Cong., 2d. sess., May 8–9, 1974) [hereinafter cited as *PSRO Oversight Hearings*], at 152 and 479.

35. The swift introduction and passage of the PSRO amendment has been criticized from a general policy planning perspective:

> The Congress decided, with only minimal support from the Administration, and with opposition from the AMA and other providers, that the state of the art of review of utilization and quality was sufficient to institute a national system for such reviews and that these reviews would have beneficial effects on both controlling utilization and costs of care as well as its quality. The Congress basically used as its substantiating evidence, not basic and objective research, but the experience of a few medical society-sponsored foundations which are now carrying out such reviews.

Myers, "Health Services Research and Health Policy: Interactions," XI *Medical Care* 352 (July–August 1973), at 356. Whether the experience of those foundations was in fact a valid model is itself questionable. The usual voluntary physician membership, cost determination functions, and closed system nature of foundations is not analogous to the power given to PSROs. See Chapter Three at 89 *supra.*

36. See *Hearings* at 2415 and 2421 for example.
37. See Chapter Two at 32 *supra.*
38. 39 FR 10204, March 18, 1974. Interim guidelines have been issued. See *PSRO Program Manual,* March 15, 1974, Chapter I, §116.10 and §300 *et seq.* For basic information on the development of the Support Center concept the following documents are relevant:
    1. *PSRO Letter* (McGraw-Hill publication): August 15, 1973 at 5; September 1, 1973 at 1–3; September 15, 1973 at 1–2; October 1, 1973 at 4; October 15, 1973 at 1–4; November 1, 1973 at 2–6; November 15, 1973 at 4–6; December 1, 1973 at 1–2; December 15, 1973 at 3–4; January 1, 1974 at 3–4; February 1, 1974 at 1–2; March 1, 1974 at 1–2; March 15, 1974 at 1; April 1, 1974 at 3.
    2. *Consumer Clearinghouse for PSRO Action* (published by Health Research Group, 2000 P St., N.W., Washington, D.C. 20036) no. 2, August 8, 1973, and no. 3, April 5, 1974.
    3. *American Medical News,* "More Time Asked for PSRO Comment," January 21, 1974 at 1; "Reaction to PSRO Area Designations is Mixed," March 25, 1974 at 1; "PSRO Chief Explains How Program Will Work," April 1, 1974 at 1; "Senator Bennett Tells His Views on PSRO," June 18, 1973 at 1; "Senator Hits PSRO Panic," November 19, 1973 at 1.

4. Remarks of Senator Bennett, 119 *Cong. Rec.* S20439, November 15, 1973.

5. Letter from Senator Bennett to Ernest Howard, M.D., executive vice-president, American Medical Association, June 21, 1973 (available from Senate Finance Committee).

6. *OPSR Memo No. 3,* March 1974 (published by OPSR, HEW).

39. For a discussion of other issues raised by statewide PSRO designations, see testimony of Alice Gosfield, *PSRO Oversight Hearings* at 490.

40. See Chapter Three at 68 *supra* for a discussion of the consumer organizing potential in a local focus.

41. §1159; 42 USC §1320c–8.

42. Federal Advisory Committee Act, P.L. 92–463 (October 6, 1972), §10(a)(1) and (2). For more information on the act, see Markham, "The Federal Advisory Committee Act," 35 *U. Pitt. L. Rev.* 557 (1974).

43. 5 USC §552(b)(5). See letter from Robert E. McGarrah, Jr., Esq. to Caspar W. Weinberger, December 5, 1973 and reply of Sidney Edelman, Esq., December 27, 1973, on file with the author.

44. Tancredi and Barsky, n. 4 *supra.*

45. *Id.* at 851–852.

46. *Id.* at 856.

47. The consumer's other function is self-education. Patients who have little knowledge of health care and its limitations expect far too much of the provider. They can react with hostility when the healing arts don't heal. But it is in the quality assurance process that the capabilities and limits of health care are best revealed. Consequently, participation by consumers in quality assurance, particularly perceptive consumers who play leadership roles in the community, will ultimately help to close the gap between public expectations and provider performance.

Advancing the Quality of Health Care (Washington, D.C.: Institute of Medicine, National Academy of Sciences, August 1974) at 35.

48. For other reasons to disseminate information to consumers see letter from Alice Gosfield to Secretary of HEW, July 11, 1974, published in "PSROs and Medical Information—Safeguards to Privacy," OPSR/HEW (1974).

49. It was more than a year after the passage of the PSRO amendment before the general press gave some attention to the program. See, for example, Hicks, "Nation's Doctors Move to Police Medical Care," *New York Times,* October 28, 1973, at 1, col. 4; (an earlier article reporting the AMA national convention made brief reference to PSRO. See Lyons, "AMA Exhorted to Back Reform," *New York Times,* June 28, 1973, at 19.) See Winsten, "Imposing Controls on Doctors," *Wall Street Journal,* December 6, 1973, at 14; "Review and Outlook, 'No Time for Patients'," *Id.*; Cant, "Patient's Rights and The Quality of Medical Care," *Time,* December 17, 1973, at 56.

None of the articles cited examined the significance of the program for patients or the public by more than passing reference. Subsequent articles continued to focus only on the response of organized medicine. See, for example, Lyons, "Doctors Revolt Over AMA Stand," *New York Times,* December 2, 1973, at 1, col. 4; Lyons, "Physicians Oppose Monitoring Plan," *New York Times,* December 5, 1973, at 1, col. 3; Schmeck, "Medicare Review Planned by HEW," *New York Times,* December 20, 1973, at 34; and Clark, "How Good is Your Doctor?", *Newsweek,* December 23, 1974 at 46. See also the author's letters to the editors, to the *New York Times,* November 5, 1973; to the *Wall Street Journal,* December 12, 1973; and to *Time,* December 17, 1973, on file with the author.

50. The AMA attempted to inform physicians about PSROs by distributing to them a kit labeled "PSROs, Deleterious Effects" (including a speech titled "Excorcising the Devil from PSRO") to 400 state and county medical societies and 500 physician members of the AMA's House of Delegates. "Our purpose was to alert the public to PSRO and its potential impact on their lives," the Vice Chairman of the AMA board of trustees was reported to say. HEW health chief Edwards called the kit "factually incorrect, incomplete and misleading." Senator Bennett claimed the kit reached "new heights of distortion and misrepresentation." Quotations taken from "New Weapon for PSRO's Enemies: AMA Packet," *Medical World News,* April 19, 1974, at 13. In that article Edwards was quoted as saying, "Many doctors and the public know very little about the PSRO law. . . It behooves government and the medical profession to increase their understanding and not aggravate the situation with misinformation." *Id.* The use of the kit was suspended shortly after it was issued. See also *PSRO Letter* (no. 17), April 15, 1974, at 3–5; "AMA Suspends PSRO Kit Use," *American Medical News,* April 15, 1974, at 25; and Schmeck, "AMA is Assailed by HEW Official," *New York Times,* March 29, 1974, at 38. Distribution of the kit was resumed about one and a half months after its use was suspended. The most inflammatory pieces had been removed; but the kit was still the subject of heated debate in the Senate Finance Committee's hearings on implementing PSROs. *PSRO Oversight Hearings* at 65–69.

51. For evidence of support for this from a coalition of consumer-concerned groups, see generally "PSROs and Medical Information—Safeguards to Privacy," OPSR/HEW (1974).

52. *PSRO Program Manual,* Chapter I, §107 at 4. Chapter IX of the *Manual* will set forth guidelines on "Data Needs and Processing." At this writing, the chapter had not been issued. For an early study of data requirements of PSROs, see, "Projections of Anticipated Data Requirements for [PSROs]," *Medical Record News,* April 1973, at 33–38. Secretary Weinberger stated that data needs would be met by building on existing systems. *PSRO Oversight Hearings* at 10. *PSRO Letter* (no. 19), May 15, 1974, at 3.

Whether claims data used by paying agents will be reliable has already been discussed. See Chapter Four at xx *supra*. But there is also a question as to whether existing systems will be sufficient for generating other required data. See Roghmann, "Use of Medicaid Payment Files for Medical Care Research," XII *Medical Care* 131 (February 1974).

53. For a comprehensive summary of existing health information systems on federal, state, and local levels, see Murnaghan, "Health Services Information Systems in the US Today," 290 *NEJM* 603 (March 14, 1974).

    The Medicaid program now includes specific financial incentives to the states to create centralized mechanized claims processing and information retrieval systems. The regulations implementing §1903(a)(3) [42 USC §1396b(a)(3), §235, P.L. 92–603] with specific application to information systems (45 CFR §250.90) appear at 39 FR 17763, May 20, 1974. For a description of the "Medicaid Management Information System" for which the federal government will reimburse the states 90 percent of installation costs, see Godmere, "Medicaid Management Information System," 1 *Soc. & Rehab. Record* 30 (March 1974).

54. See *Records, Computers and The Rights of Citizens*, Report of the Secretary's Advisory Committee on Automated Personal Data Systems, HEW No. (OS) 73–97 (July 1973) [hereinafter cited as *Records and Computers*]. An inquiry in June 1974 by the author to the HEW reference library revealed that the guidebook was never produced.

    Also relevant is the Comptroller General's recent report to Congress that data systems in the Social Security Administration should be more efficient if redesigned to meet the potential of its advanced computers. See Comptroller General's Report to the Congress, "Increased Efficiency Predicted if Information Processing Systems of Social Security Administration are Redesigned," B–164031(4), April 19, 1974.

55. For an overview of these data systems, see "An Overview of Existing Quality Review Systems and Programs," *Medical Record News*, April 1973, at 40–46. The reliability of the data analyzed by these programs has been criticized. See Hendrickson and Myers, "Some Sources and Potential Consequences of Errors in Medical Data Recording," 12 *Methods of Information in Medicine* 38 (January 1973). The large role for computers in PSROs has been demonstrated in seminars for health care data processing specialists. See "Health Field Faces Regulation," *Computer World*, June 12, 1974 at 8.

56. For a discussion of the various computerized medical information systems available for use in individual institutions, see Ball, "Financial Manager's Guide to Medical Data Processing in the USA," 4 *Hosp. Fin. Mgt.* 10 (January 1974).

57. Murnaghan, *supra* n. 53, at 609.
58. See "Officials Envision Future Role as Source of Data for PSROs," *American Medical News,* March 11, 1974, at 8. In discussions around the issue, Blue Shield executives have attempted to play down the importance of the source of data to physicians, emphasizing to them that development of specifications is a more appropriate role for them. "It matters little to medicine who performs the collection and storage tasks, so long as they are competent ... the specifications for output include deciding what data, how often and how it should be organized. Whoever develops those specifications controls the data." James D. Knebel, Executive Vice-President, National Association of Blue Shield Plans, in "PSROs Data Roles Outlined," *American Medical News,* January 21, 1974, at 15.
59. See "Announcement of Medical Care Evaluation Seminar, February 28, 1974, Sponsored by the Hospital Utilization Project," on file with the author.
60. "Confident FMCs all set to become PSROs," *Medical World News,* September 14, 1974, at 18.
61. *Id.*
62. Densen, "Public Accountability and Reporting Systems in Medicare and Other Health Programs," 289 *NEJM* 401 (August 23, 1973).
63. *PSRO Transmittal No. 9* (BQA), October 18, 1974 sets forth the basic, base line data requirements conditional PSROs must meet.
64. §1156(c)(1); 42 USC §1320c–5(c)(1).
65. *Id.*
66. *Program Manual,* Chapter VII, §790.3 at 20.
67. §1155(a)(4); 42 USC §1320c–4(a)(4).
68. *Program Manual,* Chapter VII generally.
69. §1155(a)(4); 42 USC §1320c–4(a)(4).
70. *Sen. Fin. Comm. Rpt.* at 262.
71. *Id.*
72. See this chapter at 177 *supra.*
73. §1155(b)(3); 42 USC §1320c–4(b)(3).
74. §1155(b)(4); 42 USC §1320c–4(b)(4).
75. §1157; 42 USC §1320c–6.
76. *Id.* This reporting requirement is separate from and additional to the penalties and fines process. See Chapter Seven at 232 *infra.*
77. §1155(d); 42 USC §1320c–4(d).
78. §1163(e)(4); 42 USC §1320c–12(e)(4).
79. §1163(f); 42 USC §1320c–12(f)
80. *Id.*
81. See comments of Robert E. McGarrah, Jr., Esq., reported in Turner, "Health Report/HEW Begins Medical Review; AMA Hospitals Mount Opposition," *National Journal Reports,* January 19, 1974, at 90–102.
82. §1166(a); 42 USC §1320c–15(a). The statute does, however, provide for "interchange of data and information... (including but not limited to

usage of existing mechanical and other data-gathering capacity)" among PSROs and other appropriate agencies or providers. §1165; 42 USC §1320c–14.

83. §1166(b); 42 USC §1320c–15(b). At the same time, there is no liability for generating information and passing it on within the system. §1167(a); 42 USC §1320c–16(a).

84. *Sen. Fin. Comm. Rpt.* at 57–58.

85. §1864; USC §1395aa.

86. The full provision is as follows:

> Within 90 days following the completion of each survey of any health care facility, laboratory, clinic, agency or organization by the appropriate State or local agency described in the first sentence of this subsection, the Secretary shall make public in readily available form and place the pertinent findings of each such survey relating to the compliance with (1) the statutory conditions of participation imposed under this title and (2) major additional conditions which the Secretary finds necessary in the interest of health and safety of individuals who are furnished care or services by any such facility, laboratory, clinic, agency or organization.

> *Id.;* there is a similar Medicaid provision. §1902(a)(37); 42 USC §1396a(a)(37).

87. Rogatz, "In the light of public scrutiny," 47 *Hospitals JAHA* 46 (August 16, 1973).
> Some analysts favoring policies against disclosure cite consumers' inability to understand technical information in order to preclude its release to them. As Rogatz implies, the better course is to assure that the information will be understood by supplying with it additional material indicating its limitations and appropriate uses.

88. §1160(b)(1); 42 USC §1320c–9(b)(1).

89. §1160(b)(2); 42 USC §1320c–9(b)(1).

90. See *Advancing the Quality of Care, supra* n. 47, at 33 where it is suggested that disclosure itself is a sanction.

91. See n. 52 and n. 55 *supra.*

92. §1167(c); 42 USC §1320c–16(c). See Chapter Seven at 235 *infra.*

93. See Chapter Two at 45 *supra.*

94. Unfortunately, remedying underutilization in an individual case does not seem to be contemplated by norms as the statute and *Program Manual* define them. For example, if a patient were admitted to a hospital with a heart attack (myocardial infarction) and the standards permitted coverage for three chest X-rays during the course of treatment, and the patient received only one chest X-ray, what could the individual patient do to get the other X-rays? If there is anything he can do to enforce a "right" to the additional studies in a compensatory sense, he must know what that "right" entails—to what the norm entitles him.

95. This possibility has been limited by the "hold harmless" provisions. See Chapter Five at 145 *supra*.
96. Another provision of the Social Security Act supports nondisclosure principles. §1106(a); 42 USC §1306(a) is a general provision against disclosure of information within HEW. It provides that no information may be disclosed which is not in accordance with regulations. It gives the Secretary very broad discretion to withhold information acquired by HEW. Criminal penalties attach for its violation. The statute, however, does not appear to be applicable to PSROs. The legislative history indicates that Congress considered PSROs non-government agencies, and therefore not technically part of HEW. *Sen. Fin. Comm. Rpt.* at 266. See *Schechter* v. *Weinberger,* n. 99 *infra.*
97. PSRO disapproval of the medical necessity for continued hospital care beyond the norms for that diagnosis will not mean the physician must discharge the patient. The physician's authority to decide the date of discharge as well as whether his patient should be admitted in the first place cannot be and are not to be taken from him by the PSRO. The review responsibility of the PSRO is to determine whether the care should be paid for by medicare and medicaid. By making this determination in advance, the patient, the institution and the physician will all be forewarned of the desirability of making alternative plans for providing care or financing the care being contemplated.

    Sen. Fin. Comm. Rpt. at 264.
98. 5 USC §552.
99. *Dellums* v. *HEW,* Civil Action No. 181–72, D.D.C. *mem. ord.* filed July 11, 1973. See also, *Schechter* v. *Weinberger,* No. 73–1797, D.C. Cir., October 3, 1974, reported in *CCH Medicare and Medicaid Guide* ¶27,089.
100. "Whatever in connection with professional practice, or not in connection with it, I see or hear in the life of man, what ought not to be spoken abroad, I will not divulge, thinking that all such should be kept secret."
101. At least 36 states specifically recognize a physician-patient privilege, The Federal Rules of Evidence look to the common law (in which there is no privilege) or to the law of the state when there is a privilege in that jurisdiction. There were proposed changes which implied elimination of the physician-patient privilege under the federal rules. See letter from the Health Law Project and National Health Law Program, *Hearings on Proposed Rules of Evidence Before the Special Subcommittee on Reform of Federal Criminal Laws of the House Committee on the Judiciary* (93d Cong., 1st sess. 1973) at 586.
102. See Roedersheimer, "Action for Breach of Medical Secrecy Outside the Courtroom," 36 *U. Cin. L. Rev.* 103 (1967).
103. Mental illness records are often considered an especially difficult problem

because of the extreme intimacy of disclosures made in the course of treatment and the particularly damning effect of any revelation of those statements outside the physician-patient relationship.

For example, in *State ex. rel. Carroll* v. *Junker,* 79 Wn.2d 12, 282 P.2d. 775 (1971) the court considered a lower court order permitting research by a law professor and students into civil commitment proceedings through access to 189 current and active cases. Washington has a statute specifically ordering such court records closed, subject to examination on court order granted under judicial discretion. RCWA §71.02.160, §71.02.250, Ch. 51, §1 (1959) Wash. Sess. Law 418. (Similar limitations on research on mental patient files exist in New York [Art. *N.Y. Mental Hygiene Law* §20 (McKinney 1971)] and California, [*Cal. Welfare & Institutions Code,* §5328 (West 1971)] among other states.) The reasons for these exceptions were outlined by the court:

Apparently the legislature—consistent with due process of law and avoidance of the Star Chamber—believed that one way to encourage a clinical approach, maintain a clinical atmosphere, and sublimate any penal aspects of mental illness, is to avoid making public spectacles of the mentally ill and to close the files. There are other reasons, too, for directing that the files be closed, not the least of which is that witnesses, members of the family, and others interested in the proceeding may act and speak with candor and forthrightness under the statutory theory that in most instances the proceeding is undertaken for the good of the subject and with the intention of getting a sick person into a hospital where he may receive medical care, and that the benefits of confidentiality and privacy far outweight the dangers of Star Chamberism. (482 P.2d. 775, 782)

After weighing the interests of the researchers against those of the patients, the court overturned the lower court's grant of permission for the research. See "Right to Privacy—Confidentiality of Mental Illness Files," 7 *Gonzaga L. Rev.* 106 (Fall 1971).

104. *PSRO Oversight Hearings* at 97, 112, 121, 132, 349, 352, 362, 388, 407.
105. Among the bills which have been offered to repeal the PSRO law are several which were introduced with expressions of fear that the program would undermine the confidentiality of the doctor-patient relationship.

The legislation allows PSROs to examine a doctor's patient care records. This is totally offensive. Also, the Secretary of Health, Education and Welfare can request review records. It would seem that the confidential nature of the doctor-patient relationship for those relying on medicare and medicaid could be seriously compromised.

Remarks of Rep. John Ashbrook (R–Ohio) introducing H.R. 11394, 119 *Cong. Rec.* H9952, November 13, 1973.

This radical concept of Government intervention into medicine would accomplish what the "plumbers unit" failed to do in the celebrated burglary of Dr. Ellsberg's psychiatrist's office. PSRO will enable the Government to "legally burglarize" the confidential medical records of every patient treated under any of the many government-sponsored health care programs.

Remarks of Rep. John Rarick (D–La.) on his bill H.R. 11444, 119 *Cong. Rec.* E7593, November 29, 1973. See also Sheridan, "The Alarming New Assaults on Doctor-Patient Privacy," *Medical Economics,* April 15, 1974, at 31–45.

106. §1155(b)(3); 42 USC §1320c–4(b)(3).
107. Quoted in Sheridan, n. 105 *supra* at 32.
108. *Id.* at 35.
109. See Porter, "Computer Raped by Telephone," *New York Times Magazine,* September 8, 1974, at 33.
110. Since the days of the Founding Fathers we have recognized that organized society must obtain considerable information from its members to facilitate the governmental functions and private services. We have also accepted the need for some tightly limited government surveillance of criminals and antisocial activities, in order to protect lives, property and the public peace.

Westin, "We Can't Blame Everything on the Machines," *Prism,* June 1974, at 66.
111. See, for example, *Hague* v. *Williams,* 37 NJ 328, 181 A. 2d. 345 (1962) where a physician was held not liable for disclosing medical information to a life insurance company. There is no legal obstacle to disclosure in those states which do not recognize a physician-patient privilege. But see *Hammond* v. *Aetna Casualty and Surety Co.,* 243 F. Supp. 793 (N.D. Ohio, 1965) which upheld an action for breach of confidentiality by relying on medical codes of ethics, public policy, and the nature of the doctor-patient relationship.
112. See testimony of Lowell E. Bellin, M.D., M.P.H., Commissioner of Health and Acting Services Administrator, New York City:

The typical chart in the typical hospital today goes through at least 10 to 15 hands, which I can identify: One, the nurse on the ward, the practical nurse, the messenger who brings the chart, the insurance company that reviews the chart, Blue Cross, Blue Shield, so on.

PSRO Oversight Hearings at 349.

I do not think we should perpetuate the illusion that we can devise a foolproof system assuring high quality medical care while eliminating all abuses of medical information. We must accept the reality that there is not and never will be a system guaranteeing perfect confidentiality and simultaneously providing coordinated care for an individual over a continuing period of time.

Weed, "The Public's Needs Must Be Met," *Prism,* June 1974 at 23.

113. See Westin, *supra* n. 110.

114.   This information is needed to operate the program, not for statistical purposes. However, the importance of such information to the operation of the program in no way diminishes its potential relevance to activities oriented toward other than daily operational considerations.

Densen, "Public Accountability and Reporting Systems in Medicare and Other Health Programs," 289 *NEJM* 402 (August 23, 1973).

115. "The special study approach to understand the reasons for variations in utilization and costs is cheaper, more reliable and more likely to be specifically aimed at answering a useful question." *Id.*

116. §1902(a)(7); 42 USC §1396a(a)(7).

117. 45 CFR §205.50(a)(2)(i)(d). This provision applies to Titles I, IV–A, X, XIV, XVI, and XIX of the Social Security Act; but is subject to state legislation which gives public access to records of disbursements of funds if the legislation prohibits use of names obtained through such access for political or commercial purposes. 45 CFR §205.50(b).

118. See Curran, Laska, Kaplan, and Blank, "Protection of Privacy and Confidentiality," 182 *Science* 797 (November 23, 1973) for a history of the program and its attention to confidentiality needs.

119. See "Confidentiality panel proposed," *American Medical News,* November 18, 1974, at 1.

120. Meldman, "Centralized Information Systems and the Legal Right to Privacy," 52 *Marquette L. Rev.* 335 (Fall 1969).

121. "One way to conserve physician review time is through automated screening of claims by computers...." *Sen. Fin. Comm. Rpt.* at 264.

122. *Sen. Fin. Comm. Rpt.* at 265.

123. See Morris, "The Computer Data Bank–Privacy Controversy Revisited: An Analysis and an Administrative Proposal," 22 *Cath. U. L. Rev.* 628 (Spring 1973) in which the author proposes Federal Communications Commission oversight of data banks. See especially *Records and Computers, supra* n. 54, and also "Comment–Public Access to Government-Held Computerized Information," 68 *Northwestern L. Rev.* 433 (May–June 1973) for some recent considerations of the general issue of tensions between privacy and access in computerized data banks. For similar discussions, specifically on health information, see *Prism,* June 1974, Special Issue, "Is Privacy Obsolete? The Challenge to Medicine and Society."

124. 5 USC §552.
125. 5 USC §552(a)(6). See *Records and Computers* at 273. The Freedom
of Information Act was substantially amended by the "Privacy
Act of 1974" (P.L. 93–579, 93d Cong., S.3418, December 31,
1974), adding §552a to establish safeguards and conditions on
the compilation and use of individually identifiable data by federal
agencies. Release of such information to someone other than the
subject of it, for a purpose other than that for which it was gathered,
may be made only with the written consent of the subject.
Individuals may also gain access to and ask for correction of material
gathered about them. The previously existing section on medical
information has not been affected by the new law.

126. 44 USC §§3501–3511.
127. 44 USC §3509. See *Records and Computers* at 270.
128. 44 USC §3508.
129. 15 USC §§1681–1684t. See *Records and Computers* at 66–75.
130. 15 USC §1681g(a). Contrast this policy with proposals and programs to
always give patients access to their medical records; see Shenkin and
Warner, "Giving the Patient His Medical Record: A Proposal to
Improve the System," 289 *NEJM* 688 (September 27, 1973); "How
to reduce patients' anxiety: show them their hospital records,"
Medical World News, January 13, 1975, at 48; and Weed, "The
Public's Needs Must be Met," *Prism,* June 1974, at 22.
131. §1166(a); 42 USC §1320c–15(a). See this chapter at 187 *supra.*
132. See Jackson, "Guardians of Medical Data," *Prism,* June 1974, at 38; and
Westin, "We Can't Blame Everything on the Machines," *Prism,* June
1974, at 60.
133. *OPSR Memo,* no. 4, April 1974, at 4–5. The *Program Manual* provides
that "[s]pecific data requirements and the rights of the Secretary to
data will be part of each conditional or operational agreement or
contract." Chapter V, §550.62.
OPSR/BQA has recommended release of aggregate (not individually identified) data on practitioners, and aggregate utilization data
on individually identifiable providers. Results of medical care
evaluation studies would be "privileged data" and therefore not
disclosable. "Privileged data" is defined as "medical data and
information identifiable to individual patients and practitioners."
PSRO Letter (no. 35), January 15, 1975, at 5; and National
Professional Standards Review Council, Meeting Report, October
29–30, 1974 (HEW, Office of the Assistant Secretary for Health).
134. §1154(a); 42 USC §1320c–3(a).
135. §1154(b); 42 USC §1320c–3(b).
136. *Id.* The designation process, by law, must consider seven factors to
determine if an organization "qualifies" for designation. At least for
initial designation, such an organization (1) must be a nonprofit
professional association; (2) must be composed of licensed doctors

of medicine or osetopathy engaged in practice in the area; (3) must include in its membership a substantial proportion of physicians in an area; (4) must be "organized in a manner which makes available professional competence to review health care services of the types and kinds with respect to which PSROs have review responsibilities"; (5) must be voluntary and open to all licensed physicians in the area without membership or dues-paying requirements; (6) may not restrict eligibility to serve as a PSRO officer or to be assigned review duties. If an organization qualifies as above, it (7) must further be willing to and capable of performing in an effective, timely, and objective manner and at a reasonable cost, the duties, functions, and activities of a PSRO as demonstrated in a formal plan submitted to the Secretary. §1152(b); 42 USC §1320c–1(b).

137.   §1153; 42 USC §1320c–2.

138.   §1154(b); 42 USC §1320c–3(b).

139.   §1152(b)(2); 42 USC §1320c–1(b)(2).

140.   *Sen. Fin. Comm. Rpt.* at 261.

141.   Areas to be covered in reports include administrative reports of activities which have occurred or are planned, financial reports, aggregate review findings, work plans, and evaluation data reports. *Program Manual,* Chapter V, §550.62.

142.   §1152(a)(2); 42 USC §1320c–1(a)(2).

143.   *Sen. Fin. Comm. Rpt.* at 261.

144.   §1152(f)(1) and (2); 42 USC §1320c–1(f)(1) and (2); and 24 CFR §100.001 *et seq.* on physician polling.

145.   42 CFR §100. 104.

146.   The *Program Manual* does provide for other state and local government review procedures on applications after fiscal year 1974. For conditional and final designations, notice of intent to apply must be sent to state or areawide planning clearinghouses for comment and recommendations. *Program Manual,* Chapter VI, §604. This procedure is required to meet the mandate of the Intergovernmental Cooperation Act of 1968, 42 USC §4201 *et seq.*

147.   There are, however, extensive and specific requirements for the proposals which are submitted. *Program Manual,* Chapter V, §500 *et seq.* on "Requirements for Qualification as a Conditional PSRO," and Chapter VI, §600 *et seq.* on "PSRO Selection and Agreement Process."

148.   §1162(c)(2); 42 USC §1320c–11(c)(2).

149.   5 USC §551 *et seq.*

150.   (Emphasis added.) 5 USC §551(8).

151.   5 USC §551(9).

152.   Some of these requirements include the right of a party to present his case, submit rebuttal evidence, and cross-examine others, and the agency's responsibility to offer findings and conclusions on which the determination is made. The provisions of each section do not necessarily operate together.

153. 5 USC §§556, 557.
154. 5 USC §558(b).
155. §1154(b); 42 USC §1320c–3(b).
156. §1152(a)(2); 42 USC §1320c–1(a)(2).
157. Technically, the relationship between the PSRO and the Secretary is one of "agreement" rather than contract. This designation is a way of eluding the strictures of the Government Contracts Act (41 USC §§35–45), which conditions the process of awarding contracts. The change from technical contracts to technical agreements was made after fiscal 1974 to facilitate implementation of the program. Weinberger testimony, *PSRO Oversight Hearings* at 20; and *PSRO Letter* (no. 19), May 15, 1974, at 4.
158. §1154; 42 USC §1320c–3.
159. §1152; 42 USC §1320c–1.
160. §1154(b); 42 USC §1320c–3(b).
161. §1152(b)(2); 42 USC §1320c–1(b)(2).
162. Gellhorn, "Public Participation in Administrative Proceedings," 81 *Yale L. J.* 359 (January 1972) [hereinafter cited as Gellhorn]. For a discussion of the practical problems with public participation in the administrative process, see 60 *Georgetown L. J.* 525 (February 1972); and Clagett, "Informal Action–Ajudiciation–Rule Making: Some Recent Developments in Federal Administrative Law," 1971 *Duke L. J.* 51.
163. Gellhorn at 379.
164. 429 F. 2d. 725 (D.C. Cir. 1970). See also Comment, 6 *Harv. Civ. Rights – Civ. Lib. L. Rev.* 559 (1971).
165. Gellhorn at 379.
166. In *NWRO* v. *Finch,* 429 F. 2d. 725 (D.C. Cir. 1970), the court permitted intervention only in formal compliance hearings. This position underscores the need for a hearing requirement in the PSRO final designation process. It would be more difficult to open any informal Secretarial decision.
167. 326 US 327 (1945).
168. *Id.* at 330.
169. See also *Delta Airlines Inc.* v. *Civil Aeronautics Board,* 275 F. 2d. 632 (D.C. Cir. 1959) *cert. den.* 362 US 969 (1960).
170. 5 USC §558(c)(1).
171. 5 USC §558(c)(2).
172. *Sen. Fin. Comm. Rpt.* at 261.
173. For related arguments in the context of broadcast licenses see *Citizens Communication Center* v. *FCC,* 447 F. 2d. 1201 (D.C. Cir. 1971) where a policy statement issued by the FCC would have required an initial determination of the licensee's record of service to the community. At that proceeding, challengers could only present evidence of the licensee's failure to serve. If the weight of the evidence nonetheless demonstrated substantial service, the license would be renewed automatically. If the agency found failure of

service, a full comparative hearing would be held. The court held that a new applicant must always be given the chance to make the comparative showing to displace the existing license.

174. For a discussion analyzing the reaons for each requirement and their interrelations, see "Note—Recent Changes in the Scope of Judicial Control Over Administrative Methods of Decisionmaking," 49 *Ind. L. J.* 118 (Fall 1973).

175. See, for example, *SEC* v. *Chenery Corp.*, 332 US 194 (1947).

176. See *Hornsby* v. *Allen,* 326 F. 2d 605 (5th Cir., 1964), *Holmes* v. *N.Y. City Housing Authority,* 398 F. 2d 262 (2d. Cir., 1968); *ABC Air Freight* v. *CAB,* 391 F. 2d 295 (2d. Cir. 1968); and *Environmental Defense Fund* v. *Ruckelshaus,* 439 F. 2d. 584 (D.C. Cir. 1971).

177. See Chapter Two at 32 *supra;* Chapter Three at 68 *supra;* Chapter Four at 116 *supra;* and this chapter at 196 *supra.*

178. §1163(b); 42 USC §1320c–12(b).

179. *Sen. Fin. Comm. Rpt.* at 268.

180. *American Medical News,* June 11, 1973, at 3. The members of the Council when it was first named were the following: Clement R. Brown, M.D., Director, Medical Education, Mercy Hospital and Medical Center, Chicago, Illinois; Ruth Covell, M.D., Assistant to the Dean, School of Medicine, University of California at San Diego; Merlin K. DuVal, M.D., Vice President for Health Sciences, University of Arizona at Tucson; Thomas J. Greene, M.D., surgeon, Detroit, Michigan; Robert J. Haggerty, M.D., Professor of Pediatrics, University of Rochester, Rochester, New York; Donald C. Harrington, obstetrician-gynecologist, and Medical Director, San Joaquin Foundation for Medical Care, Stockton, California, Robert B. Hunter, M.D., family physician, Sedro Woolley, Washington; Alan R. Nelson, M.D., internist, Salt Lake City, Utah; Raymond J. Saloom, D.O., osteopathic physician, Harrisville, Pennsylvania; Ernest W. Saward, M.D., Professor of Social Medicine, University of Rochester, Rochester, New York; William C. Scrivner, M.D., obstetrician-gynecologist, Belleville, Illinois. *Background Material Relating to Professional Standards Review Organizations* (PSROs), Staff of the Senate Finance Committee, May 8, 1974 at 9. Dr. Greene died in a car accident during his first year of service. In July 1974, Dr. Cornelius L. Hopper was named to replace Dr. Greene. Dr. Hopper is a neurologist and Vice-President for Health Affairs and Director of the Andrew Clinics at Tuskegee Institute, Alabama. *HEW News Release,* July 28, 1974.

181. *American Medical News,* June 11, 1973, at 3.

182. William Connor, Deputy Secretary for Regulatory Affairs (under the Assistant Secretary for Health) at HEW, formerly Deputy Director of PSROs, speaking at a meeting sponsored by the Federal Bar Association and the National Health Lawyers Association, June 8,

1973, Washington, D.C. At that meeting a representative of a Regional Comprehensive Health Planning Agency (RCHP) complained that RCHPs were unaware of any of the processes and planning going on around PSROs. See Chapter Two n. 158 at 64 *supra.*

183. "Meet the Professional Standards Review Council," *Health-PAC Bulletin* (no. 59), July–August 1974, at 16.

184. *Id.*

185. See this chapter at 179 *supra.*

186. "It shall be the duty of the Council to advise the Secretary in the administration of this part." §1163(e)(i); 42 USC §1320c–12(e)(i).

187. "The Professional Standards Review Organization may apply such norms in such area as are approved by the National Professional Standards Review Council." §1156(a); 42 USC §1320c–5(a).

188. §1163(e); 42 USC §1320c–2(e).

189. Statement of Merlin K. DuVal, M.D., reported in *Health-PAC Bulletin* (no. 59), July-August 1974, at 17.

190. Although the Council members may, on any single issue, express positions concurring with consumers' interests, there has been no affirmative attempt to seek consumer views. During fiscal year 1974, of 19 organizations with which the National Council sought to develop working relationships, not one was an organization representing consumers or their advocates. See *National Professional Standards Review Council, Second Annual Report* (July 30, 1974), at 25–27.

On only one occasion, as a result of pressure from the Nader-affiliated Health Research Group, was a coalition of consumer-oriented groups permitted to make an organized presentation to the Council. See "PSROs and Medical Information—Safeguards to Privacy," HEW/OPSR (July 1974).

191. §1163(c); 42 USC §1320c–12(c).

192. §1159; 42 USC §1320c–8. See Chapter Five at 146 *supra.*

193. §1160(b),(c); 42 USC §1320c–9(b),(c). See Chapter Seven at 232 *infra.*

194. §1162(c)(1); 42 USC §1320c–11(c)(1).

195. §1162(c)(2),(3); 42 USC §1320c–11(c)(2),(3).

196. §1162(b); 42 USC §1320c–11(b).

197. *Sen. Fin. Comm. Rpt.* at 268.

198. *Consumer Clearinghouse for PSRO Action Newsletter* (published by Health Research Group, 2000 P St. NW, Wash., D.C. 20036) (no. 3), April 5, 1974, at 2. See also *PSRO Letter* (no. 1), August 15, 1973, at 6–7.

199. *Consumer Clearinghouse Newsletter, supra* n. 198.

200. §1162(e); 42 USC §1320c–11(e). The expenses of this group are to be considered expenses of administration of the Statewide Council. §1162(e)(3); 42 USC §1320c–11(e)(3).

201. *Program Manual,* Chapter XV (draft), §1502.21 (October 24, 1974). This chapter was published in draft form while the Office of General Counsel determined if Advisory Groups are subject to the Federal Advisory Committee Act, 5 USC App. I. See n. 42 *supra.* If it is

determined that the act does apply, Advisory Groups will be expected to meet its requirements on meetings, reporting and record keeping. Other provisions will not be changed. *OPSR Issuance No. 3,* December 5, 1974.

202. *Id.,* Chapter XV, §1506.40.

203. *Id.*

204. *Id.*

205. *Id.* at §1506.60.

206. American Nurses' Association, *Peer Review in PSRO,* September 5, 1974, (HEW, Office of the Assistant Secretary for Health, OPSR), at 22; National League for Nursing, *Id.* at 26.

207. American Association of Nephrology Nurses and Technicians, *Id.* at 29.

208. American Society of Hospital Pharmacists, *Id.* at 31; American Pharmaceutical Association, *Id.* at 3–4.

209. National Association of Social Workers, *Id.* at 36. See also *The Advocate* (published by the National Association of Social Workers), vol. 3, no. 8, April 1974, at 2–3.

210. American Society of Medical Technology, *Peer Review in PSRO, supra* n. 206, at 40; American Medical Technologists, *Id.* at 41; The International Society for Clinical Laboratory Technology, *Id.* at 45.

211. American Association of Bioanalysts, *Id.* at 42.

212. American Association for Respiratory Therapy, *Id.* at 46.

213. American Dietetic Association, *Id.* at 49.

214. American Society of Radiologic Technologists, *Id.* at 52.

215. American Occupational Therapy Association, *Id.* at 53.

216. American Physical Therapy Association, *Id.* at 55.

217. American Speech and Hearing Association, *Id.* at 56.

218. American Optometric Association, *Id.* at 60.

219. National Rehabilitation Association, *Id.* at 58; American Society of Allied Health Professionals, *Id.* at 63.

220. *Program Manual,* Chapter XV (draft), §1506.80 at 9.

221. The *Program Manual* asserts that the authority for Statewide Support Centers exists under three separate sections of the act: (1) §1156(a); 42 USC §1320c–5(a) which provides that the National Council and the Secretary "shall provide such technical assistance to the [PSRO] as will be helpful" in using norms; (2) §1163(c); 42 USC §1320c–12(c) which provides for technical and consultative assistance to the National Council; (3) §1169; 42 USC §1320c–18 which provides for technical assistance to potential PSROs. *Program Manual,* Chapter II, §300.1 at 2. Considering that the statute provides for the creation of two state level entities, and one local entity for each local PSRO area, the creation of statewide PSRO Support Centers was not contemplated by the law and runs contrary to its local thrust.

222. *Id.* §302.30 at 4.

223. *Id.* §304(h) at 5.

224. *Id.* §306 at 5–6.
225. *PSRO Transmittal No. 8* (HSA/BQA), September 30, 1974.
226. *Id.*
227. *Program Manual,* Chapter II, §308(a) at 6.
228. See "Pennsylvania MDs get PSRO contract," *American Medical News,* April 15, 1974, at 25; and *HEW News Release,* April 17, 1974. Mrs. Frankie M. Jeters, of the Welfare Rights Organization, Pittsburgh, Pa., sits on the board of directors of the Pennsylvania Medical Care Foundation.
229. "No Professional Standards Review Organization shall utilize the services of any individual who is not a duly licensed doctor of medicine and osteopathy to make final determinations in accordance with its duties and functions under this part with respect to the professional conduct of any other duly licensed doctor of medicine or osteopathy, or any act performed by any duly licensed doctor of medicine or osteopathy in the exercise of his profession." §1155(c); 42 USC §1320c–4(c).
230. *Program Manual,* Chapter V, §550.13(a) at 14.
231. *Id.*
232. *Id.* §510.16–36 at 8–10.
233. (Emphasis added.) *Id.* §550.11 at 14.
234. *Id.* §550.17 at 15.
235. Unless the nonphysicians responsible for these types of care are especially oriented toward consumer participation, as social workers might be, they, too, may seek to limit consumer involvement in issues subject to their technical expertise.
236. See *Sen. Fin. Comm. Rpt.* at 262 for the implication of program change based on profile analysis.
237. *Program Manual,* Chapter V, §550.41(c) at 16.
238. See Chapter Five at 153 *supra.*
239. *Program Manual,* Chapter V, §550.41(e) at 16.
240. *Id.* §550.42 at 17.
241. (Emphasis added.) *Id.* §540 at 13.
242. Because reimbursement for organizations is available, as a practical matter, this provision could serve to organize consumers around PSRO issues.
243. §1152(b)(1)(B); 42 USC §1320c–1(b)(1)(B).
244. *Sen. Fin. Comm. Rpt.* at 259–260.
245. §1152(c)(2)(A)(i); 42 USC §1320c–1(c)(2)(A)(i).
246. §1152(c)(2)(A)(ii); 42 USC §1320c–1(c)(2)(A)(ii).
247. §1152(c)(2); 42 USC §1320c–1(c)(2).
248. (Emphasis added.) *Id.*
249. Upon designation of a specific group to be a PSRO, if 10 percent of the local doctors claim the group is not sufficiently representative of them, a poll must be conducted. If 50 percent so claim, the Secretary may not, under any circumstances, enter into an agree-

ment with that group. §1152(f)(2); 42 USC §1320c–1(f)(2). Regulations have been issued. See 39 FR 16202, May 7, 1974; 42 CFR §101.101 *et seq.*

250. State and local affiliates of the American Public Health Association might be organizations which could qualify.

251. §229(a),(b), P.L. 92–603; amending §§1862 and 1866 of the Social Security Act; 42 USC §§1395y and 1395cc.

252. *Sen. Fin. Comm. Rpt.* at 200.

253. §1862(d)(1); 42 USC §1395y(d)(1).

254. (Emphasis added.) §1862(d)(4); 42 USC §1395y(d)(4).

255. (Emphasis added.) *Id.*

256. §1862(d)(1)(C); 42 USC §1395y(d)(1)(C).

257. §1862(d)(4)(A); 42 USC §1395y(d)(4)(A).

258. §1862(d)(4)(B); 42 USC §1395y(d)(4)(B).

259. §1862(d)(4)(D); 42 USC §1395y(d)(4)(D). See 20 CFR §405.315a *et seq.*; and 20 CFR §§405.614, 405.502, 405.1519, 405.1530, 405.1543. Appeals from determinations under §229 are provided for.

260. §1157; 42 USC §1320c–6.

261. *Sen. Fin. Comm. Rpt.* at 201.

262. *Id.* at 261.

Chapter Seven

Sanctions and Enforcement

The preceding chapter on accountability did not discuss the concept of enforcement—those processes which create the compliance and cooperation of participants in the program, thereby assuring their accountability to the program itself. Enforcement generally, and sanctions as one aspect of enforcement, embody principles of accountability in a unique way: they guarantee that there will be a structure and system to perform other obligations. If those on whom the system is predicated—providers and physicians—choose to violate the statute, or choose not to participate in the program at all, there can be no system.

Enforcement can be achieved through sanctions (involuntary penalties imposed) or incentives (positive inducements to comply); and both elements are included to some degree in the PSRO statute. Clearly an incentive to physicians to use PSRO norms, criteria, and standards arises from the financial clout wielded by PSROs. An individual physician will perform according to the program's dictates to avoid a reduction in income which can result from disallowances of coverage. Because no federal money will be available as payment for services which have not been granted PSRO approval,[1] physicians and providers are encouraged to seek that approval. The malpractice exemption[2] offered by the statute is another incentive to doctors and institutions to apply PSRO norms, criteria, and standards, and to bring their cases to the PSRO for review. But as the discussion below will demonstrate, although the statute appears to have strong sanctions built into it to guarantee cooperation, several aspects of program operation which will be most vulnerable to abuse have no sanctions which attach to them (e.g., rotation of participation among physician reviewers, patient complaints, and nontechnical aspects of care).

Effective enforcement is essential to the systemic accountability of the PSRO program because the law does attempt to force the compliance of physicians and providers with the goals of the program. In addition, the

Secretary of HEW is required to ensure the proper implementation of PSROs within HEW, as well as throughout the system generally. Whether enforcement is effective is important to consumers in a practical way, because without conscientious activity by those charge with enforcement obligations there can be no program to serve consumers.[3] If the program is ever to work in the consumers' interests, it must be given a chance to exist first; and enforcement is, therefore, a legitimate object of consumer concern.

In the PSRO program, the success of the enforcement effort is especially critical because the physicians whom the program seeks to regulate are also relied on for basic regulatory administration. They are expected to enforce the program's goals and values among their fellow physicians (and providers). Some commentators have characterized this phenomenon as an example of the capture of regulatory agencies by the regulated industry.[4] That analysis does confront the fundamental problem of effective enforcement in an "industry-oriented" program, but it fails to categorize accurately the severity of the dilemma in the PSRO context. Where a program is industry-oriented and accepted by the regulated industry, (or the regulated industry captures the regulation process), the program's provisions are enforced at the discretion of the regulators, or, through industry lobbying, enforcement provisions are diluted to prevent stringent efforts. In the PSRO program, physicians will not and have not captured the regulatory body; they are identical with it. In fact, as a practical matter, the PSRO law organizing physicians into locally controlled, exclusively physician-membership entities, and then subsidizing them directly with government funds, inherently strengthens political vested interests and their ability to seek their own ends. Given the massive lobbying and campaign financing activities of organized medicine,[5] it is legitimate to ask whether individual PSROs, and the program as a whole, once organized and subsidized, will ever be made accountable or answerable to elements outside the program.[6] In the PSRO program, the choice may be full (or at least substantial) physician compliance with program goals or the complete collapse of the PSRO system, with eventual substitution of a non-physician-controlled program. Effective enforcement, then, will be critical to overcoming the industry-oriented aspects of the program which undermine its purpose.

Expectations of vigorous physician enforcement efforts, where there is little enthusiasm for the program, are unrealistic. Superimposing an HEW enforcement mechanism on top of individual PSRO responsibilities may also be ineffective considering HEW's difficulties in beginning implementation of the program.[7] In the face of HEW's inadequacies, whether enforcement mechanisms as designed in the PSRO law can work may depend on demand from consumers and others whose interests are affected by the program and who therefore seek its proper implementation. Otherwise there may be no effective way to enforce the enforcement system. And, if consumers are to influence the enforcement process, the law must give them an ability to participate in that process. In that way, enforcement mechanisms themselves must be consumer accountable. Obviously the system will not function if there is no reason for it to do so. The existence of the law—words on paper—is inadequate to assure the program's operation. If the words are given meaning through effective enforcement— sanctions and incentives which operate in meaningful, practical ways—the PSRO program will work.

LIABILITY

An affirmative requirement to conform to the system's demands, including compliance with specific norms and guidelines, is prescribed by the statute.

> It shall be the *obligation* of any health care practitioner and any other person (including a hospital or other health care facility, organization or agency) who provides health care services for which payment may be made . . . to assure that services or items ordered or provided . . . under this Act—
> (A) will be provided only when, and to the extent, medically necessary;
> (B) will be of quality which meets professionally recognized standards of care; and
> (C) will be supported by evidence of such medical necessity and quality in such form and fashion and at such time as may be reasonably required by the [PSRO] . . .[8]

A second obligation proscribes violation of the duties to comply: Each practitioner and institution has the "obligation, within reasonable limits of professional discretion, not to take any action which would authorize any individual to be admitted as an inpatient or to continue as an inpatient in any hospital or other health care facility," unless the in-patient care is determined by the physician or institution to be "consistent with professionally recognized health care standards" and not able to be provided more economically in a different facility.[9]

The obligations as stated are independent of the sanctions available to be imposed for violation of them. On one hand they merely set forth a basic good faith standard for those who would serve Medicare and Medicaid patients. On the other hand, however, they could be used to establish actionable legal duties to perform according to standards, and a breach of any of those obligations would make the obligated party liable to suit. Conceivably, the obligation to be sure services are rendered according to standards, and by implication to assure that coverage will be availale, could make a physician or provider liable in tort for the costs of services not covered. This would mean that an individual patient who was injured because of the physician's or provider's failure to fulfill his obligations could sue. The damages would be the costs he or she incurred as a result of the failure. This type of analysis has been used to hold a physician liable for the cost of services he ordered for his patient which were not covered;[10] it is also very similar to the concept of "waiver of liability" or "hold harmless" which has been discussed several times in this book.[11]

The PSRO statute does provide for other specific and direct sanctions for failure to meet the specified obligations. Those penalties are the following: (1) exclusion from eligibility to provide services on a reimbursable basis (i.e., exclusion from participation in Medicare and Medicaid);[12] or, in lieu of such exclusion, (2) reimbursement to the government in the amount of the cost of the medically improper or unnecessary services,[13] or (3) if such services amount to more than $5000, then $5000.[14] Despite the apparent severity of these penalties, the process which must be exhausted before they can be used is a long and attenuated one and will itself discourage their application.

Complaints of violation of obligations are evaluated initially by the PSRO. It may discover abuses or violations on its own in the general course of its duties[15] or "on the basis of [further] investigations of situations of possible abuse identified in its own review or referred to it by the Secretary or his administrative agents."[16] There is no provision for initiation of complaints by, or acceptance of them from, others in the system—from a practitioner against an institution, a providing institution against a practitioner, or, most important, a patient against a provider or practitioner.[17] The wording of the Finance Committee's report implies that these complaints must be channeled through some element of the HEW bureaucracy or must be discovered by the PSRO on its own. For a PSRO to respond to complaints with effective enforcement and meaningful systemic change, where necessary, it must have the ability to accept complaints from all elements of the system, not just the government. The statute does not so restrict the PSRO's right to adjudicate complaints, nor should a narrow construction be applied.

The PSRO must offer "reasonable notice and opportunity for discussion with the practitioner or provider concerned."[18] The Senate Finance Committee would hold the PSRO to a specific standard in initially evaluating complaints. "In determining responsiblity for overuse of services, uneconomical use of services, or the provision of substandard services, the PSRO would take into account actual ability of the provider or physician to control the activities in question."[19] If the complaints are still viable after such evaluation, the PSRO reports the matter to the Statewide Council together with its recommendations for sanctions.[20] The Statewide Council then reviews the matter, makes its recommendations,[21] and sends the case to the Secretary for further action.

The Secretary decides whether penalties will be imposed. The Secretary must make two findings before holding the doctor or institution in violation of statuatory obligations: (1) that the offense indicated "fail[ure] in a substantial number of cases substantially to comply with obligations"[22] or gross and flagrant violations of any obligation in one or more instances;[23] and (2) that by the offense the provider or physician demonstrated an "unwillingness or lack of ability substantially to comply"[24] with obligations imposed by the PSRO statute. The provider or physician who is dissatisfied with the Secretary's determination is afforded the opportunity for a hearing following the same procedures that apply generally in the PSRO scheme.[25] If the Secretary elects to impose exclusion from Medicare and Medicaid on the offender, the exclusion becomes effective after reasonable notice to both the provider and the public.[26] If, on the other hand, the Secretary imposes a fine, the amount of the fine may be deducted from any amounts the government would otherwise have to reimburse.[27] (Significantly, there is no requirement of notice to the public when the Secretary chooses the fine sanction.) These sanctions are in addition to any other sanctions provided under law.[28]

Exclusion from participation in the publicly financed programs is the more serious of the two penalties. The fine process, when put into effect, is actually nothing more than a determination that the physician must absorb the cost of the services which violated the obligations. If payment has not yet been made, then the fine process would mean only that the physician or provider could not expect payment for those services. If payment for those services has already been made, it would mean only that the physician or provider would return the money already paid. In neither instance does the fine process necessarily entail the physician paying new moneys out of his pocket to cover the amount of the services. If the physician's payment was not forthcoming, the law would permit the government to deduct that amount from any other moneys it might owe the violator, including, for example, potential refunds from income tax overpayments.

From a quality perspective, the consumer's interest would be best met through the exclusion of practitioners or providers who have failed to meet their obligations. Their failure would be evidence of patterns of poor practices. But to exclude poor performers would limit the pool of physicians and institutions available and willing to serve Medicare and Medicaid patients. How, then, should the Secretary's choice of sanctions be made? Because it is their interests which will ultimately be adjudicated through the available sanctions, consumers must have the ability to affect the Secretary's determination. Program Review Teams, with consumer members, have been given authority to confer with the Secretary on the exclusion of providers from the Medicare program,[29] and they may be more effective in this process than PSROs in overcoming the prejudice of physicians in favor of their colleagues.[30]

The standards for imposition of penalties are narrow. They present problems of proof; for example, what is "substantial" lack of compliance? Moreover, the "actual ability to control" standards set forth by the Senate Finance Committee may provide big loopholes for those who would otherwise be subject to penalties. This emphasis on the importance of using the sanctions available to be applied is not to suggest that they must be uniformly and rigidly imposed in every instance. In medical care the need for flexibility is critical to absorb medical deviations which cannot rightfully be considered overutilization or substandard care.[31] In addition, by evaluating the physician's or provider's actual ability to control the circumstances, the system provides for reasonability; it would be obviously unfair to penalize a physician practicing medicine in an underfinanced, understaffed hospital in a medically underserved area because he is willing to serve patients there but cannot meet the PSRO's standards. The basic point of the enforcement process, however, is to establish a mechanism which, accepting the general context and the particular circumstances of a case, will effectively deal with those who abuse the system or refuse to cooperate with it for reasons other than those dictated by principles of high quality medical care.[32]

The single greatest obstacle to enforcing existing PSRO sanctions is the willingness of physicians to discipline each other. The "conspiracy of silence" of which physicians are often accused,[33] or the perils of cronyism— "There but for the grace of God go I"[34] —have become matters of serious concern in the face of expanding nonphysician roles in the regulation of medical care. As physician-supportive commentators have come to understand,

> [p]rofessional self-help is a privilege extended by society.... Society believes it lacks the knowledge and expertise to evaluate professional service and judgment. But beliefs can and do change. The public can be stampeded into believing that its rights are impinged, that medicine isn't policing its own ranks, that the privilege of self-government should be abridged, and that the public should participate with medicine in its self-government.[35]

Physicians are now faced with greater demands to improve their poor disciplinary records. Existing disciplinary mechanisms have not been used conscientiously; and examination of medical practice license revocation procedures indicates the low frequency with which physicians have disciplined each other. License revocation is also, in some ways, analogous to the PSRO sanction process.

In most such procedures, after a complaint is initiated the local medical society holds a hearing, and if warranted, refers the matter to the state medical society or state licensure board for further action against the doctor. There has been unusually little data published on the results of these processes. Two primary studies over the last 10 years reveal some increase in the frequency with which physicians are disciplined. During the five year period from 1963 to 1967, only 938 actions were taken by all state licensing boards against physicians in the United States.[36] During a more recent five year period (1969–1973), the number of state board actions increased 50 percent to 1437, with California acting more often than any other state.[37] In the earlier study, the penalty most often imposed was probation; revocation was reserved for only the most extreme circumstances. Most of the revocations during that period were for narcotics offenses, and the majority of them were for personal addiction of the physician. The second most common ground for revocation was mental incompetence due to mental illness. Other disciplinary proceedings—suspension, reprimands—followed criminal convictions (many for illegal abortions), or charges of "unprofessional conduct," defined differently in each state.[38] There was, in this study, no indication that disciplinary actions were initiated because of complaints of poor quality practice, other than as practice was affected by other factors (narcotics addiction, mental incompetence). The later study demonstrated the same basic patterns.

It is significant that the major reasons for actions taken by licensing boards in 1963-1967 relied on determinations by other bodies—courts and mental hospitals, for example. Three trends have been cited as contributing to the later increase in disciplinary activity: (1) the inclusion of lay members on state boards; (2) an increase, in some states, in voluntary surrender of licenses; and (3) the influence of consumer activities.[39] In considering the consumer accountability of these and PSRO processes, it is important to note that in California, with the highest level of activity, the head of the state board believes the consumer trend is directly responsible for California's comparatively good discipline.[40]

There are two basic differences between PSROs and state licensing boards which may give PSROs greater ability to discipline errant physicians. PSROs may initiate their own investigations, unlike licensing boards which only can respond to complaints from others. In addition, while licensing boards claim to be hampered by court decisions which overturn their penalties,[41] PSROs have direct legislative authority to impose limited sanctions directly related to the purposes of the program. The ultimate determinants of the effectiveness of PSRO enforcement efforts will be physicians' acceptance of norms and the PSROs' willingness to view deviations from them as sufficiently serious to warrant penalties. If the PSRO fails to enforce the program, the Secretary may yet have the final say through termination of the PSRO's agreement. [42]

MALPRACTICE EXEMPTION

An incentive to PSRO physicians to comply with PSRO standards is provided in the malpractice exemption. Under that provision

> no doctor of medicine or osteopathy and no provider (including directors, trustees, employees, or officials thereof) of health care services shall be civilly liable to any person under the law of the United States or any State ... on account of any action taken by

him in compliance with or reliance upon professionally developed norms of care and treatment applied by a PSRO.[43]

The insulation from liability, however, is not complete. A practitioner or provider must exercise "due care" in his professional activities which are "reasonably related to and resulting from, the actions taken in compliance with or reliance upon" such norms of care and treatment.[44] That means that a practitioner or provider generally complying with the PSRO system, relying on its norms, criteria, and standards, cannot be held liable for injuries as the result of his actions if he was appropriately careful in his reliance on norms, criteria, and standards.

The standard for due care is that "a physician following practices which fall within the scope of those recommended by a PSRO" would not incur liability "in the absence of negligence in other respects" for having followed PSRO prescribed practices.[45] Under the malpractice exemption, neither physician nor provider acting in compliance with PSRO norms can be held civilly liable "on account of" such action (1) if it was performed in the course of his exercising his profession or role as a provider; and (2) if he (or she) exercises "due care in all professional conduct" relating to reliance on or compliance with PSRO norms. The real effect of the due care proviso will be determined by judicial interpretation. Congressional intent is to extend the limitation on liability, thereby restricting the circumstances when a physician or practitioner could successfully be sued: "The intention of this provision in the amendment is to remove any inhibition to proper exercise of PSRO functions, or the following by practitioners and providers, of standards and norms recommended by the review organization."[46]

In no case can the exemption prevent the filing of any malpractice complaint. The patient can allege anything.[47] But once the complaint is filed, if the practitioner (or provider) has exercised due care, the malpractice exemption will prevent a judgment against him. Part of the determination of due care will be based on consideration of the physician or provider's application of norms, criteria, and standards.[48] There are essentially two circumstances where application of PSRO norms, criteria, and standards will still not protect the physician from malpractice liability: (1) if he selects an inappropriate standard, but follows it correctly; and (2) if he selects an appropriate norm but applies it negligently. In addition, there will be other issues in the delivery of care (e.g., informed consent, abandonment) which will not be the subject of norms (although PSROs optimally would examine these psychosocial, nontechnical aspects of the quality of medical care[49]). The scope of the norm which *was* used in each case, then, will be at issue in a malpractice action to determine whether the exemption appropriately may be used.

The legislative history specifies how much evidentiary weight is to be attached to the norm itself: "Failure to order or provide care in accordance with norms employed by the PSRO is not intended to create a legal presumption of liability."[50] Although the AMA has expressed fear of the use of norms as the exclusive and ultimate standards in any case,[51] it is clear they are not intended to create any legal presumption, let alone an irrebuttable presumption. If the norms are properly developed, they will, by their nature, reflect appropriate standards of reasonable care, and should be considered with all other evidence of extenuating circumstances or other mitigation of liability. For a court to look solely to norms in considering a malpractice action under the PSRO scheme would run contrary to the legislative intent: "The intent is not conformism in medical practice—the objective is reasonableness."[52] To do so would violate the statute, which requires the use of norms only as "principal points of evaluation."[53] However, the determinations of the PSRO, its findings and reasons, are, as pieces of evidence, competent (if presented by the PSRO or its official recordkeeper), material (having something to do with the issue under litigation), and relevant (tending in logic to prove the fact for which it is introduced).[54]

Proper application of a norm, despite consequent injury, will shield a provider or practitioner from liability. In that instance, the patient might find himself with the sole recourse of attacking the norm itself. Such an attack would probably be best directed at the PSRO for having promulgated the standard. To challenge the norm itself the patient would have to assert two facts: (1) that the care and services deemed to be covered by the norm were insufficient or incorrect for the diagnosis and age group to which the norm applied; and (2) that there was no other norm available to be applied in his case. The second allegation is necessary to preclude a defense by the PSRO that the physician was responsible for having misapplied the norm or chosen the wrong norm. The situations in which such actions would be possible would be rare because the maintenance of any such suits would depend heavily on the patient's ability to find a physician to testify against both the norm under litigation and the process by which it was established. Because norms will be established by physicians themselves, it would be unlikely such a witness could be found.

A suit predicated on misapplication of a norm, in contrast with a suit contesting the norm itself, could properly be directed at the physician, the institution, and the PSRO. The Senate Finance Committee has specifically provided, "[i]t is not intended however, that this (malpractice exemption) preclude the liability of any person who is negligent in performing PSRO functions or who misapplies or causes to be misapplied the professional standards promulgated by a review organization."[55] Examining one example of misapplication, the Committee stated its intention: "A physician or provider should not be relieved of responsibility where standards or norms are followed in an inappropriate manner or where an incorrect recommendation by the PSRO is induced through provision of erroneous or incomplete information."[56]

The AMA is correct in its assertion that due care will be at issue in any malpractice action under PSROs or otherwise.[57] Where absence of due care cannot be proved, despite the patient's injury, he will not recover any damages. But the malpractice exemption which codifies that principle, and thereby seeks to limit litigation, may encourage PSROs to seek other forms of dispute resolution which can save the plaintiff and the defendant time and money.[58]

Besides the incentive effect within the PSRO system, the malpractice exemption will have impact on other aspects of the health care delivery system. Because of increasing suits and high damage awards, the problem for physicians of obtaining and retaining malpractice insurance has reached crisis proportions in many states. In New York, the company serving the State Medical Society canceled its coverage after 25 years. Six months later the society found a replacement plan which offered coverage at rates 93.5 percent higher than the old plan.[59] After 15 years, the plan covering 3000 internist members of the American College of Physicians canceled its coverage.[60] Several no fault malpractice insurance bills have been introduced since these developments.[61] In light of the crisis, reports from the Utah Professional Review Organization (Senator Bennett's model for PSROs) are interesting. Alan Nelson, M.D., UPRO's president, told the Senate Finance Committee:

> I will not say that our peer review program is responsible for these changes, but coincidence [sic], in the same timeframe we have been operating our program, there has been no increase in the premiums for our group liability program versus the 10% per year increase nationwide, and up to 120% increase in neighboring states.
> A 5% dividend was declared for physicians participating in the MASA group liability program. It amounted to $33,000 in liability premiums returned, and the decreased liability insurance premiums for higher risk categories decreased up to $155.[62]

The federal malpractice exemption may be made stronger still as medical societies faced with exorbitant increases in malpractice insurance premiums search for a way to lower those premiums. The New York State Medical Society has asked its state legislature to grant immunity from civil liability to physicians who use PSRO standards.[63] The overall systemic effect of malpractice exemptions is still open to speculation; but the use of objective and essentially impartial standards for judging negligence in medical care will undoubtedly be extended.

ROTATION

One of the fundamental ways of assuring the educational and peer pressure value of PSROs[64] is the requirement that all physicians be able to participate in the PSRO duties on a rotating basis. The statute provides that fostering rotation be an important aspect of a PSRO's duties and functions. To "promote acceptance of PSRO functions and activities by physicians and patients and other persons,"[65] the PSRO is to "encourage" all physicians in its area to participate as reviewers, "to provide rotating physician membership of review committees on an extensive and continuing basis," and to assure that membership on review committees has "the broadest representation feasible in terms of the various types of practice" in which physicians engage in that area.[66] More specifically, the Senate Finance Committee set this standard: "To be approved, a PSRO applicant must provide for the broadest possible involvement, as reviewers on a rotating basis, of physicians engaging in all types of practice in an area, such as solo, group, hospital, medical school and so forth."[67] The broad participation requirement is a method to preclude PSRO exclusionary practices such as dues, or other membership criteria, or domination in other ways by organized medical societies.[68] Although membership must be open, PSRO review responsibilities are restricted in the statute to "only those [physicians] having active hospital staff privileges in at least one of the participating hospitals in the area served by the PSRO."[69] The Senate Finance Committee justifies this stipulation and conditions physician review in one other important way:

> The purpose here is to assure that only doctors knowledgeable in the provision and practice of hospital care will review such care. To the extent feasible, it is intended that a physician not be involved in decisionmaking in the review of care for the PSRO which was provided in a hospital where he has active staff privileges (except to the extent of his involvement with "in-house" review acceptable to the PSRO).[70]

Other provisions exclude physicians for professional and financial conflicts of interest.[71]

The *Program Manual* reiterates the statute's requirements for broad participation in its criteria for evaluating a conditional PSRO application.[72] Organizations must, "when they apply, have as members of their organization at least 25 percent of the physicians eligible for membership. . . ."[73] Planning grants can be awarded to an organization which shows the potential to achieve that level of membership;[74] and conditional PSROs are mandated to increase their membership: "Each PSRO must devise and implement an approved plan for recruiting, on a continuing basis, physicians of all types and levels as members and reviewers."[75] However, no suggestions are offered as to how to accomplish successful recruitment.

The fundamental criticism of all these provisions is that each PSRO has no ability to enforce them, nor does the system as a whole. With no way to enforce rotation, there can be no guarantee of either the educational value of the PSRO program or of the widespread participation it seeks. To understand the magnitude of the problem, it is necessary to consider the different, diverging, sometimes dissident, sometimes self-serving groups who must be wooed to join the PSRO if its efforts are to be successful.

Physician Attitudes

Two major surveys on acceptance of PSROs have been done. One which examined only the issue of PSROs found that 53.1 percent of all doctors are against the PSRO program.[76] One-fifth of practicing general practitioners say they will refuse to treat Medicare and Medicaid patients rather than have a PSRO monitor their performance; one-fourth of all practitioners fear PSROs will cut their incomes; and one-third of all practitioners fear PSROs will trigger more malpractice suits.[77] Geography, type of practice, and age were significant factors in determining acceptance.[78] That study was undertaken in September of 1974, when most physicians had heard of PSROs and were relatively sensitized to the issues they raise. The sample included 951 responses of 2,337 questionnaires sent—a response rate of 40.7 percent.[79]

A second study gathered material in September 1973 and focused primarily on physician acceptance of national health insurance.[80] Of 2,713 "senior" physicians (those beyond the residence level), 1,303 interns and residents, and 3,419 medical students, 75 percent favored a national health insurance program "under which the work of doctors is routinely reviewed by a panel of practicing doctors"[81] and 57 percent felt strongly that physician review should be included in a national health insurance plan.[82] Despite the fact that "peer review" and PSROs are not necessarily the same thing, Senator Bennett cited the findings of the second study, on the Senate floor, saying:

> I am delighted with the improved climate that seems to be developing around the PSRO program and happy to be able to share with my colleagues a recent news release from the Columbia University College of Physicians and Surgeons, which demonstrates a grassroots physicians' support for the PSRO concept.[83]

Although the later, 1974 study probably more accurately reflects an increased political awareness of PSROs,[84] hardcore resistance[85] is apparently not uniformly intransigent. Dr. Nelson of UPRO reports:

> ... [D]evelopment of UPRO was met with some apprehension, as might be expected. However, hardcore resistance has generally given way to a reasonable position, as physicians, hospital administrators, carriers and patients have come to understand the program's goals. In fact, cooperation has been such that the program has tripled its scope during the period of operation going from a review of 12,000 hospital patients in the first year to 35,000 this year.[86]

But another obstacle to broad participation is the PSRO system's predication on leadership by organized medical groups, by implication those which are American Medical Association affiliates. Although the national organization is vociferous in its activities, there is some question as to whether it is representative of most physicians. The AMA's own claims of membership are one source of information. In 1970 it claimed as members 64.1 percent of all American physicians.[87] The statewide affiliates of the AMA claimed 64.7 percent of all American physicians;[88] but only 88.9 percent of the state medical society members belonged to the national organization.[89] In 1971 AMA membership decreased significantly and the national group claimed only 59.3 percent of all physicians in the United States;[90] and that year state medical society membership fell slightly to 63.9 percent.[91] Some estimates have placed AMA membership as low as 45 percent of those eligible to join.[92] The organization emphasizes the membership of office-based practitioners among its regular members; in 1970 that figure was 82 percent but by 1971 it had declined to 75 percent.[93] This decline in AMA participation resulted in a vigorous membership campaign, offering financial incentives to state and local societies which contribute to increased AMA membership.[94] In 1971 the organization raised dues by 57 percent and lost nearly 12,000 members; between 1970 and 1972, dues-paying memberships dropped by 7 percent.[95] Dues-paying status, however, is not a true reflection of the representativeness of any society. In 1973, a survey found that 23 percent of physicians felt the AMA represented their opinion "on hardly any issues in the organization of health care," and a full 55 percent felt they were represented only on "some" issues.[96]

In addition to the AMA affiliates' difficulties in attracting members, another problem arises from the fact that the AMA and its affiliates do not represent two other major physician groups—black doctors and osteopaths. The National Medical Association (NMA), the black physicians' organization, initially passed a resolution generally supporting "the overall concept of peer review and PSROs as a means or mechanism for achieving peer review and quality control of medical care," but with reservations.[97] Significant to the rotation concept was the resolution that each constituent NMA association file

> ... its own PSRO application as an attempt to gain designation as the PSRO for their district where there are as many as 300 or more black physicians. NMA regards this as a potentially successful approach in the Los Angeles area, Washington, D. C. and possibly New York City.[98]

A later proposed resolution called on the NMA to seek an injunction barring further PSRO expenditures until black physicians were assured of a vote in their proceedings.[99] This was deemed necessary by some NMA members because of the "built-in disenfranchisement for black MDs, since due to their numerical smallness they can never muster enough MDs to run a PSRO." [100] Also of note is the statement by past NMA president Emory N. Rann, M.D. "I cannot see how the physician from the Ivory Towers—no matter how sincere, how dedicated, how honest—can be considered exactly a peer to those who fight the battles of ghetto and rural health." [101]

There are approximately 15,000 osteopathic physicians in the United States, 250 osteopathic hospitals providing 25,000 patient beds, and eight existing schools of osteopathic medicine. [102] The American Osteopathic Association (AOA) does not claim to speak for every individual osteopath, [103] but the organization's position on PSROs reflects concerns for autonomy similar to those expressed by the National Medical Association;

> The autonomy of the osteopathic profession may well be threatened by the legislation in allowing an admixture of physicians (D.O. and M.D.) reviewing each other when in fact the M.D. may not be qualified by philosophy or training to review osteopathic medical care distinctive to the osteopathic profession. [104]

Though urging compliance with the law, and expressing support for concepts of peer review, osteopathic associations will be seeking representation of their membership on PSRO bodies.

> ... [T]here are only 15,000 osteopathic physicians in the country. Some States with large osteopathic populations have minimal or a paucity of DOs or where there may be only 7 to 10. It is our position, of course, that only one osteopathic physician is a significant number. And we are concerned of the possibility that these physicians, maybe 10 to 12 in one State, may not even have any type of recognition into this PSRO structural arrangement. [105]

The AOA's position on PSROs would have osteopaths seek "equal D.O. and M.D. representation on the final appellate body of state or local PSROs when final adjudication of particular osteopathic medical care procedures or osteopathic care distinctive to the osteopathic profession." [106]

Dentists are another professional group whose services will be reviewed by PSROs. [107] The apparent intention is to treat dentists as non-physician health care practitioners, like physical therapists, nurses, social workers, and others. [108] In addressing the American Dental Association's Council on Dental Care Programs—Conference on PSRO and Peer Review, Dr. Henry Simmons of the Office of Professional Standards Review said:

> It's expected then that the local PSRO will consult with your Association's state and local chapters to obtain their recommendations concerning those in your profession who would be best able to participate in the review activities of the PSRO as they affect your profession. In addition, those same local dental groups would be involved in the development of standards and criteria of care to be used in dental care in that area. [109]

It is obvious that physicians are entirely unqualified to review dental services.[110] If dentists were not satisfied with established relationships between PSROs and local dental societies, their dissatisfaction could seriously hamper efforts to review Medicare and Medicaid dental services.

Each PSRO must contend not only with non-AMA-affiliated medical societies, but also with growing physician unions,[111] some of which are already working against PSROs.[112] These and other organized groups which have not received PSRO contracts may have an interest in refusing to cooperate with a PSRO in the hope of thereby causing it to lose its agreement for failure to meet the rotation requirements.[113] Other organizations which have agreed to support the PSRO system may seek to mold its activities in ways that further their own interests. Medical schools and teaching hospitals, for example, have chosen norms as the area of particular concern to them, presumably in order to prevent their being drawn so narrowly as to stifle innovative academic medicine.[114] Confidentiality of medical records is an issue of special concern to psychiatrists.[115] The American Academy of Pediatrics feels that PSROs should "be given every opportunity to prove their effectiveness in assuring better quality pediatric care through the cooperation of all physicians delivering child health care ... . The Academy will continue ... in seeking changes that would maximize the acceptability of the PSRO system with both patients and providers of child health care."[116] Participation by diverse groups with their own perspectives on the program can benefit the program and consumers only if there is true rotation. Without continually changing emphases in the program, one group may become able to dominate the system, and, in seeking its own ends, would pervert the review process.

The various groups noted above are essentially national organizations which engage in lobbying efforts on behalf of their members. Because the PSRO system will operate primarily on a local level, some consideration should be given to the representative nature of locally organized medical societies.

Even though membership in local medical societies (AMA affiliates) appears proportionately higher still than participation in state medical societies,[117] such figures, where locally available, are not necessarily valid indicators of participation. Many physicians belong to local medical societies because they must in order to gain admitting privileges to certain local hospitals.[118] Such physicians regard their membership more as a necessary formality than as a vehicle through which they can influence the health care services or politics surrounding them in their area. Because of such differences both in the level of membership status and the members' commitment to participate, there is created the tendency for a stable group of physicians to dominate local medical society activities, and therefore, in the PSRO system, to "capture" review responsibilities. These political factors, as well as the time requirements and sacrifices of income that will have to be made in order to engage actively in PSRO functions, will preclude some physicians (and maybe many) from participating. Remuneration to physicians for their review is available under the statute as part of the administrative costs of carrying out the duties and functions required in the agreement between the Secretary and the local PSRO.[119] Whatever the rate HEW is willing to pay, however, it cannot in many instances compare favorably with what many doctors can earn in their practices. If the reimbursement rate were high enough, some doctors wavering in their support for the program might be persuaded to participate; but where significant disagreement with the program exists, money may not provide sufficient incentive.[120]

Faced with organized medicine's conflicting motivations—(1) to control the local PSRO to influence its activities in order to serve the specialized interest of particular groups and (2) to ignore the PSRO in the hopes it will fail—some designated PSRO areas may have no organization available to assume review duties, or those physicians who are willing to take on the responsibility will become so entrenched because of lack of interest by others that the educational purpose of the program would be vitiated. Nor does the statute confront the problem that might be created where there are no physicians with active hospital practices who choose to review care, but other eligible physicians (nonpracticing medical school professors, or program administrators, for example) seek PSRO designation. Should such a situation arise, the Secretary would be torn between two options: (1) designate the group a PSRO despite possible challenge to it as unrepresentative of the majority of physicians; or (2) wait until after 1976 to designate an alternate PSRO. Then areas where no organization would assume PSRO duties at first would be without a PSRO until an alternate designation could be made. Presumably the ultimate threat of naming another entity which need not be representative of practicing physicians will inspire participation among those physicians who should be sought under the law in the first instance.

Los Angeles County is one area of the country where this theoretical problem became real. When proposed area designations were published, it was proposed that all of Los Angeles County be one PSRO area (Area XVIII).[121] At approximately the same time the Los Angeles County Medical Association (LACMA) voted not to support PSROs at all, and to seek repeal of the law establishing them. Los Angeles County as a whole has approximately 12,000 practicing physicians, and, on reconsideration, HEW decided the single designation for the whole county was too large; they designated, in the final regulations, eight separate areas in Los Angeles County.[122] In the resulting divisions was an area in East Central Los Angeles having an unusually high percentage of poor and old people, blacks, chicanos, and other racial minorities.[123] When the medical establishment in the area made no move to organize a PSRO, the interns and residents decided to apply and were awarded a $78,750 planning contract by the Secretary.[124] The head of the East Central Los Angeles PSRO (ECLAPSRO) estimated there were about 2,300 practicing physicians eligible to practice in the area, and that about 800 or 30 percent were physicians-in-training.[125] Despite ECLAPSRO's attempt to win their support, the medical society steadfastly refused to join, help, or otherwise participate in ECLA-PSRO's activities; but one senior member of the association broke ranks and joined the ECLAPSRO board of directors. The medical society then agreed to offer restricted, qualified support to the housestaff organization despite a basic belief that the "student" doctors had no business reviewing the care rendered by their teachers.[126] In their approach to PSROs, ECLAPSRO had sought consumer participation and accountable processes of review—including consideration of a patient's advocate system and dissemination of information which might be beneficial to consumers.[127] When the organization applied for conditional status, LACMA decided finally to join with them, faced with the possibility that ECLAPSRO might actually win a conditional designation, (although some reports said that of 3,400 eligible physicians, ECLAPSRO had enrolled only 125 members).[128] In order to be designated they would have had to show they had 850 members. The new entity is now called Area 24 PSRO, and within one month of its formation (and assumption of the remaining planning contract moneys) they had enrolled 750 members.[129] The former head of ECLAPSRO remains, at this writing, the executive director of the Area 24 PSRO.

The basic lesson of the ECLAPSRO experience is political; but it is critical to the issue of broad representation of physicians in local PSROs. One interpretation would have HEW using the Interns and Residents Association at the University of Southern California–Los Angeles County medical Center to act as a fundamental economic threat to the recalcitrant medical establishment, forcing them to accept the program—thereby molding it to a spectrum of interests—or be faced with review by a more hostile process. Another interpretation would see the antiestablishment political aspects of ECLAPSRO's activities (consumer accountability) as the threat to physicians which led them to stop resisting the program; and that analysis holds a sad lesson for consumers. Although domination by any one organized group can only stagnate the review process, ECLAPSRO's policies sought to include consumer accountability. That orientation was unacceptable to the physicians who later joined and formed Area 24 PSRO, and the resulting entity, while more representative of area physicians, is a weakened organization from the consumer's perspective.

Practical Considerations

The political climate in which PSROs are developing will hamper enforcement efforts. Obstacles to broad participation, both on a continuing basis and by a large cross section of physicians, are best overcome by focusing the enforcement prerogatives first on the most local element of the system—the hospital. The sanctions offered by the statute can only deal with massive individual failures; they cannot effectively manage incremental failures. If enforcement activity is centered around the hospitals, doctors who would ordinarily be involved in organized activities could be expected to continue their participation, and those physicians who might otherwise eschew active participation in organized medical society activities would be included.

HEW sees the major educational force of the PSRO program as emanating from more intimate peer pressure—that is, when doctors who are on familiar terms with their colleagues confront them in a constructive way, the effect is better than a sanction system where unknown "peers" deliver determinations from on high. [130] In addition, each PSRO has great leverage over its constituent hospitals through the delegation of case by case review authority to the institutional utilization review committee. [131] If rotation were made a requirement for delegation of that authority, hospitals would have to move actively to encourage participation. [132] While the Senate Finance Committee and the *Program Manual* specifically restrict PSRO acceptance of utilization review committees to those institutions whose physicians participate in PSRO activities, [133] neither document imposes on the hospital the requirement of assuring rotation. Making it the hospital's responsibility to impose rotation requirements as a condition of participation as a Medicare and Medicaid provider should be a more effective incentive to rotation because hospitals depend so heavily on Medicare and Medicaid moneys for basic support. [134]

Practical enforcement efforts in the PSRO structure and in American health care delivery generally must confront the "free enterprise" system of American medicine. It is difficult for the federal government to control the activities of physicians who, but for servicing those people whose health care is dependent on government financing, function independently. Attempts to force participation on such practitioners may result in their refusal to participate in the system at all. The outcome has been threatened and would only further injure disadvantaged Medicare and Medicaid patients who face the greatest difficulties in obtaining quality medical services. For example, in the Medicaid system, unrealistic reimbursement schemes [135] make it possible for physicians to ignore an undesirable program without suffering undue loss of income. It is this factor which enables one-fifth of general practitioners to say they will not treat Medicare and Medicaid patients rather than endure PSRO review. [136] Under Medicare Part B, even if reimbursement levels are unacceptable, physicians can effectively avoid them through the assignment option. [137] Under that mechanism, a physician can choose to step into the shoes of the beneficiary, thereby agreeing to accept as payment for his services only what the government is willing to reimburse him. If he does not accept assignment—and nothing forces him to—government payment is made to the beneficiary directly, but the patient remains liable for whatever the physician charges. It is significant to the acceptance of the PSRO system that the rate at which Part B physicians and suppliers accept assignment has been steadily declining since 1969; so that in 1969 at various times as many as about 68 percent (down to a low in December of about 64 percent) of physicians accepted assignment, but in 1973 that rate fell to between about 55.4 percent and 59.2 percent. [138] The Social Security

Administration considers these rates as "a general indication of medical community satisfaction with the Supplementary Medical Insurance program especially with the level of amounts paid by the program for specific services and the promptness of payment." [139] Because of these reimbursement mechanisms, while cooperation of hospitals is assured, cooperation by individual practitioners is not. Because the functioning of the program may not be sufficient impetus to broad participation, other affirmative incentives may be necessary. Guaranteed reduction in malpractice premiums to participating physicians should be considered; [140] and exemption from case by case review for physicians with demonstrated records of compliance with the program (subject to periodic review) has been suggested, [141] but should be widely publicized to encourage physician acceptance.

Other approaches could also further physician cooperation with the PSRO program. National health insurance with universal entitlement would give the federal government the lever necessary to impose controls. State licensure of hospitals and physicians requiring participation in a PSRO as a condition to practicing medicine or running a hospital would further help to resolve the problem of participation. Expansion of PSRO jurisdiction, either voluntarily by private insurers, or through state regulation mandating PSRO review for all health care, would encompass a sufficiently large portion of the population to penalize effectively those physicians who refused to participate in PSROs. Federal regulation of those insurance programs as part of the PSRO process would serve the same purposes. Although these alternatives would require some change in existing mechanisms, they are feasible within the context of current medical practice. Other possibilities which would go well beyond today's system—e.g., a national medical service in which all physicians are employed by the federal government—would assure PSRO operations or that of some other cost control and quality review mechanism. Such reforms would be so extensive as to be inappropriate merely to assure PSRO enforcement.

But unless some additional techniques for creating incentives to cooperation are built into the system, the essentially independent structure within which American physicians deliver health care will respond only voluntarily to the program or not at all. Begrudging participation by those who are dissatisfied with the program may result in a reorientation of the initial thrust of the PSRO scheme to meet the needs of the physicians in this seller's market. [142] Until publicly subsidized consumers are given sufficient buying power to create a buyer's market, or at least equity between the bargaining groups, the ultimate fate of programs like PSROs will rest with physicians.

OTHER ENFORCEMENT ISSUES

The preceding discussion examined enforcement problems in the PSRO system as created by the statute. There are other issues which require cooperation and compliance by physicians that the statute does not confront. For example, there is no specific provision under which a PSRO may directly impose a sanction for fraud; the intentional misrepresentation of services rendered in order to be reimbursed at a higher level is beyond the PSRO's specified authority. The only attention given to fraudulent situations is included in the section on the limitation of liability for persons who provide information to a PSRO. [143] Under that provision, no one giving information to a PSRO shall be civilly liable for having done so. The statute, however, prohibits use of the apparently broad exemption if the information is unrelated to the performance of the duties and functions of a PSRO, or if "such information is false and the person providing such information knew or had reason to believe that such information was false." [144] The rest of the statutory provisions, as well as the Senate Finance Committee report, [145] imply that these provisions are intended as safeguards against personal vendettas where malice would subvert the validity of information given to the PSRO for its use in the course of performing its duties. The limitation on liability restriction, then, is not directly applicable to fraud perpetrated for financial gain. Nor does financial fraud literally violate any obligation as a practitioner or provider. Although every participant in the PSRO process is under an obligation to assure that care will be given according to PSRO norms, criteria, and standards, and that it is medically necessary, there is no specific obligation to give true information. A situation could conceivably arise where care actually met appropriate standards and did not in its delivery violate any obligation under the PSRO statute, but the information given about it was false. For example, giving information which would indicate that the patient's condition was more serious than it actually was so that more services would be covered, especially in an advanced determination situation, would not necessarily lead to any PSRO sanction. No sanctions, under the PSRO scheme, can apply to a single, individual fraudulent incident. The PSRO is charged only with a duty to

> ... use such authority or influence it may possess as a professional organization, and to enlist the support of any other professional or governmental organization having influence or authority over health care practitioners ... [and providers] ... in assuring that each comply with all obligations imposed on him. [146]

The 1972 Social Security Amendments created, for the first time, provisions for punishing these frauds in the Medicare and Medicaid programs. [147] Under those provisions, single incidents of fraud like that described above would be punished as misdemeanors with fines of up to $10,000 or imprisonment for no longer than a year or both. [148] The section which created Program Review Teams to review excessive services or charges under Medicare [149] also provides that no payment can be made if the Secretary determines there was fraud or falsification of statements for purposes of reimbursement. [150] Both these mechanisms contrast sharply with the PSRO's lack of authority to penalize such activity. Although it is true that cases of falsified information could be dealt with under the Medicare and Medicaid fraud provisions, it is also true that the PSRO will first discover where information does not coincide with services rendered. Only if exchange of information between the PSRO and the enforcement agencies under Medicare and Medicaid is ongoing, complete, and accurate will those penalties be able to be applied to fraud in the PSRO system. Considering the infrequent discipline physicians are known to impose on their colleagues, the absence of penalties within the PSRO structure for fraud may not make any practical difference. Total analysis of the system, however, reveals the absence of this type of enforcement mechanism.

One final enforcement problem is implicated in the advance determination situation, particularly where care is proposed to be delivered in a long term care setting. As has already been discussed, the statute does not provide for PSRO sanctions to be imposed as a result of patient complaints (although ideally they would be taken into consideration in the PSRO's investigation of abuse). Nor is there a mechanism created to monitor advance determinations for consistency with services ultimately rendered. Patient complaints would be especially important in the context of long term care. Where services are of long duration, specific episodes of PSRO review (prospectively to determine in advance what medical services should be approved or retrospectively for reimbursement) are infrequent in the course of the total length of stay or number of services rendered to an individual patient. In some circumstances, review need only be performed every 30 days, every 60 days, or even every 90 days. [151] In reviewing a request for services in a nursing facility, if approved, the PSRO will certify the case for specific services and a specific length of stay. After that review the case will not reappear for PSRO consideration until the length of stay has expired or some other action must be taken (transfer to a different facility, for example). During the period between the initial review and subsequent review for appropriate purposes, the services actually delivered to the patient may not be those for which his case was approved. For example, physicians' orders, approved by the PSRO, for special diets or special nursing care may no longer be followed during the interim. Other issues will arise relating to both the technical quality of care and nontechnical aspects of quality. If the PSRO is to assure the quality of the services it approves prospectively, the patient himself may have to be heard, where that is possible. Unless the PSRO system can accommodate complaints from patients in such situations, PSRO review will leave unchecked some critical elements in health care delivery. Although the Senate Finance Committee sees PSROs as having the authority through their sanction-leveling power to determine responsibility for the "provision of substandard services," [152] that supposition must be given specific force through regulations mandating PSROs to assure the quality of the services they approve.

Notes for Chapter Seven

1. §1158; 42 USC §1320c–7.
2. §1167(c); 42 USC §1320c–16. See this chapter at 235 *infra.*
3. If consumers were to conclude that the program does not serve them and should, therefore, be dismantled, the extent of enforcement efforts would be relevant to the program's vulnerability to consumer attack.
4. See Cohen, "Regulatory Politics: The Case of Medical Care Review and Public Law 92–603" (Paper presented at the Annual Meeting of the American Political Science Association, New Orleans, Louisiana, September 5, 1973).
5. For a vivid demonstration of the extent of AMA campaign spending efforts, see Common Cause, *Federal Campaign Finances, 1972– Interest Groups and Political Parties,* vol. 1, Business, Agriculture and Dairy, Health (Washington, D.C., 1974).
6. Two vested interest groups are effectively created: (1) organized medicine is strengthened through direct subsidy of physicians who are not required to include nonphysicians in their activities (but see n. 120 *infra*); and (2) PSRO staffs—primarily executive directors who receive salaries of about $25,000 a year—perform essentially management functions only (they have no substantive authority under the law) and have a vested interest in maintaining their jobs. See, for example, advertisement for "PSRO Executive Director," *New York Times,* February 16, 1975, §4, at 12. The creation of these vested interests leads to real political and financial effects.

   The American Association of Foundations for Medical Care, an organization of prepaid practice groups, formed the American Association of PSROs, an information and lobbying group having as its members PSROs. It performs coordination and information services through conferences and other activities. But in health care politics, these types of organizations inevitably use public moneys for lobbying efforts to justify their own existences. See, for example, McFadden, "State Studying Health Unit Dues," *New York Times,* February 16, 1975, Sec. 1, at 47, col. 1., where it was reported that New York State had asked seven such organizations to account for expenditures of dues paid by Medicaid. These organizations (the New York State Nursing Home Association, the Metropolitan New York Nursing Home Association, the New York State Association of Homes for the Aged, the Greater New York Hospital Association, the Hospital Association of New York State, the New York State Association of Private Hospitals, and the New York State Guild of Nursing Homes) lobby, advertise, and litigate on behalf of their members. Legal fees and travel to conventions were items charged to the government which New York State will no longer pay for. The public money is obtained when the members of the associations include the cost of the disputed items among the appropriate costs of delivering services which the government *will* reimburse. Because PSROs obtain their funds directly from the federal government, determining reasonable and appropriately reimbursable costs will be a function with far-reaching consequences. If it is justifiable to subsidize AAPSRO activities through reimbursements to its PSRO members, it is only equitable to subsidize consumer interests as a legitimate vested interest as well.

7. See Chapter One at 17 *supra.*
8. §1160(a)(1); 42 USC §1320c–9(a)(1). Essentially the same obligations are imposed on providers except that, in addition to medical necessity and economy standards, a provider must be sure that "(in the case of a patient who required care which can, consistent ... with standards, be provided more economically in a health care facility of a different type) there is in the area in which such individual is located, no such facility or no such facility which is available to provide care to such individual at the time when care is needed by him." §1160(a)(2)(B)(ii); 42 USC §1320c–9(a)(B)(ii).
9. §1160(a)(2): 42 USC §1320c–9(a)(2).
10. See *Albert Einstein Medical Center v. Lipoff,* Civ. No. 3872x (C.P., Phila. April 23, 1973); and "Malpractice: Expanding the Physician's Scope of Duty to Render Him Liable for Unwarranted Hospital Costs Incurred by His Patient," 3 *Capital U.L. Rev.* 156 (1974). In the lower court, where Blue Cross refused to pay for unnecessary services and the hospital sued the patient, the physician was held liable for the amount of uncovered services. On appeal the court held for the patient but against Blue Cross.
11. See Chapter Five at 145 *supra.*
12. §1160(b)(1); 42 USC §1320c–9(b)(1).
13. §1160(b)(3); 42 USC §1320c–9(b)(3).
14. *Id.*
15. §1157; 42 USC §1320c–6.
16. *Sen. Fin. Comm. Rpt.* at 266.
17. The *Program Manual* does suggest that each PSRO have a standing Grievance Committee "to receive and consider complaints on non-review related matters." *Program Manual,* Chapter V, §550.41(c) at 16. But the complaints referred to as part of the enforcement process are conceptually different from grievances. Grievances are complaints about particular situations affecting individuals. Grievances should be handled through individual accountability mechanisms. See Chapter Five at 144 *supra* for a discussion of the PSRO grievance process; and Chapter Six at 177 *supra* for a definition of individual accountability.
18. §1160(b)(1); 42 USC §1320c–9(b)(1).
19. *Sen. Fin. Comm. Rpt.* at 266.
20. §1157; 42 USC §1320c–6.
21. §1160(b)(1); 42 USC §1320c–9(b)(1).
22. *Id.*

23. §1160(b)(1)(A); 42 USC §1320c–9(b)(1)(A).
24. §1160(b)(1)(B); 42 USC §1320c–9(b)(1)(B).
25. §1160(b)(1); 42 USC §1320c–9(b)(1).
26. §1160(b)(4); 42 USC §1320c–9(b)(4).
27. §1160(b)(3); 42 USC §1320c–9(b)(3).
28. §1160(b)(1); 42 USC §1320c–9(b)(1). Those could be criminal penalties, damages from malpractice actions, or even continuing education requirements established under regulations.
29. §229, P.L. 92–603; §§1862(d), 1866(b)(2); 42 USC §§1395y(d), 1395cc(b)(2). See Chapter Six at 207 *supra.*
30. Their membership is similar, however, to Statewide Councils, and their substitution for those Councils in this process might yield no significantly different results.
31. The Senate Finance Committee recognized that need: "Failure to order or provide care in accordance with the norms employed by PSRO is not intended to create a legal presumption of liability." *Sen. Fin. Comm. Rpt.* at 267.
32. If PSRO norms would cover only the most minimal services for cost control reasons only, then a physician seeking to practice good quality medicine would presumably be justified in violating the system.
33. Clark, "How Good is Your Doctor?", *Newsweek,* December 23, 1974, at 49.
34. See comments of Robert P. Fry, M.D., in "Are You Ready to Blow the Whistle on Bad Doctors?" *Medical Economics,* November 11, 1974, at 79.
35. Edwin J. Holman, Secretary of AMA Judicial Council, quoted in "From 'Disciplinary Inertia' to 'Peer Plus Review'," 8 *Hosp. Practice* 199 (April 1973).
36. Derbyshire, *Medical Licensure and Discipline in the United States* (Baltimore: Johns Hopkins Press, 1969) at 77.
37. The study did not include Louisiana, Missouri, Pennsylvania, and South Carolina, which refused to supply figures. "How Well Does Medicine Police Itself?" *Medical World News,* March 15, 1974, at 68.
38. Derbyshire, *supra* n. 36, at 77–90.
39. "How Well Does Medicine Police Itself?" *supra* n. 37, at 72. "Sick doctor" legislation (giving the licensing board authority to act against a physician who is unable to practice for a variety of physical and mental conditions) and relicensure based on continued competency are other incipient trends. *Id.* See also Altman, "AMA Urges Discipline of Incompetent Physicians," *New York Times,* Ocrober 29, 1973 at 1, col. 2; and "The Public Won't Stand for Any More Doctor Cover-Ups!", *Medical Economics,* October 28, 1974, at 31.
40. He has reportedly said, "The consumer movement is perhaps stronger here than anywhere else. Our own board operates under the Department of Consumer Affairs—in fact we're the department's biggest user." "How Well Does Medicine Police Itself?" *supra* n. 37, at 72.

41. *Id.* at 71.
42. §1152(d)(2); 42 USC §1320c–1(d)(2).
43. §1167(c); 42 USC §1320c–16(c).
44. *Id.*
45. *Sen. Fin. Comm. Rpt.* at 267. Similar interpretations presumably would apply to institutions.
46. *Id.*
47. As Dr. Derbyshire (*supra* n. 36) has said, "Sure anyone with $10 can sue, but he won't win." "How Well Does Medicine Police Itself?" *supra* n. 37, at 69.
48. See Chapter Six at 190 *supra* for a discussion of consumer information needs in malpractice litigation under the PSRO system.
49. See Chapter Two at 32 *supra*.
50. *Sen. Fin. Comm. Rpt.* at 267.
51. See the AMA's proposed amendment #8 at Chapter One, n. 31, at 22 *supra*. The AMA has also proposed repeal of the malpractice exemption.

    Section 1167(c) should be repealed. Section 1167 purports (in subsection (c)), to limit the liability of an individual furnishing items or services when such individual has acted in compliance with norms of care applied by a PSRO, provided that he exercised due care in his conduct. This provision could have the unintended and undesirable effect of pressuring practitioners to adhere to norms. Moreover, the provision is at best meaningless because on its face it is applicable only when the practitioner has exercised due care—the very issue at the heart of the malpractice issues.

    PSRO Oversight Hearings at 76–77.
52. *Sen. Fin. Comm. Rpt.* at 263.
53. §§1156(a),(c)(2); 42 USC §1320c–5(a),(c)(2).
54. For other considerations of the effect of the malpractice exemption, see Kleinman, "PSRO: Malpractice Liability and the Impact of the Civil Immunity Clause," 62 *Georgetown L. J.* 1499 (1974).
55. *Sen. Fin. Comm. Rpt.* at 263.
56. *Id.*
57. See n. 51 *supra*.
58. See Thompson et al., "Patient Grievance Mechanisms in Health Care Institutions," Report No. SCMM–FC–PG for the Secretary's Commission on Medical Malpractice, Appendix to the *Report of the Secretary's Commission on Medical Malpractice,* January 16, 1973, at 758. See generally *Report of the Secretary's Commission on Medical Malpractice* and *Appendix,* January 16, 1973, Reports, Studies and Analysis, DHEW, Publication No. (OS) 78–89. See also Health Outcomes Commission proposal which would employ binding arbitration, Chapter One at xx *supra*. Cohen, "Manpower and Social Controls," 48 *Hospitals, JAHA* 105 (April 1, 1974) surveys

recent malpractice trends in the context of licensure and PSROs as general trends in health regulation.

59. "Medical Liability Outlook Bleak: Rising Premiums, Fewer Insurers, and More Suits," *American Medical News,* November 14, 1974 at 18, 20.

60. *Id.*

61. *Id.* and S. 215 (94th Cong., 1st sess) (Inouye-Kennedy); and S. 188 (94th Cong., 1st sess) (Nelson).

62. *PSRO Oversight Hearings* at 358–359.

63. See "Liability proposals include PSRO clause," *American Medical News,* January 27, 1975, at 5. The proposal was made after the state society, which insures 20,000 physicians, found a replacement carrier at an increase in rates of 93.5 percent. Six months later, the new carrier asked for an additional increase of almost 200 percent. The society's president said the increase would have meant premiums of $45,000 to $50,000 a year for some physicians. The new insurer agreed to fulfill its contract, but then will discontinue all malpractice coverage. *Id.* For some of the insurance companies' arguments, see "Malpractice insurers cite problems," *American Medical News,* November 4, 1974, at 23. Primarily they cite increasing costs and frequency of claims.

64. See "PSRO: An Educational Force for Improving Quality of Care" (HSA/BQA), October 1, 1974.

65. §1155(d); 42 USC §1320c–4(d).

66. *Id.* The section also provides for publication of notices about PSRO activities. §1155(d)(4); 42 USC §1320c–4(d)(4). See Chapter Six at 187 *supra.*

67. *Sen. Fin. Comm. Rpt.* at 259.

68.   Participation in a PSRO would be voluntary and open to every physician in the area. Existing organizations of physicians should be encouraged to take the lead in urging all their members to participate and no physician could be barred from participation because he is or is not a member of any organized medical group or be required to join any such group or pay dues or their equivalent for the privilege of becoming a member or officer of any PSRO nor should there be any discrimination in assignments to perform PSRO duties based on membership or nonmembership in any such organized group of physicians.
    Id.

69. §1155(a)(5); 42 USC §1320c–4(a)(5).

70. *Sen. Fin. Comm. Rpt.* at 260.

71. No physician may review the care of a patient in whose treatment he participated directly or indirectly; nor may he review services provided by an institution in which he (or his family) has a financial interest. §1155(a)(6); 42 USC §1320c–4(a)(6).

72. Membership must be open and voluntary. *Program Manual,* Chapter V, §510.16(e) at 9.

73. *Id.* §500 at 2.

74. *Id.*; and Chapter IV, §400 at 2.
75. *Id.*, Chapter V, §510.2 at 9.
76. "Are You in Favor of PSRO?" *Medical World News,* October 25, 1974, at
     71.
77. *Id.*
78. Fifty-four and nine tenths percent of all practitioners less than 45 years
     old accept PSROs, but only 34.6 percent of those over 45 accept
     them. Physicians in the Northeast were more accepting than others. *Id.*
79. *Id.*
80. Colombotos, Kirchner, Millman, *Physicians View National Health Insur-
     ance, A National Study,* a preliminary report of findings presented
     to Health Staff Seminar, September 23, 1974. (available from John
     Colombotos, Ph.D., Associate Professor, Columbia University,
     School of Public Health, Division of Sociomedical Sciences). See also
     "Poll Shows MD support for NHI," *American Medical News,*
     September 30, 1974, at 1; and "If Health Plan Comes, Doctors
     Favor PSROs," *Medical Tribune,* August 21, 1974, at 2.
81. Colombotos, et al., *supra* n. 80, at 12.
82. *Id.*
83. 119 *Cong. Rec.* S12214, July 11, 1974.
84. Basic information about the program was a long time coming. See,
     Chapter Six at 183 and 184 *supra.*
85. See Chapter One at 17 *supra.*
86. Nelson, "PSRO—Alive and Well in Utah," 3 *Medical Opinion* 56 (October
     1974).
87. Haug, "AMA Membership," *The Profile of Medical Practice, 1971,* Center
     for Health Services Research and Development, American Medical
     Association, at 24–26.
88. *Id.*
89. *Id.*
90. Haug, "AMA Membership," *The Profile of Medical Practice, 1972,* Center
     for Health Services Research and Development, American Medical
     Association, at 24–26.
91. *Id.*
92. Cleary, "AMA Agress to Cleaning Up Blood Transfusions," *Evening
     Bulletin* (Philadelphia), December 5, 1973, at 20.
93. Haug, *supra* n. 90.
94. See "State, county societies get AMA membership incentives," *American
     Medical News,* November 5, 1973, at 22.
95. See "AMA membership levels off," *American Medical News,* June 4,
     1973, at 1.
96. Colombotos et al., *supra* n. 80, at 7.
97. *National Medical Association News,* November 1973, at 4.
98. *Id.*
99. The Detroit Medical Foundation and Old North State PSRO which
     applied for planning grants are affiliated with the NMA. Neither of
     them was funded during the first cycle, in part because rival

organizations applied from the same areas. See also "Problems hamper efforts of NMA," *American Medical News,* August 12, 1974, at 1.

100. *Id.*

101. See Rann, "Inaugural Speech, NMA Convention 1973," *Urban Health,* February 1974 at 23. See also Cooper and Thompson, "PSROs and Minority Physicians," *Id.* at 22.

102. Testimony of Dr. John C. Taylor, president, American Osteopathic Association, *PSRO Oversight Hearings* at 91.

103. *Id.*

104. American Osteopathic Association, Professional Standards Review Organizations (PSRO)—Position Statement, Memo B/H July/73–119.

105. Testimony of Dr. Taylor, *supra* n. 102, at 93.

106. See n. 104 *supra.*

107. For consideration of PSROs and dentistry, see Friedman, "PSRO in Dentistry" (Paper presented at the 102d Annual Meeting of the American Public Health Association, New Orleans, LA., October 20–24, 1974). See also Barish and Collins, "Peer review for quality care in private solo dental practice," 89 *JADA* 866 (October 1974); Bailit et al, "Quality of dental care: development of standards" 89 *JADA* 842 (October 1974); and Jago, "Issues in assurance of quality dental care," 89 *JADA* 854 (October 1974).

108. Neither fish nor fowl in PSROs, dentists seem to be considered on a par with a variety of ancillary medical professions. See Chapter Six at 203 *supra.*

109. Simmons, "PSRO and the Law," *Conference on PSRO and Peer Review,* February 26–27, 1974 sponsored by the ADA Council on Dental Care Programs, at 145.

110. See testimony of Dr. Sidney R. Francis, American Dental Association, *PSRO Oversight Hearings* at 144.

111. There are at least two national physician union federations, the American Federation of Physicians and Dentists, and the National Physicians Council. See "Unions 'still here, growing'," *American Medical News,* September 9, 1974, at 1. Union supporters claim 55,000 practitioners belong to groups styling themselves as unions. *Id.* See "Las Vegas MDs form AFL-CIO union," *American Medical News,* April 3, 1972, at 1. And now the interns and residents union, Physicians National Housestaff Association, has joined the Coalition of American Public Employees. See "Housestaff group moves toward national union," *American Medical News,* October 14, 1974, at 1.; and "PNHA joins union coalition," *American Medical News,* January 27, 1975, at 5.

112. "Union moves to halt Iowa PSRO," *American Medical News,* June 10, 1974, at 9.

113. Attacking a potential PSRO as "unrepresentative" is another strategy dissatisfied groups might employ. See Chapter Four at 118 *supra.*

114. Editorial (based on a policy statement approved by the American

Association of Medical Colleges), 48 *Journal of Medical Education* 457 (May 1973).

115. "Despite political distrations, psychiatrists stress care delivery," *American Medical News,* May 20, 1974, at 26.

116. See *PSRO Oversight Hearings* at 505. Other professional organizations which have offered qualified support for the program include the American College of Physicians, American Society of Internal Medicine, American Association of Foundations for Medical Care, and American College of Surgeons. See *PSRO Oversight Hearings* at 52, 83, 140, 159.

117. These figures are not centralized. The AMA does not compute them, nor do state societies. State society officials do often agree, however, that local membership is often higher than state society membership.

118. The requirement of medical society membership as a precondition to hospital admitting privileges is a phenomenon recognized by local society officials. But the condition is imposed by individual hospitals. Neither medical societies nor the American Hospital Association and its affiliates maintain statistics on this.

119. §1155(f)(2); 42 USC §1320c–4(f)(2).

120. This is not to say that reimbursement for participation in PSRO activities is not essential for the initial stages of implementation. The chairman of the PSRO group in Philadelphia reported that when the group was negotiating its planning contract, the HEW grant officer negotiating with them asserted that HEW would not reimburse physicians for time spent in initial implementation activities. The grant officer indicated it was assumed that nonprofessional administrative staff would perform most of the initial activities needed to implement the program. The theory behind this policy, he was reported to have said, was that HEW did not believe it was necessary to reimburse physicians for activities they had always engaged in, like attending meetings. After considerable discussion with a member of the National Council and Dr. Henry Simmons, Director of the Office of Professional Standards Review (OPSR), the chairman leanred that the "policy" was in fact "negotiable." Report of Sidney Krasnoff, M.D., to the Proposed Area 12 PSRO Pro-Tem Board of Directors, meeting, June 12, 1974 (Philadelphia).

Independent inquiry to OPSR revealed that the "interim policy" used in negotiation for grants would not permit reimbursement to physicians for planning activities (or other activities) not directly related to grant responsibilities. Further clarification indicated reimbursement would be available for physician "consultants" on activities required under an agreement. Apparently the burden is on the negotiating group seeking the contract to discover that the policy is negotiable. Telephone interview with Information Officer OPSR, June 20, 1974.

If the HEW philosophy is based on a notion that the effect of the law is such that physicians have no choice but to participate without remuneration, PSRO implementation will only be grudgingly undertaken by physicians, with poor results for everyone.

121. Proposed 42 CFR §101.7 (38 FR 34945, December 20, 1973).
122. 42 CFR §101.7 (39 FR 10206–07, March 18, 1974).
123. Of the 1.5 million residents of the area, some 60 percent are estimated to be eligible for Medicare and Medicaid. See "PSRO in LA County—a generation gap," *American Medical News,* October 28, 1974, at 1, 18.
124. Copy on file with the author.
125. See n. 123 *supra.*
126.   These people are still in training; they are our students and we are their teachers. They just don't have the experience to certify hospital admissions or review lengths-of-stay, or judge patterns of care. Yet this is what they propose to do. And I believe most practicing physicians are against it.

Sanford F. Rothenberg, M.D., President, Los Angeles County Medical Association, quoted in "PSRO in LA County—a generation gap," *supra* n. 123, at 1.
127. The author had several conversations with one of ECLAPSRO's legal counsel on practical issues of consumer accountability when their planning grant was in its draft stages. Interviews with Kenneth Wing, Esq.
128. *PSRO Letter* (no. 36), February 1, 1975, at 7.
129. *Id.*
130. See "PSRO: An Educational Force for Improving Quality of Care" (HSA/BQA), October 1, 1974.
131. See Chapter Three.
132. For example, the California State Medical Association has included participation in utilization review committee activities among its "Guiding Principles for Physician—Hospital Relationships," California Medical Association, 1967 at 6. Under the designation "Control of Medical Care," the principles set forth the role of the utilization review committee:

This committee is established within the medical staff of a hospital to assure that all of the inpatient service given is necessary and could not be provided as effectively in the home, office, or other available facility. The committee analyzes and identifies factors that may contribute to unnecessary or ineffective use of inpatient services and facilities and makes recommendations designed to minimize ineffective utilization.

Id. at 5. The principles further provide: "Each physician has a responsibility to be an active participant in the work of any of the committees to which he has been appointed. Of equal importance each physician must make it his personal responsibility not only to comply with decisions made by the staff on recommendation of its

committees, but to insist that all other physicians also comply." *Id.*
at 6–7. The association directly links this responsibility to Section 4
of the AMA Principles of Medical Ethics, elevating the California
requirements to the level of an ethical standard. *Id.* at 7.

133. *Sen. Fin. Comm. Rpt.* at 262. See *Program Manual,* Chapter V,
§520.04(c) at 1.

134. See figures in Pettengill, "The Financial Position of Private Community
Hospitals, 1961–1971," 36 *Social Security Bulletin* 4 (no. 11)
(November 1973), Table 1.

135. In Pennsylvania, for example, all office (and clinic) visits, and treatment in
an emergency room which does not result in a hospital admission,
are reimbursed at flat rates of $6 and $10 respectively, regardless of
the services provided or treatment performed. The $6 fee was raised
in 1973 from $4 for all out-patient care. *Medical Assistance Memo
No. 4,* Commonwealth of Pennsylvania, Harrisburg, January
15, 1973.

136. See n. 76 *supra,* and accompanying text.

137. §1842(b)(3)(B)(ii); 42 USC §1395u(b)(3)(B)(ii). See Chapter Five at
143 *supra.*

138. The rates fluctuate seasonally and the term "supplier" includes independent clinical laboratories, ambulance services, firms renting or selling
durable medical equipment, sellers of prosthetic services and other
appliances, and medical supply houses. See Waldhauser, "Assignment
Rates for Supplementary Medical Insurance Claims, Calendar Year
1973," *Health Insurance Statistics,* HI–63, December 5, 1974,
DHEW Pub. No. (SSA) 75–11702, SSA, Office of Research and
Statistics.

139. *Id.* at 1

140. See this chapter at 238 *supra.*

141. The *Program Manual* does permit exemption from admission certification
and continued stay review for certain proficient physicians and
providers. *Program Manual,* Chapter VII, §705.14(a)(2) at 6, and
§720.1(b) at 23.

142. Statewide Support Centers are an example. See Chapter Seven, at xxx
supra.

143. §1167; 42 USC §1320c–6.

144. *Id.*

145. *Sen. Fin. Comm. Rpt.* at 267.

146. §1160(c); 42 USC §1320c–9(c).

147. §242(a), (b), P.L. 92–603; §1877, §1909 of the Social Security Act; 42
USC §§1395nn, 1396h.

148. *Id.*

149. §229, P.L. 92–603; §§1862(d)(1), 1866(b)(2); 42 USC §§1395y(b)(1),
1395cc(b)(2). See Chapter Six at 207 *supra.*

150. §229(a), (b), P.L. 92–603; §§1862(d)(1)(A), 1866(b)(2)(D); 42 USC
§§1395y(d)(1)(A), 1395cc(b)(2)(D).

151. See Chapter Three at 80 *supra.*

152. *Sen. Fin. Comm. Rpt.* at 266.

Index

accountability: admissions certification, 73; and AMA proposals, 12; concept of, 4, 173; confidentiality, 196; consumer, lack of in PSRO, 18; enforcement, 230; hearings, 145; hearings and review, 159; physician role in review, 117; and prior authorization, 168; and PSRO data availability, 188; utilization review, 70

Administrative Procedure Act, 197

Advisory Committee on Medicare Administration, 119

AMA: criteria and norms, 56; fear of norms, 237; malpractice and norms, 252; national treatment guidelines, 66; and PROs, 11, 12; PSRO kit, 213; standards for delegation of authority, 83; state society control, 180

American Academy of Pediatrics, 56, 243

American Association of Comprehensive Health Planners, 64

American Association of Foundations for Medical Care, 17

American College of Physicians, 56

American Dental Association, 242

American Hospital Association, 17; hospital budgets, 28; Quality Assurance Program, 102

American Nurses Association, 56

American Osteopathic Association, 242

American Podiatary Association, 56

American Public Health Association, 179, 211

appeals: and PSRO decision, 49

Ashbacker Radio Corp. v. FCC, 199

Ashbrook, Rep., 20, 219

Associated Hospital Services, Inc., 129

Association of American Physicians and Surgeons et al v. Weinberger, 27

Barrett v. United Hospital, 170

Bell v. Heim; 42, 150; conditions, 61

Bellin, L.E., 219

benefits package, 18; artificial, 62; defined, 46; and hospital utilization review, 75

Bennett, Wallace: accountability, 174; AMA kit, 213; cost control, 21; cost, quality and physician control, 104; on health care cost, 4; on overutilization, 43; on physician PSRO support, 240; role as sponsor, 2

Blue Cross/Blue Shield: control of PSRO, 17; as fiscal agents, 112; utilization review, 97

Boddie v. Conn., 156

Bohlen v. Richardson, 161

bureaucracy: and advocacy, 168; and hierarchy review, 137; and utilization review, 74

Bureau of Quality Assurance, 73, 103

care: case by case review, 73; evaluation studies, 58; and flexibility, 64; judicial review, 146–149; patients and the courts, 165, 166; pattern analysis, 78; paying agents, 124; sanctions and liability, 236

Caudelle v. Weinberger, 165

Charlottesville, Va., 56, 63

Citizens Communication Center v. FCC., 223

claims: and judicial review, 149

Wilson Coe, Admr. v. Sec. of HEW., 161

Cohen, W., 128

communication: and care delivery, 37; and consumer accountability, 178; doctor-patient, 32, 53; social service depts., 69; Professional and Hospital Activities, 102

Commission on the Quality of Health Care, 14

261

conflicts of interest, 99, 100
confidentiality, 7, 191, 100; patient-
physician priviledge, 217; provision for,
21
Connor, W., 224
consumer: accountability, 174; court
decisions, 165; enforcement process,
230; entitlement, 44; evaluation and
quality assessment, 52; hearings and
review provision, 147; improper utilization, 79; interests, 6; and norms, 32;
ombudsman program, 206; patient advocacy program, 153; and paying agents,
110; and PSRO data availability, 187;
responses to physician treatment, 38;
and statute for PSRO structure, 200; and
utilization reivew, 68
Contract Performance Review Team, 131
cost: control, 6; control and PSRO, 47;
fee setting mechanism, 92; and health
care delivery options, 178; and norms,
37; and paying agents, 111; payments,
109; and physicians authority, 217; post-
payment review, 79; and prior authorization, 168; PSRO and institutional change,
67; reimbursements, 65; utilization, 50;
utilization review, 74
critieria, 76
Curtis, Carl, 54

data: Blue Shield, 215; and consumer
service, 18; and disclosures, 131; health
care delivery, 182; insulation and AMA,
12; medical records and review process,
39; for norms, 57; and paying agents,
110; processing and paying agents, 124;
provider, patient profiles, 120; reorganization, 96; San Joaquin and Sacramento
Medical Foundations, 106; statutory
provisions, 187
decisionmaking: AMA model, 14; competence, 113; equitable representation,
175; PSRO trial period, 199; statute lack
of provision for consumer, 205
Dillums, R.W., 190
Doe v. Bellin Memorial Hospital, 170
due process, 154

Edwards, 213
Eisen v. Carlisle and Jacquelin, 160
elderly: analysis of condition, 53; in
Bennett, 5; service utilization, 105
enforcement: overview, 229
entitlement, 10; concept of, 62, 161;
disputes, 143
equal protection: concept, 170

Fair Credit Reporting Act, 195

Federal Reports Act, 194
fraud, 130, 248
Freedom of Information Act, 182, 194, 221
funding: paying agents, 123; PSRO utilization review, 72; and reimbursement
strategy, 251

Gellhorn, Prof., 199
Georgia, 56
Goldberg v. Kelly, 141, 151, 153
government: and case by case review, 74;
confidentiality procedure, 195; and
control of health industry, 246; data
system, 184; due process rights, 154, 167;
EMCROs, 55; and HMO procedure, 90;
intervention, 2; legislation, 15; long-term
care facilities, 53; medicaid total utilization review, 81; and Medicare hearing
rights, 142; and notion of public representatives, 203; patient advocacy program, 153; and reimbursement, 93; review
system, 53; state action, 170; waiver and
liability, 69
Hague v. Williams, 219
Hamilton v. Blue Cross of North Dakota
and HEW, 161
Hammond v. Aetna Casualty and Surety
Co., 219
Hamon v. Weinberger, 167
Harrell v. Harder, 160
Harris v. Richardson, 165
Harska, Rep., 20
Havighurst, Clark, 93, 170
health care: access, 49; quality, 14
Health Insurance Plan, 89
Health Security Act, 14, 16
hearing: mechanism, 141
HEW: audits, 119; cost control, 116; and
development of PSRO, 17; enforcement
mechanism, 230; and Los Angeles Courts,
244; and PSRO compliance, 95; sanctions,
20
Hill v. State Dept. of Welfare, 160
HMO: act, 16; capitation fee, 90; incentive
to low utilization, 61; physician fees,
92; and PSRO tensions, 52; in Social
Security Amendment Act, 26
hospitals: evaluation studies, 78; role in
utilization review, 76
Hultzman v. Weinberger, 165

Ingram v. Weinberger, 165
innovation: government medical care
review organization, 55; implementation
phase, 118; and norms, 29, 114; predetermined criteria, 64; and review, 52
insurance companies, 130
InterStudy, 11, 25

Joint Commission on Accreditation of Hospitals, 102
judicial review, 165, 166; and class action, 160; and PSRO hearings, 200

Kaiser Health Plan, 89
Kennedy, Senator, 16
Knickerbocker Hospital v. Downing, 140
Kunstler v. Occidental Life Insurance, 161

Lee v. Weinberger, 167
Liability: *Bell v. Heim,* 150; decisions, 165, 166; *Knickerbocker Hospital v. Downing,* 140; and obligations, 231; physician, 251; and physician payment, 144; "state action," 170; waiver, 68
localism: concept of, 8
Los Angeles County, 244

malpractice, 236; exemption, 235; and PSRO norms, 33; and statute, 10
Martinez v. Richardson, 150
Medicaid/Medicare, 10; confidentiality, 193; coverage expansion, 33; data and norms, 37; fraud, 86; hearings, 139; hearings and appeals, 143; HMO procedure, 90; institutional review committee, 74; long-term care, 80; physician extension, 54; and PSRO authority, 95; review failure, 75; sanctions, 122; utilization review, 53; utilization review failure, 70
Medical Services Administration, 95
medical society, 8; as PSRO, 22
methodology: accounting and review, 71; "discharge planning," 81; EMCRO, 56; of review, 77
monitor: confidentiality, 194; function analysis, 79; and government in Bennett, 4; performance, 118; physician attitude, 240; PSRO delegation authority, 88; responsibility definition, 134
MSIS, 193

National Council: norms, 50
national health insurance, 106, 240; and government control, 247; proposals, 16; unified review, 62
National Medical Association, 241, 255
National Professional Standards Review Council, 9, 34, 119
National Urban Coalition, 210
National Welfare Rights Organization v. Finch, 199, 223
Nelson, Alan, 238, 240
New Mexico Foundation for Medical Care, 42
New York, 130; State Medical Society, 238

norms: *Bell v. Heim,* 42; concept of, 29; consensual, 57; establishment, 34; as liability shield, 237; and nonphysician personnel, 41; planning capabilities, 47; "regional," 50; selection and criteria, 36
nursing facilities, 82; national data, 57

Ogilvie, Richard, 179
Oregon, 56
Ortwein v. Schwab, 158
overutilization: and Bennett, 43; quality, 21

patients: as a class vs. as an individual, 62; profile and norms, 34
payment: retroactive denial, 114
peer review: concept of, 4
Pennsylvania: reimbursement, 65
physicians: authority in review, 117; and carrier ties, 132; and court decisions, 165, 166; enforcement efforts, 230; and government intrusion, 29; norms and incentives, 43; payment and misdiagnosis, 65; performance and care quality, 52; prepaid health care, 91; and PSRO system, 202; role in case by case review, 74; unions, 256
policy: Institute of Medicine, 90; statutory structure, 7
poverty: analysis of condition, 53; in Bennett, 5; *Boddie v. Conn.,* 156; medically needy, 159; and service utilization, 105
prepaid group practice, 106
profile: PSRO delegation guidelines, 83
Program Review and Evaluation Project, 133
PSRO: advisory groups, 203; appeals structure, 138; authorization, 115; autonomy, 86; contracts for norm development, 56; and delegation authority, 83; discipline, 22; and effect on HMO in Havighurst, 179; and jurisdiction over HMO, 92; lobbying group, 250; Los Angeles county, 245; manual, 54; medical necessity, 44; monitor procedures, 70; norms and review, 30; orientation, 4; overview, 8; paradox, 1; and paying agents, 126; payments, 109; payment provision, 145; performance evaluation, 197; physician attitude, 240; professional supporters, 257; program implementation and confidentiality, 192; proposal hearings, 179; provider/patient profiles, 120; review methodology, 77; review process, 38; role of Blue Shield, 134, 136; sanctions, 232; selection, 118; and Senate Finance Committee, 17; and service providers, 95; and state action, 170; variant norms, 63; voluntary participation, 254

public interest, 6, 21; and case by case
review, 74; judicial review, 147; nondisclosure, 190; role of paying agents, 123;
Somers, 176; utilization review, 68

quality: aspect, 25; assessment and utilization review, 99; assurance process, 212;
in Bennett, 5; and norms, 33; PSRO and
changing role, 67; and PSRO parameters,
30; sanctions, 232, 233; underutilization,
91; utilization review, 75

Rann, E.N., 241
Rarick, J., 20, 219
recordkeeping, 58; and utilization review,
76
reimbursement, 74; and carriers, 135; and
conflict of interest, 116; and control,
247; foundation, 106; fraud, 79; Medicaid, 49; Medicare, 60; place in cycle, 41;
practice of, 8; vital for participation,
257
review: competence, 112; court decisions,
165; determination criteria, 9; end result,
38; implications, 44; and long-term care,
80; and medical audit, 103; paying agents
and utilization patterns, 130; and payments, 111; and potential fraud, 79, 80;
prepaid health care delivery, 89; utilization and failure, 70; process and end
result, 52; program goals, 67; PSRO, 58;
and reimbursement, 79; sanctions, 121;
San Joaquin and Sacramento Medical
Foundations, 105; statutes, 107; waivers,
82
Richardson v. Perales, 167
Ridgely v. Secretary of HEW, 166
Ridgeway, James, 191
Rogatz, 216

Sacramento, Calif., 56
San Joaquin and Sacramento Medical
Foundations, 105
Senate Finance Committee: admission, 49;
Blue Cross/Blue Shield and data collec-
tion, 194; data availability and quality of
service, 188; on implementation effort,

117; on norms, 43; norms and review,
51; and paying agents, 122; peer review
course, 37; penalties and liability, 233;
preadmission review, 45; and PSRO
acceptance, 197; and PSRO and professional code, 99; PSRO proposal, 17;
PSRO review activities, 72; PSRO review
authority, 127; recordkeeping, 58;
regional norms, 54; review procedure,
40; utilization review evaluation, 70
Simmons, Henry, 53, 242
Social and Rehabilitation Service, 97
Social Security Act: amendments, 10; and
Associated Hospital Services Inc., 129;
and Blue Cross Association, 120; and
Bureau of Hearings and Appeals, 143;
coping with review failure, 75; judicial
review, 161; Medicare reimbursements,
60; nondisclosure, 217; Program Review
Teams, 207; survey of review practices,
128
Society of New York Hospital v. Mogensen,
140
Somers, A., 176, 209
Sowell v. Richardson, 166
standards: on review, 76
Statewide Professional Standards Review
Councils, 119
Stephens v. Weinberger, 167
Supreme Court, 150, 156, 199

Tancredi and Barsky, 183
Todd, Malcolm, C., 192
Turner v. Wohlgemuth, 168

underutilization, 216; concept of, 48
U.S. v. Kras, 157
utilization: priorities, 55; review committee
criteria, 72; service, 13

waivers, 102
Watkins v. Mercy Medical Center, 170
Weinberger, C., 101; norms for PSRO, 55
Word v. Peoker, 167

Zahn v. International Paper Co., 160

About the Author

Alice Gosfield is a principal analyst at Health Policy Perspectives, Inc., a non-profit public health law and policy consulting group in Philadelphia. She received her BA from Barnard College of Columbia University and her JD from New York University Law School. In addition to writing this book, she has participated in a variety of health care related projects including drafting hospital licensing regulations for a state health department, advising Blue Cross subscribers on achieving their rights in corporate governance, assisting Medicare and Medicaid patients with grievances arising from those programs and researching conflicts of interest in the practice of university medical centers staffing municipal hospitals. She is a member of the Pennsylvania Bar.